CONTEMPORARY TOPICS
IN IMMUNOBIOLOGY
VOLUME 8

CONTEMPORARY TOPICS IN IMMUNOBIOLOGY

A Continuation Order Plan is available for this series. A continuation order will bring delivery of each new volume immediately upon publication. Volumes are billed only upon actual shipment. For further information please contact the publisher.

CONTEMPORARY TOPICS IN IMMUNOBIOLOGY

VOLUME 8

EDITED BY

Noel L. Warner
University of New Mexico
Albuquerque, New Mexico

and

Max D. Cooper
University of Alabama in Birmingham
Birmingham, Alabama

PLENUM PRESS • NEW YORK AND LONDON

The Library of Congress cataloged the first volume of this title as follows:

Contemporary topics in immunobiology. v. 1–
    1972–
New York, Plenum Press.
    v. illus. 24 cm. annual.

    1. Immunology–Periodicals.
QR180.C632   574.2'9'05   79-179761
ISSN 0093-4054

Library of Congress Catalog Card Number 68-26769

ISBN-13: 978-1-4684-0924-6   e-ISBN-13: 978-1-4684-0922-2
DOI: 10.1007/978-1-4684-0922-2

Contributors

Erika R. Abney
: *Department of Zoology*
  University College London
  London, England

Robert C. Burton
: *Transplantation Unit*
  Massachusetts General Hospital
  Harvard University
  Boston, Massachusetts 02114

Stanley E. Chism
: *Division of Radiation Oncology*
  University of California
  San Francisco, California 94122

Max D. Cooper
: *Departments of Pediatrics and Microbiology*
  and the Comprehensive Cancer Center
  University of Alabama Medical Center
  Birmingham, Alabama 35294

Manlio Ferrarini
: *The Rockefeller University*
  New York, New York 10021
  Present address: Institute of Biological Chemistry
  University of Genoa
  Genoa, Italy

James W. Goding
: *The Walter and Eliza Hall Institute of Medical Research*
  The Royal Melbourne Hospital
  Melbourne, Victoria 3050 Australia

Otto Haller
: *Department of Immunology*
  Uppsala University Box 582,
  S-751 23 Uppsala, Sweden

J. Stephen Haskill
: *Department of Obstetrics and Gynecology*
  University of North Carolina at Chapel Hill
  Chapel Hill, North Carolina 27514

Pekka Häyry
: *Transplantation Laboratory*
  Department IV of Surgery
  University of Helsinki
  Helsinki, Finland

John F. Kearney
: *Department of Microbiology*
  and the Comprehensive Cancer Center
  University of Alabama Medical Center
  Birmingham, Alabama 35294

Rolf Kiessling

Department of Tumor Biology
Karolinska Institute
S-104 01 Stockholm 60, Sweden

J. F. A. P. Miller

The Walter and Eliza Hall Institute of Medical Research
Royal Melbourne Hospital P.O.
Melbourne, Victoria 3050, Australia

Graham F. Mitchell

Laboratory of Immunoparasitology
The Walter and Eliza Hall Institute of Medical Research
Royal Melbourne Hospital P.O.
Melbourne, Victoria 3050, Australia

Lorenzo Moretta

Institute of Microbiology
University of Genoa
Genoa, Italy

Leslie A. Radov

Department of Pharmacology
Pennwalt Corporation
Rochester, New York 14603

Noel L. Warner

Immunobiology Laboratories
Departments of Pathology and Medicine
University of New Mexico School of Medicine
Albuquerque, New Mexico 87131

Preface

In this current volume of *Contemporary Topics in Immunobiology* we have chosen to continue with the multiple-theme approach that was developed in Volumes 1, 3, and 5 of this series. Immunobiology still shows little sign of decreasing its active growth rate, but rather is continuing to broaden its range of interests and applications, particularly as new techniques and methods are adapted from other fields of medical research.

This present volume reflects both several of the more classical areas of immunology now addressed in the light of contemporary immunology, and several newer directions that have been taken in other fields.

The general subject of T-cell heterogeneity and functions of T-cell subpopulations is addressed in Chapters 1 and 2. The potential role of genes of the major histocompatibility complex in controlling the immune functions of T lymphocytes still remains a major unresolved issue in immunogenetics, and the current status of this problem is excellently reviewed by J. F. A. P. Miller. The further elucidation of functional subpopulations of human T lymphocytes has been particularly hampered by the lack of available markers for characterizing and isolating such subpopulations. A major step in this direction has been made by L. Moretta, M. Ferrarini, and M. D. Cooper, who review their experience with Fc-receptor-bearing human T-lymphocyte populations.

Although the predominant interest in lymphocyte subpopulations has centered on the T-cell series, the subject of B-cell heterogeneity has become a considerably escalating field of research in immunobiology, in part through studies of the role or roles of membrane immunoglobulins as antigen receptors for immunity or tolerance. Progress in this field has also been considerably aided by the discoveries of murine IgD and allotypes of murine IgM and IgD, and these aspects are extensively covered by J. W. Goding in Chapter 7 and J. F. Kearney and E. R. Abney in Chapter 8.

Of considerable current interest in many areas of the world is the potential benefit to be gained from a better understanding of the role of the immune response in protection against parasitic infections. This field desperately requires the application of "newer" immunobiological approaches and one facet of this, namely, studies with athymic nude mice, is well reviewed in Chapter 3 by G. F. Mitchell.

The remaining three chapters of this volume are devoted to the field of tumor immunology and reflect the still considerable uncertainty of the relative roles played by various cell types in immune responses to different tumor antigens. In addition to the anti-tumor response of T cells, B cells, and macrophages, a new cell type—termed the natural killer cell—has recently been recognized as another potential cell type that may be capable of lysing many tumor cell lines. In Chapter 6, R. Kiessling and O. Haller comprehensively review the evidence that these natural killer cells may play a major role in immunological surveillance. On a broader level, J. S. Haskill, P. Hayry, and L. A. Radov have considered the potential role of various cell types in allogeneic and anti-tumor immunity, but have particularly concentrated in Chapter 5 on a major aspect that is frequently overlooked and ill defined, namely the *in situ* tumor response, as contrasted with systemic immunity. The analysis of mechanisms of T-cell-mediated immunity to tumors is relatively difficult to assess in *in vivo* studies; as in many other systems, considerable efforts have been made to develop primary immune responses *in vitro*, and the experience in this field of R. C. Burton, S. E. Chism, and N. L. Warner is reviewed in Chapter 4, with particular emphasis on the potential to further analyze the nature of tumor antigens as recognized by T lymphocytes.

Thus, in this volume, we feel that the multiauthor multitheme approach may provide a cross-sectional view of the range of topics in contemporary immunobiology 1977–78, and we gratefully acknowledge the cooperation of all authors in the preparation of this volume.

Noel L. Warner
Max D. Cooper

Contents

Chapter 3

Metazoan and Protozoan Parasitic Infections in Nude Mice

Graham F. Mitchell

Chapter 6

**Natural Killer Cells in the Mouse: An Alternative Immune
Surveillance Mechanism?**

Rolf Kiessling and Otto Haller

Chapter 7
Allotypes of IgM and IgD Receptors in the Mouse: A Probe for Lymphocyte Differentiation

James W. Goding

Chapter 8

Immunoglobulin Isotype Expression

John F. Kearney and Erika R. Abney

Chapter 1

Influence of Genes of the Major Histocompatibility Complex on the Reactivity of Thymus-Derived Lymphocytes

J. F. A. P. Miller

The Walter and Eliza Hall Institute of Medical Research
Royal Melbourne Hospital P.O.
Melbourne, Victoria 3050, Australia

I. INTRODUCTION

In the mouse the MHC (major histocompatibility complex, or *H-2*) is situated on chromosome 17 about 15 centimorgans from the centromere (Klein, 1975, 1976). It spans a distance of about 0.5 centimorgan and may be divided into five regions: *K*, *I*, *S*, *G*, and *D*. The *K* and *D* gene products were the first to be recognized since they control acceptance or prompt rejection of allografts. They can readily be detected by antisera produced by immunizing members of one inbred strain with histoincompatible cells from another inbred strain. The antigens detected by such antisera are found on all tissues after birth. By using different antisera many alleles were discovered at each locus. The *G* region determines alloantigens present on erythrocytes. The *S* region regulates the level of some complement components and codes for C4. The *I* region determines products of major importance for the genetic control of specific immune responses (*Ir*, or immune responsiveness, genes) (Benacerraf, 1973). It is divided into several subregions, *I-A*, *I-B*, *I-J*, *I-E*, and *I-C*, and these determine membrane glycoproteins known as *I*-associated (*Ia*) antigens. Products of the *I-A*, *I-C*, and *I-E* subregions are expressed on B lymphocytes, macrophages, epidermal cells, and spermatozoa (Shreffler and David, 1975), and products of the *I-J* subregion control determinants present on a subpopulation of T lymphocytes with suppressive functions (Murphy *et al.*, 1976). In addition, the *I* region codes for cell interaction molecules (Katz and Benacerraf, 1975) and components involved in stimulating mixed lymphocyte reactions (Shreffler and David, 1975).

1

The human genetic complex corresponding to the mouse MHC is known as HLA and is situated on chromosome 6. Among its products are alloantigens determined by the regions *HLA-A*, *HLA-B* (analogous to *K* and *D* in mice), and *HLA-C* and serologically detectable on all nucleated cells after birth. The *HLA-D*-region determinants have been defined by cell culture techniques and are mainly responsible for stimulation in mixed lymphocyte cultures. They also code for alloantigens expressed mainly on B lymphocytes, macrophages, epidermal cells, spermatozoa, and endothelial cells (Kissmeyer-Nielson, 1975).

The MHC exerts a profound influence on many aspects of T-cell (thymus-derived cell) functions. At least four effects deserve special mention:

1. The frequency of T cells reactive to cell surface alloantigens coded by the MHC is 100 to 1000 times that of T cells reactive to other antigens (Simonsen, 1967; Wilson *et al.*, 1977).
2. The control of the extent of a T-cell response to a variety of antigens is exerted by genes which have been localized to the *I* region of the MHC (Benacerraf, 1973).
3. The MHC imposes restrictions on the activities of sensitized T cells (see Section II).
4. Soluble factors, which bear MHC-coded determinants, influence the activation of a variety of T-cell subsets (Tada, 1978; Feldmann *et al.*, 1977; Munro and Taussig, 1975).

The aim of this chapter is to review briefly some of the recent work performed in mice which allows the formulation of a hypothesis that may be used to explain tentatively the relationships among MHC gene products, T-lymphocyte activation, and immune reactivity.

II. CONSTRAINTS IMPOSED ON T-CELL ACTIVITIES BY GENES OF THE MAJOR HISTOCOMPATIBILITY COMPLEX

Activation of some T lymphocytes requires antigen presentation by other cells, e.g., macrophages (Feldmann *et al.*, 1977). This has been well documented for helper T cells (T_H) involved in cooperating with B cells (bone-marrow-derived cells) to enable optimal production of IgG antibody (Basten *et al.*, 1975) and for T cells (T_D) involved in delayed-type hypersensitivity (DTH) (Oppenheim and Seeger, 1976). Some T cells, e.g., cytotoxic T lymphocytes (T_C), may be activated optimally when antigen is presented in association with "accessory" cells (Julius and Herzenberg, 1973). In the last few years it has become very clear that MHC gene products play a critical role in the sensitization of many of these T-lymphocyte subsets (Table I).

Table I. MHC-Imposed Constraints on the Reactivity of T Lymphocytes

Species	Experimental system	MHC region	T-cell subset and phenotype[a]	Reference
Guinea pig	Specific antigen-induced	I	–	Rosenthal et al. (1975)
Mouse	proliferation of sensi-tized lymphocytes	I	–	R. H. Schwartz et al. (1976)
Mouse	in vitro	I	–	Peck et al. (1977)
Man		HLA-D	–	Bergholtz and Thorsby (1977)
Mouse	Optimal cooperation be-tween primed T and B lymphocytes for in vivo antibody responses	I-A	T_H (Ly-1)	Katz and Benacerraf (1975)
Mouse	Optimal induction of T_H cells by macrophage-associated antigen in vitro	I-A	T_H (Ly-1)	Erb and Feldmann (1975)
Mouse	T cells cytotoxic to:			
	(a) virus-infected target cells	K or D	T_C (Ly-2,3)	Doherty et al. (1976)
	(b) chemically modi-fied target cells	K or D	T_C (Ly-2,3)	Shearer et al. (1975)
	(c) non-H2-alloantigen	K or D	T_C	Bevan (1975)
	(d) H-Y antigen	K or D	T_C	Gordon et al. (1975)
Man	T cells cytotoxic to H-Y antigen	HLA-A	T_C	Goulmy et al. (1977)
Mouse	Transfer of delayed-type hypersensitivity to:			
	(a) proteins and polypeptides	I-A	T_D (Ly-1)	Miller et al. (1975, 1977)
	(b) contact chemicals	I, K, or D	T_D (Ly-1 and Ly-2,3)	Miller et al. (1976)

[a]For the phenotypes, see Vadas et al. (1976) and Feldmann et al. (1977).

It was initially demonstrated that the activation of proliferation of sensitized guinea pig T lymphocytes required that the antigen-presenting macrophages had the same I-region determinants as the T cell (Rosenthal et al., 1975). This was subsequently shown to apply to mouse (R. H. Schwartz et al., 1976) and to human lymphocytes (Bergholtz and Thorsby, 1977). For example, the activation of T-lymphocyte proliferation in man in response to purified protein derivative of tuberculin was strongest when macrophages in the culture had the same *HLA-D* determinants as those of the donor of the sensitized T lymphocytes. Essentially comparable findings have been obtained in studies of collaboration between primed T_H and B lymphocytes *in vivo* (Katz and Benacerraf, 1975) and in the induction of T_H cells for *in vitro* antibody responses (Erb and Feldmann, 1975).

Cytotoxic T lymphocytes derived by conventional immunization procedures and specific for virus-specified antigens (Doherty *et al.*, 1976) or chemically modified membrane antigens (Shearer *et al.*, 1975) expressed their cytotoxic potential effectively only when antigenic target cells and killer cells were of the same *H-2K* or *H-2D* type. The same restriction applied to T cells cytotoxic for cells bearing minor histocompatibility antigens (Bevan, 1975; Gordon *et al.*, 1975). Conversely, cells lacking *H-2K* or *H-2D* molecules on their surface (e.g., the teratocarcinoma line, F9) are apparently not recognized by cytotoxic T lymphocytes (Forman and Vitetta, 1975; Goldstein *et al.*, 1976; Doherty *et al.*, 1977).

MHC-imposed constraints have also been reported in the transfer of DTH in mice, the region involved being *I-A* for protein and polypeptide antigens (Miller *et al.*, 1975, 1977) and *I*, *K*, or *D* for contact chemicals, such as dinitrofluorobenzene (Miller *et al.*, 1976) and for some virus-infected cells (Zinkernagel, 1976a).

As has recently been realized, the MHC-imposed constraints on T-cell functions can, in some cases, arise as a result of sensitization (see Section III). Thus there need be no constraints on the activities of unprimed T cells, with the possible exception of the activation of T cells to antigens the response to which is under strict MHC-linked *Ir* gene control (see Section V). The restrictions imposed by the MHC on functioning of sensitized T cells have clear implications for the means by which T cells are activated and recognize antigen.

III. IMPLICATIONS OF MHC-IMPOSED RESTRICTIONS FOR ANTIGEN PERCEPTION BY T LYMPHOCYTES

The transfer of DTH to protein antigens in mice was shown to be possible only in *I-A*-compatible recipients (Miller *et al.*, 1975; Vadas *et al.*, 1977). Various experiments made it unlikely that the inability to transfer DTH in MHC-incompatible recipients could be attributed to rejection of the injected cells, their total recruitment into areas such as the spleen, or their engagement in a mixed lymphocyte reaction (Vadas *et al.*, 1977). For example, DTH was successfully transferred from sensitized F_1 hybrid mice to naive mice of the parental strain which are competent to reject the F_1 cells (Table II). The possibility that suppressive influences were generated in an allogeneic environment found no

Table II. MHC-Imposed Constraints on the Transfer of DTH in Mice

Group	Source of sensitized T cells	Naive recipient	L/R ^{125}I-UdR uptake in recipients[a]
1	BALB/c mice sensitized to FGG by footpad inoculation	BALB/c	2.6 ± 0.2
		CBA	1.1 ± 0.1
		F$_1$ (CBA X BALB/c)	2.1 ± 0.1
2	F$_1$ (CBA X BALB/c) mice sensitized to FGG by footpad inoculation	BALB/c	2.2 ± 0.1
		CBA	1.6 ± 0.1
		F$_1$ (CBA X BALB/c)	2.3 ± 0.1
3	F$_1$ (CBA X BALB/c) mice sensitized to FGG-pulsed BALB/c macrophages intraperitoneal injection	BALB/c	1.6 ± 0.2
		CBA	1.1 ± 0.1
		F$_1$ (CBA X BALB/c)	1.8 ± 0.2

[a] The naive recipients were tested for DTH by the radioisotopic ear method, using 5-iodo-2'-deoxyuridine-^{125}I (^{125}I-UdR) as described previously (Vadas et al., 1975). Briefly, the mice were challenged with antigen in the left (L) ear, injected intraperitoneally with 2 μCi of ^{125}I-UdR, and the ears removed 24 hr later for counting in a Packard Gamma Spectrometer. The results are expressed as the ratio of radioactivity in the left ear to that in the right ear (L/R ^{125}I-UdR uptake). It is unusual to obtain a ratio of >1.2 in nonsensitized mice or in naive mice not receiving sensitized cells. Arithmetic means ± standard error of five to six mice per group.

supporting evidence in most strain combinations. The explanation we favor to explain the MHC-imposed restriction is that sensitized T cells are not able to perceive antigen when this is presented on MHC-incompatible stimulator cells, presumably macrophages (Vadas et al., 1977).

By using three different experimental systems, we showed that T-cell sensitization in DTH to protein antigens was directed both to the antigen and to the MHC product responsible for restriction and presumably displayed on antigen-presenting macrophages. The models involved chimeric mice, athymic nude mice, and antigen-pulsed macrophages (Miller et al., 1976). For example, macrophages from CBA or BALB/c mice were pulsed with fowl gammaglobulin (FGG) in vitro, washed, and injected into (CBA X BALB/c)F$_1$ mice. Lymphoid cells from mice sensitized with such macrophage preparations were tested for their ability to transfer DTH into parental naive recipients. Transfer was possible provided that the macrophages used for sensitization were of the same genotype as the recipient (exemplified in group 3 of Table II). This strongly supports the notion that sensitization is directed not to the antigen as such but to cell surface structures on the macrophage determined partly by the I-region product and partly by processed antigen. Sensitization of T cells in an F$_1$ would lead to the activation of two subsets of F$_1$ T cells with respect to the specificity of their antigen-combining sites: one with sites directed toward the antigen and I-region product of one parental strain, the other with sites directed toward the antigen and I-region product of the other parental strain. Sensitization of F$_1$ T cells by antigen-pulsed macrophages of one parental strain would thus lead to the activation of only one of these two subsets of T cells. Whether the specificities involved are encompassed in one or two genetically independent molecules per T cell (Wilson *et al.*, 1977) cannot be determined on the basis of the present experimental design.

The conclusion that the MHC imposes constraints only as a result of sensitization has also been reached in experiments involving helper T cells (von Boehmer and Sprent, 1976; Pierce *et al.*, 1976; Kappler and Marrack, 1976), cytotoxic T cells (Pfizenmaier *et al.*, 1976; Zinkernagel, 1976*b*; von Boehmer and Haas, 1976), and T cells proliferating in response to antigenic stimulation (Paul *et al.*, 1977). Reactivities of sensitized T cells of many types seem therefore to be directed not to antigen as such but to antigen and a particular MHC gene product. This may account for a variety of observations which were interpreted to indicate that T and B cells differed in the spectra of their pattern of reactivities to antigen (e.g., Schirrmacher and Wigzell, 1972). Such a difference in antigen reactivity would be expected if T cells could react only if antigen were presented in association with cell membrane MHC gene-specified products. The recognition molecule on T and B cells may thus be the same or very similar. Only the requirements for antigen processing and presentation may differ.

An obvious candidate for the T-cell receptor for antigen is a molecule identical to B-cell immunoglobulin, referred to as IgT (Marchalonis, 1974). In view of the difficulty that some investigators have had in isolating IgT, it has been suggested that the antigen-specific receptor on T lymphocytes may not be classical immunoglobulin but a different molecule. This may in part be coded by *C*-region genes located in the MHC and thus different from the *C* genes of classical immunoglobulin (Munro and Taussig, 1975). The molecule must, however, use the same *V*-region genes as immunoglobulin, since receptors for certain antigens on T and B cells have identical *V*-region idiotypes, as do circulating antibodies directed against the same antigens (Binz and Wigzell, 1975; Eichmann and Rajewsky, 1975). Although a DNA translocation model for sharing of *V*-region genes by various *C* regions linked on the same chromosome is quite likely (Gally and Edelman, 1972), it is more difficult to envisage translocation between unlinked *V*-region genes and MHC genes. It seems more reasonable to assume that the MHC is involved, not in coding for part of the T-cell receptor, but as a necessary force in the activation of T lymphocytes to *some* antigens, as discussed in this chapter.

IV. MHC-LINKED *Ir* GENE CONTROL OF IMMUNE RESPONSIVENESS

Certain individuals within a species fail to respond to a specific antigen. This deficiency was found to map in the *I*-region. In mice, defects have been found in the response to more than 40 antigens (Benacerraf and Katz, 1975). In each case the failure to respond is recessive, i.e., the response is dominant, and an F_1 hybrid between a responder (R) strain and a nonresponder (NR) strain is capable of responding. Responsiveness is generally manifest in T-cell functions, not in B-cell potential. For this reason, it was at one time suggested that the MHC-linked immune responsiveness (*Ir*) genes may code for the antigen recognition unit on T cells (Katz and Benacerraf, 1975).

Mice of the $H\text{-}2^{a,b,d,f,j,k,r,u,v}$ haplotypes have been classed as "responders" to the random terpolymer L-glutamic acid^{60}-L-alanine^{30}-L-tyrosine^{10} (GAT), because they can produce specific antibodies after the injection of the antigen. Mice of the $H\text{-}2^{n,p,q,s}$ haplotypes are "nonresponders," as they produce no detectable antibodies. It was therefore of interest to determine whether DTH responsiveness to GAT could be elicited in NR strains. As shown in Table III, DTH to GAT could not be elicited in mice of $H\text{-}2^s$ or $H\text{-}2^q$ haplotypes, although it could be readily produced in strains known to be responders on the basis of antibody production.

We also examined whether there might be constraints on the transfer of DTH to GAT. As may be seen from Table IV, identity between donors and recipients at the *I-A* region alone (e.g., A.TL $\longrightarrow$ B10.A(4R) and B10.A(4R) $\longrightarrow$ A.TL) was sufficient to allow DTH transfer to GAT. Identity at *I-B* alone (B10.A(4R) $\longrightarrow$ B10.A(5R)), at *D* alone (A.TL $\longrightarrow$ BALB/c), or at *K* alone (A.TL $\longrightarrow$ A.SW) did not allow transfer. DTH transfer to GAT from sensitized responder strain mice was thus possible if donors and recipients were identical at the *I-A* region of the MHC, just as had been previously observed with FGG (Vadas *et al.*, 1977). One implication is that DTH transfer to all protein and polypeptide antigens requires *I-A* identity. Alternatively, the MHC region imposing constraint on DTH transfer may conceivably also control responsive-

Table III. Mouse Strain Differences in DTH Responsiveness to GAT

Strain of mice sensitized to GAT	MHC[a]	L/R ^{125}I-UdR uptake[b]
CBA	k k k k k k k k	3.4 ± 0.4
BALB/c	d d d d d d d d	2.2 ± 0.2
A.TL	s k k k k k k d	2.2 ± 0.2
A.TH	s s s s s s s d	1.1 ± 0.1
A.SW	s s s s s s s s	1.2 ± 0.1
SJL	s s s s s s s s	0.8 ± 0.2
DBA/1	q q q q q q q q	1.0 ± 0.1

[a]Regions indicated are *K*, *I-A*, *I-B*, *I-J*, *I-E*, *I-C*, *S*, and *D*.
[b]Values are arithmetic means ± S.E.M. Five to six mice per group. Data from Miller *et al.* (1977).

Table IV. MHC Restriction of the Transfer of DTH to GAT

Donor of sensitized lymphoid cells	Recipient strain	MHC of recipients[a]	L/R ^{125}I-UdR uptake in recipient mice[b]
A.TL	A.TL	s k k k k k k d	2.1 ± 0.2
	B10.A(4R)	*k k b b b b b b*	1.6 ± 0.2
	BALB/c	*d d d d d d d d*	0.9 ± 0.2
	A.SW	*s s s s s s s s*	1.1 ± 0.1
B10.A(4R)	B10.A(4R)	k k b b b b b b	1.5 ± 0.04
	A.TL	*s* k k k k k k *d*	1.6 ± 0.2
	B10.A(5R)	*b b* b k *d d d*	1.0 ± 0.02
	CBA	k k *k k k k k* k	1.5 ± 0.1

[a]Regions indicated are K, I-A, I-B, I-J, I-E, I-C, S, and D; letters in italics point to differences in regions between donor and recipient mice.
[b]Arithmetic means ± S.E. Five mice per group. Data from Miller *et al.* (1977).

ness to that antigen. If this is the case, restrictions with certain antigens should be imposed by different I subregions corresponding to those in which the Ir genes governing responsiveness to those antigens have been mapped.

V. RELATIONSHIP BETWEEN MHC-IMPOSED CONSTRAINTS AND MHC-LINKED Ir GENE CONTROL OF IMMUNE RESPONSIVENESS

Since the MHC-linked Ir genes have so far been mapped in the I region, it seemed relevant to inquire into the nature of the possible relationship between MHC-imposed constraints on the activities of sensitized T cells and MHC-linked Ir gene control of T-cell sensitization. A clue to this relationship was obtained in experiments on the transfer of sensitivity to fowl gamma globulin (FGG) and dinitrofluorobenzene (DNFB) in mice (Vadas *et al.*, 1977). Cells from (CBA × C57BL)F$_1$ and (CBA × BALB/c)F$_1$ mice sensitized to FGG were able to transfer DTH to both parents, but did so more efficiently to C57BL or BALB/c than to CBA. It is unlikely that this was due to a special property of the CBA recipients, since the difference was not seen if the F$_1$ cells were sensitized not to FGG, but to DNFB (Table V). Transfer into mice congenic with the parents showed that this effect was, at least partially, governed by the MHC. Thus transfer to FGG, but not to DNFB, was weaker into H-2^k (CBA, C3H, B10.BR) than into H-2^b (C57BL, C3H.SW) mice, regardless of their backgrounds. One possibility is that FGG is less immunogenic when processed by H-2^k than by H-2^b mice. Thus in an F$_1$ there would be more cells generated reactive to FGG-H-2^b than to FGG-H-2^k.

We wondered whether the same phenomenon, albeit more extreme, may hold for responsiveness to antigens under strict MHC-linked Ir gene control.

Table V. Transfer of DTH to FGG and DNFB from (CBA × C57BL)F$_1$ Mice into Various Recipients[a]

Recipients	H-2 genotype of recipients	L/R ^{125}I-UdR uptake in recipients of:	
		FGG-sensitized cells	DNFB-sensitized cells
(CBA × C57BL)F$_1$	k/b	2.8 ± 0.2	3.0 ± 0.2
C57BL	b	1.9 ± 0.1	2.3 ± 0.2
C3H.SW	b	2.1 ± 0.2	1.8 ± 0.2
CBA	k	1.5 ± 0.1	2.3 ± 0.2
C3H	k	1.5 ± 0.1	2.0 ± 0.2
B10.BR	k	1.2 ± 0.04	2.1 ± 0.2

[a]Data from Vadas *et al.* (1977)

DTH to GAT was transferrable from sensitized (R × NR)F$_1$ mice to naive recipients of the R but not of the NR haplotype (Table VI). In fact, the situation here is analogous to that already observed in (CBA × BALB/c)F$_1$ mice sensitized to FGG-pulsed macrophages derived from one parental strain. As mentioned in Section III, transfer of DTH from these F$_1$ mice was possible but only to naive recipients of the parental strain of the same genotype as that from which the macrophages used for sensitization were obtained (Miller *et al.*, 1976). These results can be interpreted to favor the idea that in NR strains, the macrophages fail to display the antigen under *Ir* gene control in a form immunogenic for T lymphocytes involved in DTH. The alternative possibility of a defect at the level of T-cell recognition for antigen is difficult to reconcile with these data. Thus, if the *Ir* gene coded for the T-cell receptor for antigen, an F$_1$ animal should have T cells with receptors able to recognize antigen associated with MHC products of the NR haplotype, since the *Ir* gene coding for such a receptor would be de-

Table VI. DTH Transfer to GAT by Sensitized F$_1$ (Responder × Nonresponder) Cells[a]

Naive recipients of 5 × 10^7 F$_1$ cells	L/R ^{125}I-UdR uptake[b]
(BALB/c × SJL)F$_1$	2.2 ± 0.2
BALB/c	2.6 ± 0.1
SJL	1.2 ± 0.1
(A.TL × A.TH)F$_1$	1.9 ± 0.1
A.TL	1.8 ± 0.2
A.TH	1.2 ± 0.1

[a]Sensitivity in the donors was as follows: (BALB/c × SJL)F$_1$, 9.3 ± 0.9 and (A.TL × A.TH)F$_1$ 2.5 ± 0.3. BALB/c, A.TL, and F$_1$ are responders to GAT.
[b]Values are arithmetic means ± S.E. Five to six mice per group. Data from Miller *et al.* (1977).

rived from the R parental strain. But if this were so, sensitivity from the F_1 would be transferable to naive recipients of NR haplotypes. It is, however, still possible to envisage other mechanisms based on *Ir* gene control of idiotype-specific suppressor T cells blocking expression of cells activated to the particular antigen.

With the data available so far, we can offer one mechanism by which MHC-linked *Ir* genes control T-cell responsiveness. Rather than coding for the T-cell receptor for antigen, the *Ir* genes would code for structures allowing the display of antigen on the surface of cells, such as macrophages, involved in T-cell activation. The immunogenicity of the antigen for T cells would thus be a function of the manner in which it associates with the *Ir* gene product. At this stage, there is no reason not to consider this product as being the relevant *I*-region gene determinant involved in the MHC-imposed restriction discussed above. The identity of *Ir* and *Ia* receives strong support from the concordance between *Ir* and *Ia* mapping and from the many instances in which *Ir* genes controlling responses to different antigens show a similar distribution pattern of high and low responsiveness (Klein, 1976). On the other hand, one could imagine *Ir* genes coding for components which allow interactions between particular *I*-region products and the antigen to form stable structures. These suggestions are in general agreement with ideas recently expressed by Paul and Benacerraf (1977) and by R. H. Schwartz *et al*. (1976) and based on other experimental systems.

A model based on the interactions between *I*-region gene products and antigen is supported by a variety of observations and in turn leads to a number of predictions.

1. Slight physicochemical alterations of an antigen under *Ir* gene control should allow changes in the way in which this antigen associates with the relevant *I*-region gene product on the macrophage. In some cases, therefore, a nonresponder for the original antigen should become a responder. Data suggesting that this may occur are already available (M. Schwartz *et al*., 1976).

2. Antigen unable to associate effectively with the *I*-region gene product on the macrophage should come off the cell membrane and be available as free antigen. This may tend to induce tolerance or activate suppressor T cells which are known to be readily activated by free antigen (Feldmann *et al*., 1977). Hence, antigen-specific suppressor T cells should be found in nonresponder strains, and this indeed was demonstrated in some systems (Kapp *et al*., 1974; Howie, 1977) and implicated in others (Miller *et al*., 1976).

3. It would seem probable that the MHC region imposing constraints on the activities of sensitized T cells should correspond to that region in which the *Ir* gene governing responsiveness to the antigen has been mapped. So far only the *I-A* region has been shown to restrict the activities of sensi-

tized T cells in DTH, but it would be expected that other I regions may be involved in the case of sensitivity to antigens the responsiveness to which is controlled by Ir genes mapping in regions other than I-A.

4. As a corollary, when complementing Ir genes are involved (Dorf and Benacerraf, 1975), one would expect them to function through some structure assembled at the membrane of the cell presenting antigen to T cells. One would not expect one gene to be expressed in one cell and the other in another cell, as has been suggested in studies of T- and B-cell cooperation in antibody responses to an antigen under MHC-linked Ir gene control (Munro and Taussig, 1975). Hence, even though appropriate $(NR \times NR)F_1$ combinations do complement, chimeras between the same pairs of NR strains would not be expected to show this effect. Data recently available from studies using allophenic mice tend to support this prediction (Warner et al., 1977).

5. In order to be consistent with the model offered, one would expect that the Ir genes controlling the activities of cytotoxic T lymphocytes should map in the K and D regions of the MHC, since these are the regions which restrict the activities of these cells (see Table I). Data are not generally available on this issue, although an Ir-like gene which controls the generation of cytotoxic T cells has been localized between K and I-A (Schmitt-Verhulst and Shearer, 1976).

VI. CONCLUDING REMARKS

On chromosome 17 in the mouse, and close to the MHC at the centromeric end, lies the T/t system. This is a complex region which affects embryonic development, sperm function, genetic recombination, and cell membrane structures (Bennett, 1975). It is highly probable that the T/t complex-coded cell-surface structures constitute a network of signals essential for cell–cell recognition and for the regulation of morphogenetic steps during development of the embryo. Analogies between embryonic T/t antigens and H-2 antigens have been presented and it has been suggested that the T/t complex may be an evolutionary precursor of the MHC, or that both complexes may have originated from a common ancestral gene (Artz and Bennett, 1975). To pursue the analogy still further, we would like to propose that the main function of the MHC is to control the activation and differentiation of subsets of various T lymphocytes. Once these are activated effectively, their specificity will exhibit restriction, being directed toward both the antigen and the MHC component involved in the activation. We have also proposed that the MHC-linked Ir genes exert their effects by coding for cell-surface components which allow physicochemical interactions between a given antigen and a given MHC gene product. Depending on the stability of this interaction, the combined structure will exhibit different degrees of immunogenicity for appropriate subsets of T lymphocytes. We have not excluded the possibility that the *Ir* gene product itself may, in fact, be identical to the MHC product responsible for the restriction imposed on the activities of the sensitized T cells.

The current literature abounds with examples of MHC-imposed restrictions on the activities of cytotoxic lymphocytes. In addition to the MHC itself, there are numerous histocompatibility (*H*) loci scattered throughout the mouse genome and referred to as minor *H* loci (Klein, 1976). At least 40 have been identified and the number of such loci has been estimated by some to be several hundred (Snell, 1974). Conceivably, any of these loci can act as target for cytotoxic T lymphocytes. However, if each minor *H* locus can be perceived as a target only if associated with an MHC component, then the potential number of target antigens in any MHC-incompatible strain combination must literally be enormous. This could easily account for the high frequency of alloreactive T cells. It would be of interest to determine whether this frequency is less when tested in strain combinations which differ only at the MHC and which are congenic for all other loci. Preliminary results in the DTH system indicate that good sensitivity could be achieved with allogeneic cells in mice, but only if the strain combinations used exhibited differences both at MHC and at other loci (groups 5 and 6, Table VII). By contrast, little or no sensitivity could be elicited to allogeneic cells in congenic MHC-incompatible strain combinations (group 2, Table VII).

Finally, it may be worthwhile pointing out that there are notable exceptions to the phenomenon of MHC-imposed restrictions. For example, reports of lack of *H-2* restriction are available in systems employing tumor antigens. The activities of cytotoxic T cells in some experiments were not *H-2*-restricted, either at the sensitization phase or at the effector stage (Jondal *et al.*, 1975; Ting and Law, 1977; Burton *et al.*, 1977; Holden, 1977). Various reasons have been given to account for this effect. For example, in one system, restriction was observed if cytotoxicity was tested in a 4-hr ^{51}Cr release assay but not if tested in an 18-hr assay. In another system, different degrees of restriction were noted depending on whether activation was produced *in vivo* or *in vitro*. A further notable exception to the phenomenon of MHC-imposed restriction was found in the DTH response to mouse erythrocytes parasitized by *Plasmodium berghei* (Whitelaw *et al.*, 1977). It would be interesting to determine whether lack of *H-2* restriction is found in other systems in which a stable host–parasite relationship has been established during evolution. This is because we believe that it must be more than coincidental that no MHC-imposed constraint has been observed, as stated above, with both the malaria parasite and the various oncogenic viruses responsible for tumor antigenicity, i.e., with parasitic agents that have been very successful during evolution in adapting to their hosts and evading immune

Table VII. DTH to Allogeneic Cells in C57BL Mice[a]

Group	Cells used for sensitization	Cells used for challenge	L/R ^{125}I-UdR uptake[b]
1	None	B10.D2 (H-2d, B10 background)	1.5 ± 0.1
2	B10.D2 (H-2d, B10 background)	B10.D2 (H-2d, B10 background)	1.4 ± 0.1
3	BALB.B (H-2b, BALB background)	B10.D2 (H-2d, B10 background)	1.3 ± 0.1
4	(B10.D2 × BALB.B)F$_1$ (H-2d × H-2b, B10 and BALB backgrounds)	B10.D2 (H-2d, B10 background)	1.3 ± 0.2
5	(B10.D2 × BALB.B)F$_1$ (H-2d × H-2b, B10 and BALB backgrounds)	(B10.D2 × BALB.B)F$_1$ (H-2d × H-2b, B10 and BALB backgrounds)	4.7 ± 0.6
6	(B10.D2 × BALB.B)F$_1$ (H-2d × H-2b, B10 and BALB backgrounds)	B10.D2 + BALB.B (H-2d + H-2b, B10 and BALB backgrounds)	4.8 ± 0.8

[a]C57BL is H-2b, B10 background. We have now been able to obtain DTH to allogenic cells in congenic MHC-incompatible mice using strain conditions different from those given in this table.
[b]Values are arithmetic means ± S.E.M. Six to seven mice per group. Unpublished results of J. F. A. P. Miller, J. Gamble, and M. Barg.

surveillance. It is possible that a lack of association of the antigens specified by these agents with products of the MHC is just what is required to ensure escape of the parasitized cell from what otherwise would have been a sterilizing effect of a strong T-cell-mediated immune response.

ACKNOWLEDGMENTS

The original work reported in this chapter was performed in collaboration with Dr. M. A. Vadas, Miss A. Whitelaw, and Miss J. Gamble. Support for this was obtained from the National Health and Medical Research Council of Australia and from U.S. Public Health Service Research Grant 63992 from the National Cancer Institute.

VII. REFERENCES

Artz, K., and Bennett, D., 1975, Analogies between embryonic (T/t) antigens and adult major histocompatibility (H-2) antigens, *Nature* **256**:545.

Basten, A., Miller, J. F. A. P., and Abraham, R., 1975. Relationship between Fc receptors, antigen binding sites on T and B cells, and *H-2* complex-associated determinants, *J. Exp. Med.* **141**:547.

Benacerraf, B., 1973, The genetic control of specific immune responses, *Harvey Lect.* **67**:109.

Benacerraf, B., and Katz, D. H., 1975, The histocompatibility-linked immune response genes, *Adv. Cancer Res.* **21**:121.

Bennett, D., 1975, The T-locus of the mouse, *Cell* **6**:441.

Bergholtz, B. O., and Thorsby, E., 1977, Macrophage-dependent response of immune human T lymphocytes to PPD *in vitro*. Influence of *HLA-D* histocompatibility, *Scand. J. Immunol.* **6**:779.

Bevan, M. J., 1975, The major histocompatibility complex determines susceptibility to cytotoxic T cells directed against minor histocompatibility antigens, *J. Exp. Med.* **142**:1349.

Binz, H., and Wigzell, H., 1975, Shared idiotypic determinants on B & T lymphocytes reactive against the same antigenic determinants. II. Determination of frequency and characteristics of idiotypic T & B lymphocytes in normal rats using direct visulization, *J. Exp. Med.* **142**: 1218.

Burton, R. C., Chism, S. E., and Warner, N. L., 1977, *In vitro* induction of tumor-specific immunity. III. Lack of requirement for *H-2* compatibility in lysis of tumor targets by T cells activated *in vitro* to oncofoetal and plasmacytoma antigens, *J. Immunol.* **118**:971.

Doherty, P. C., Blanden, R. V., and Zinkernagel, R. M., 1976, Specificity of virus-immune effector T cells for *H-2K* or *H-2D* compatible interactions: Implications for H-antigen diversity, *Transplant Rev.* **29**:89.

Doherty, P. C., Solter, D., and Knowles, B. B., 1977, *H-2* gene expression is required for T cell-mediated lysis of virus-infected target cells, *Nature* **266**:361.

Dorf, M. E., and Benacerraf, B., 1975, Complementation of *H-2* linked *Ir* genes in the mouse, *Proc. Natl. Acad. Sci. U.S.* **72**:3671.

Eichmann, K., and Rajewsky, K., 1975, Induction of T & B cell immunity by anti-idiotypic antibody, *Eur. J. Immunol.* **5**:661.

Erb, P., and Feldmann, M., 1975, The role of macrophages in the generation of T-helper cells. II. The genetic control of the macrophage-T-cell interaction for helper cell induction with soluble antigen, *J. Exp. Med.* **142**:460.

Feldmann, M., Beverly, P., Erb, P., Howie, S., Kontiainen, S., Moaz, A., Mathies, M., McKenzie, I., and Woody, J., 1977, Current concepts of the antibody response. Heterogeneity of lymphoid cells, interactions and factors, *Cold Spring Harbor Symp. Quant. Biol.* **41**:113.

Forman, J., and Vitetta, E. S., 1975, Absence of *H-2* antigens capable of reacting with cytotoxic T cells on a teratoma line expressing a *T/t* locus antigen, *Proc. Natl. Acad. Sci. U.S.* **72**:3661.

Gally, J. A., and Edelman, G. A., 1972, The genetic control of immunoglobulin synthesis, *Ann. Rev. Genet.* **6**:1.

Goldstein, P., Kelly, F., Avner, P., and Gachelin, G., 1976, Sensitivity of *H-2*-less target cells and role of *H-2* in T-cell-mediated cytolysis, *Nature* **262**:693.

Gordon, R. D., Simpson, E., and Samelson, L. E., 1975, *In vitro* cell mediated immune responses to the male specific (*H-Y*) antigen in mice, *J. Exp. Med.* **142**:1108.

Goulmy, E., Termijtelen, A., Bradley, B. A., and van Rood, J. J., 1977, Y-antigen killing by T cells of women is restricted by HLA, *Nature* **266**:544.

Holden, H. T., 1977, Murine sarcoma virus (MSU) induced T cell cytotoxicity lack of *H-2* restriction at the sensitization or effector phase, *Fed. Proc.* **36**:1202.

Howie, S., 1977, *In vitro* studies on *H-2* linked unresponsiveness to synthetic polypeptide antigens. II. Induction of suppressor cells in both responsive and unresponsive mice to (T,G)-A-L and GAT, *Immunology* **32**:301.

Jondal, M., Svedmyr, E., Klein, E., and Singh, S., 1975, Killer T cells in a Burkitt's lymphoma biopsy, *Nature* **255**:405.

Julius, M., and Herzenberg, L. A., 1973, A rapid method for the isolation of functional thymus-derived murine lymphocytes, *Eur. J. Immunol.* **3**:645.

Kapp, J. A., Pierce, C. W., Schlossman, S., and Benacerraf, B., 1974, Genetic control of immune responses *in vitro*. V. Stimulation of suppressor T cells in nonresponder mice by the terpolymer L-glutamic acid^{60}-L-alanine^{30}-L-tyrosine^{10} (GAT), *J. Exp. Med.* **140**:468.

Kappler, J. W., and Marrack, P. C., 1976, Helper T cells recognise antigen and macrophage surface components simultaneously, *Nature* **262**:797.

Katz, D. H., and Benacerraf, B., 1975, The function and interrelationship of T cell receptors, *Ir* genes and other histocompatibility gene products, *Transplant. Rev.* **22**:175.

Kissmeyer-Nielsen, F. (ed.), 1975, *Histocompatibility Testing*, Munksgaard, Copenhagen.

Klein, J., 1975, *Biology of the Mouse Histocompatibility-2 Complex*, Springer-Verlag, Berlin.

Klein, J., 1976, An attempt as an interpretation of the mouse *H-2* complex, in: *Contemporary Topics in Immunobiology*, Vol. 5 (W. O. Weigle, ed.), p. 297, Plenum Press, New York.

Marchalonis, J., 1974, Lymphocyte receptors for antigen, *J. Med.* **5**:329.

Miller, J. F. A. P., Vadas, M. A., Whitelaw, A., and Gamble, J., 1975, *H-2* gene complex restricts transfer of delayed-type hypersensitivity in mice, *Proc. Natl. Acad. Sci. U.S.* **72**:5095.

Miller, J. F. A. P., Vadas, M. A., Whitelaw, A., and Gamble, J., 1976, Role of major histocompatibility complex gene products in delayed-type hypersensitivity, *Proc. Natl. Acad. Sci. U.S.* **73**:2486.

Miller, J. F. A. P., Vadas, M. A., Whitelaw, A., Gamble, J., and Bernard C., 1977, Histocompatibility linked immune responsiveness and restrictions imposed on sensitized lymphocytes, *J. Exp. Med.* **145**:1623.

Munro, A. J., and Taussig, M. J., 1975, Two genes in the major histocompatibility complex control immune response, *Nature* **256**:103.

Murphy, D. B., Herzenberg, L. A., Okumura, K., Herzenberg, L. A., and McDevitt, H. O., 1976, A new *I* subregion (*I-J*) marked by a locus (*Ia*-4) controlling surface determinants on suppressor T lymphocytes, *J. Exp. Med.* **144**:699.

Oppenheim, J. J., and Seeger, R. C., 1976, Induction of cell-mediated immunity, in: *Immunobiology of the Macrophage* (D. Nelson, ed.), p. 112, Academic Press, New York.

Paul, W. E., and Benacerraf, B., 1977, Functional specificity of thymus-dependent lymphocytes, *Science* **195**:1293.

Paul, W. E., Shevach, E. M., Pickeral, S., Thomas, D. W., and Rosenthal, A. S., 1977, Independent populations of primed F_1 guinea pig T lymphocytes respond to antigen-pulsed parental peritoneal exudate cells, *J. Exp. Med.* **145**:618.

Peck, A. B., Janeway, C. A., Jr., and Wigzell, H., 1977, T lymphocyte response to *Mls* locus antigens involves recognition of *H-2 I* region gene products, Nature **266**:840.

Pfizenmaier, K., Starzinski-Powitz, A., Rodt, H., Rollinghoff, M., and Wagner, H., 1976, Virus and trinitrophenol hapten-specific T-cell-mediated cytotoxicity against *H-2* incompatible target cells, *J. Exp. Med.* **143**:999.

Pierce, C. W., Kapp, J. A., and Benacerraf, B., 1976, Regulation by the *H-2* gene complex of macrophage–lymphoid cell interactions in secondary antibody responses *in vitro*, *J. Exp. Med.* **144**:371.

Rosenthal, A. S., Lipsky, P. E., and Shevach, E. M., 1975, Macrophage–lymphocyte interaction and antigen recognition, *Fed. Proc.* **34**:1743.

Schirrmacher, V., and Wigzell, H., 1972, Immune responses against native and chemically modified albumins in mice. I. Analysis of non-thymus processed (B) and thymus-processed (T) cell responses against methylated bovine serum albumin, *J. Exp. Med.* **136**:1616.

Schmitt-Verhulst, A. M., and Shearer, G. M., 1976, Multiple *H-2* linked immune response gene control of *H-2* associated T-cell-mediated lympholysis to trinitrophenyl-modified autologous cells: *Ir*-like genes mapping to the left of *I-A* and within the *I* region, *J. Exp. Med.* **144**:1701.

Schwartz, M., Waltenbauch, C., Dorf, M., Celsa, R., Sela, M., and Benacerraf, B., 1976, Determinants of antigenic molecules responsible for genetically controlled regulation of immune responses, *Proc. Natl. Acad. Sci. U.S.* **73**:2862.

Schwartz, R. H., David, C. S., Sachs, D. H., and Paul, W. E., 1976, T lymphocyte-enriched murine peritoneal exudate cells. III. Inhibition of antigen-induced T lymphocyte proliferation with anti-*Ia* antisera, *J. Immunol.* **117**:531.

Shearer, G. M., Rehn, G. R., and Garbarino, C. A., 1975, Cell-mediated lympholysis of trinitrophenyl-modified autologous lymphocytes. Effector cell specificity to modified cell surface components controlled by the *H-2K* and *H-2D* serological regions of the murine major histocompatibility complex, *J. Exp. Med.* **141**:1348.

Shreffler, D. C., and David, C. S., 1975, The H-2 major histocompatibility complex and the *I* immune response region: genetic variation, function, and organization, *Adv. Immunol.* **20**:125.

Simonsen, M., 1967, The clonal selection hypothesis evaluated by grafted cells reacting against their hosts, *Cold Spring Harbor Symp. Quant. Biol.* **32**:517.

Snell, G., 1974, Immunogenetics: Retrospect and prospect, *Immunogenetics* **1**:1.

Tada, T., 1978, Regulation of the antibody response by T-cell products determined by different I subregions, in: *Regulation of the Immune System* (E. Sercarz and L. A. Herzenberg, eds.), Academic Press, New York (in press).

Ting, C. C., and Law, L. W., 1977, Studies of *H-2* restriction in cell-mediated cytotoxicity and transplantation immunity to leukemia associated antigens, *J. Immunol.* **118**:1259.

Vadas, M. A., Miller, J. F. A. P., Gamble, J., and Whitelaw, A., 1975, A radioisotopic method to measure delayed type hypersensitivity in the mouse. I. Studies in sensitized and normal mice, *Int. Arch. Allergy Appl. Immunol.* **49**:670.

Vadas, M. A., Miller, J. F. A. P., McKenzie, I. F. C., Chism, S. E., Shen, F. W., Boyse, E. A., Gamble, J., and Whitelaw, A., 1976, Ly and Ia antigen phenotypes of T cells involved in delayed type hypersensitivity and in suppression, *J. Exp. Med.* **144**:10.

Vadas, M. A., Miller, J. F. A. P., Whitelaw, A., and Gamble, J., 1977, Regulation by the *H-2* gene complex of delayed-type hypersensitivity, *Immunogenetics* **4**:137.

von Boehmer, H., and Haas, W., 1976, Cytotoxic T lymphocytes recognise allogeneic tolerated TNP-conjugated cells, *Nature* **261**:141.

von Boehmer, H., and Sprent, J., 1976, T cell function in bone marrow chimeras: absence of host-reactive T cells and cooperation of helper T cells across allogeneic barriers, *Transplant. Rev.* **29**:3.

Warner, C. M., McIvor, J. L., Maurer, P. H., and Merryman, C. F., 1977, The immune response of allophenic mice to the synthetic polymer L-glutamic acid, L-lysine, L-phenylalanine. II. Lack of gene complementation in two nonresponder strains, *J. Exp. Med.* **145**:766.

Whitelaw, A., Miller, J. F. A. P., and Mitchell, G. F., 1977, Studies on immune responses to parasitic antigens in mice. VI. Delayed type hypersensitivity to blood cells from *Plasmodium berghei* infected mice, *Cell. Immunol.* **32**:216.

Wilson, D. B., Heber-Katz, E., and Sprent, J., Howard, J. C., 1977, On the possibility of multiple T cell receptors, *Cold Spring Harbor Symp. Quant. Biol.* **41**:559.

Zinkernagel, R. M., 1976a, *H-2* restriction of virus-specific T-cell-mediated effector function *in vivo*. II. Adoptive transfer of delayed-type hypersensitivity to murine lymphocytic choriomeningitis. Virus is restricted by the *K* & *D* region of *H-2*, *J. Exp. Med.* 144:776.

Zinkernagel, R. M., 1976b, Virus-specific T-cell-mediated cytotoxicity across the *H-2* barrier to virus-altered alloantigen, *Nature* 261:139.

Chapter 2

Characterization of Human T-Cell Subpopulations as Defined by Specific Receptors for Immunoglobulins

Lorenzo Moretta

Institute of Microbiology
University of Genoa
Genoa, Italy

Manlio Ferrarini*

The Rockefeller University
New York, New York 10021

and

Max D. Cooper

Departments of Pediatrics and Microbiology
and the Comprehensive Cancer Center
University of Alabama Medical Center
Birmingham, Alabama 35294

I. INTRODUCTION

Receptors for immunoglobulin (Ig) molecules have been detected on mononuclear "lymphoid" cells of several animal species. Analysis of the cellular populations involved has demonstrated that Ig receptors are expressed by monocytes, macrophages, and lymphocytes (Dickler, 1976). Studies of lymphocyte subpopulations have shown that T cells (Lee and Paraskevas, 1972; Yoshida and Andersson, 1972; Soteriades-Vlachos *et al.*, 1974; Anderson and Grey, 1974; Ferrarini *et al.*, 1975a; Winchester *et al.*, 1975; Brown and Greaves, 1974), B

*Present address: Institute of Biological Chemistry, University of Genoa, Geloa, Italy.

cells (Basten *et al.*, 1972; Dickler and Kunkel, 1972), and a third subset of non-T, non-B cells, not fully characterized and often referred to as "null cells" (Frøland and Natvig, 1973; Kurnick and Grey, 1975; Horwitz and Garrett, 1977), may possess receptors for immunoglobulin. Early studies on lymphocytes revealed receptors for IgG molecules mainly, if not exclusively, but receptors for other Ig classes have been described more recently. Receptors for IgM have been found on both normal and leukemic T lymphocytes (Moretta *et al.*, 1975; McConnell and Hurd, 1976; Gmelig-Meyling *et al.*, 1976; Moretta *et al.*, 1977*a*) and B lymphocytes (Pichler and Knapp, 1977; Ferrarini *et al.*, 1977), while receptors for IgE have been detected on a subpopulation of human B cells (Gonzales-Molina and Spiegelberg, 1977).

The presence of receptors for immunoglobulins on the surface of lymphocytes poses interesting problems as to the function of these membrane structures, and provides a useful label for both identification and separation of the various cell subpopulations.

In recent years a vast amount of evidence has been collected indicating functional heterogeneity of T cells. These cells mediate a spectrum of responses, such as delayed hypersensitivity, graft rejection, antineoplastic and antiparasitic immunity, and helper and suppressor control of the antibody response (Gershon, 1974). In mice, these properties have been attributed to distinct subpopulations of T cells identified mainly on the basis of the expression of different surface alloantigens. For example, Ly-1 alloantigens are present on T cells which have helper activity, respond in mixed lymphocyte cultures, and are responsible for delayed hypersensitivity reactions. Ly-2,3 antigenic specificities are present on suppressor and cytotoxic T cells (Cantor and Boyse, 1975*a,b*; Huber *et al.*, 1976; Cantor and Boyse, 1977). In addition, differential susceptibility of murine T cells to lysis by anti-Thy-1 and complement has permitted the identification of cell subpopulations characterized by different mitogen responsiveness and homing properties, although these differences in alloantigen expression and function may be related to maturational stages of cells belonging to the same subline (Stobo, 1972; Cantor *et al.*, 1975). Mouse T lymphocytes have also been separated according to their capacity to express membrane receptors for the Fc fragment of the IgG molecule (Stout and Herzenberg, 1975*a,b*; Stout *et al.*, 1976). The subpopulation of Fc receptor-negative (FcR⁻) cells has been shown to contain "helper" cells and the precursors of cytotoxic T lymphocytes (CTL). The FcR⁺ population of cells contained differentiated CTL, but not helper T cells. Both FcR⁺ and FcR⁻ T lymphocytes were capable of a mixed lymphocyte response (MLR). More recently, using special techniques, it has been possible to demonstrate *I*-region-determined antigens (Ia) on FcR⁺ T lymphocytes, and this subpopulation of T cells may be further subdivided on the basis of differences in surface expression of Ia alloantigens (Fathman *et al.*, 1975; Stout *et al.*, 1977).

Similar analysis of human T-cell subpopulations has been more difficult to accomplish, owing to the lack of antisera specific for surface alloantigens and because certain experimental approaches used in mice obviously cannot be employed in humans. In this respect, separation of human T cells according to their capacity to bind Ig of different classes, together with functional and morphological analysis of the subpopulations so obtained, has been most valuable. The combination of this approach with others recently reported, such as separation of T cells according to the presence of cell-surface antigens recognized by appropriately absorbed heteroantisera (Evans *et al.*, 1977) or receptors for lectins (Hellström *et al.*, 1976) and to the capacity to form rosettes of different avidity with sheep erythrocytes (West *et al.*, 1977; Felsburg and Edelman, 1977), may allow a much more precise definition of human T-cell subpopulations and their functional capabilities.

This chapter will deal primarily with experiments carried out in the last few years in our laboratories to define (1) the characteristics of receptors for immunoglobulin present on human T lymphocytes, and (2) the properties of the populations carrying these receptors. We shall not attempt a comprehensive review of the extensive literature on subpopulations of T lymphocytes and on surface receptors for Ig molecules.

II. BASIC FEATURES OF DISTINCT T-CELL SUBPOPULATIONS AND THEIR RECEPTORS FOR IMMUNOGLOBULINS

A. Preparation of Purified Human T Cells

T cells present in human lymphoid cell suspensions have been identified by their capacity to bind neuraminidase-treated sheep erythrocytes (E_N) (Weiner *et al.*, 1973). Rosette formation with E_N presently represents the most reliable marker for human T cells in a variety of experimental situations (Hoffman and Kunkel, 1976). Purified T cells used in our experiments were obtained by separating E_N rosettes from nonrosetting cells on Ficoll–Hypaque density gradients as depicted in Fig. 1 (Moretta *et al.*, 1975, 1976a). The cell suspensions so obtained generally contained 99–100% E_N-RFC, and less than 1% cells with surface Ig, complement (C3) receptors, or endogenous peroxidase activity.

The T-cell preparations were also analyzed by immunofluorescence with anti-human "Ia-like" allo- or heteroantisera (Winchester *et al.*, 1976; Billing *et al.*, 1976) and anti-human B-cell-specific heteroantisera (Balch *et al.*, 1977). The antigens detected by these immunofluorescent reagents are not observed on human T lymphocytes but are on all B lymphocytes (Winchester *et al.*, 1976; Humphreys *et al.*, 1976; Hoffman *et al.*, 1977). All the purified T-cell suspensions tested in our studies had less than 1–2% cells with the B-cell antigens, and more than 99% cells had T-cell-specific antigens (Balch *et al.*, 1976).

B. Rosette Techniques for Detection of Receptors for IgM and IgG

In our experiments, receptors for IgM and IgG on T lymphocytes have been
detected by rosette formation with erythrocytes coated with purified IgM
(EA_M) or IgG antibodies (EA_G) made in rabbits (Ferrarini *et al.*, 1975a,b;
Moretta *et al.*, 1975). This method has proven very reliable and simple. In
addition, it offers the great advantage over other, in principle equally suitable,
techniques in that the cells forming rosettes can be easily separated from nonrosetting T cells. We used bovine erythrocytes as indicator cells in the rosette
system. These red cells are particularly suitable for detecting Ig receptors on
lymphocytes because, owing to their poor agglutinability, bovine erythrocytes
can be coated with relatively large amounts of antibody (Uhlenbruck *et al.*,
1967; Hallberg *et al.*, 1973). It is interesting that receptors for IgM on human
T cells have so far been detected by rosette formation with IgM-coated bovine
red cells exclusively, whereas receptors for IgG have been detected in comparable frequency using immunofluorescence to detect binding of immune
complexes (Winfield *et al.*, 1977; R. J. Winchester, personal communication)
or aggregated immunoglobulins (Stout *et al.*, 1975a) or by rosette formation
with human Rh^+ red cells sensitized with anti-Rh antibody (van Oers *et al.*,
1977) or with chicken erythrocytes coated by rabbit antibody (Samarut *et al.*,
1976).

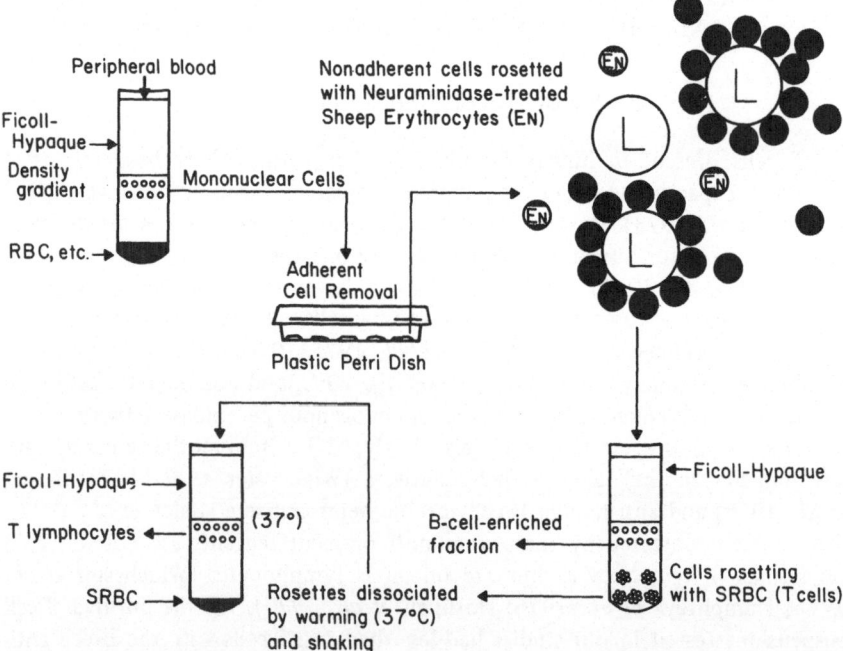

Figure 1. Schematic outline of the methods used for obtaining purified T cells and a B-cell-
enriched fraction from human blood.

The mode of expression of receptors for IgG and IgM by T cells differs in that IgG receptors can be detected on freshly isolated lymphocytes, whereas IgM receptors can only be demonstrated on cells which have been incubated *in vitro* for at least 4-6 hr under stringent culture conditions (Moretta *et al.*, 1975; McConnell and Hurd, 1976). Dulbecco's modified Eagle (DME) and TC199 media have proven equally suitable to obtain maximum expression of IgM receptors by T cells, while lower percentages of cells with receptors for IgM have been detected on cells cultured in RPMI 1640. The reason for this is unclear, and so far it has not been possible to trace the components present in DME and TC199 media which enhance the expression of the IgM receptors. The highest percentages of cells with IgM receptors have been detected in cultures supplemented with fetal calf serum (FCS) or human cord serum. Lower numbers of cells forming IgM rosettes have been found in cultures containing human adult AB or autologous serum, and generally the proportion of rosettes detected varied inversely with the percentage (from 5 to 20%) of adult human serum added. In addition, transfer of cells, which had already fully expressed the IgM receptors under optimal culture conditions, to media containing autologous serum or FCS to which small amounts of IgM had been added, resulted in a noticeable decrease in the percentage of IgM rosettes formed. These findings, together with the results of IgM rosette inhibition experiments using purified human IgM (reported in Section IIC), show that the IgM receptor is easily blocked *in vitro* by small amounts of unaggregated IgM. It is likely that receptors for IgM are present on freshly isolated T cells, but cannot be detected because normally they are occupied *in vivo* by serum IgM. This view is reinforced by studies on freshly prepared lymphocytes from patients with severe hypogammaglobulinemia with especially low or absent serum IgM. Their peripheral blood lymphocytes expressed the IgM receptor prior to incubation in culture (Moretta *et al.*, 1977*d*). The incubation of T cells from normal individuals in IgM-free media could thus allow the cells to shed both the receptors and the IgM bound to them and to resynthesize new receptors. The new receptors, free of IgM, could then be detected in the IgM rosette assay. The view that, during *in vitro* incubation, T cells release both adherent IgM and its receptor is supported by the observations (discussed in Section IIE) that receptors for IgM have a relatively rapid turnover and that their expression is blocked by cycloheximide (Moretta *et al.*, 1975).

C. Specificity of T-Cell Receptors for IgM and IgG

The specificity of the receptor for IgM on human T cells has been analyzed in a number of laboratories by studying the inhibitory capacity of purified human immunoglobulins or immunoglobulin fragments in the rosette assay. These experiments have demonstrated that the receptor has specificity for the Fc portion of the IgM molecule (Moretta *et al.*, 1975; McConnell and Hurd,

1976; Gmelig-Meyling *et al.*, 1976; Ferrarini *et al.*, 1976). More precisely, the CH₄ homology domain has been identified as the portion of the IgM molecule for which the receptor has affinity (Conradie and Bubb, 1977). Monomeric IgM seems to bind to the T-cell receptor with the same efficiency as does pentameric IgM. This was shown by experiments in which monomeric IgM molecules isolated from the serum of a patient with an 8 S monoclonal IgM spike were tested for their capacity to inhibit IgM rosette formation as compared with that of monoclonal pentameric IgM (Preud'homme *et al.*, 1977). In contrast, 8 S IgM subunits, obtained by extensive reduction and alkylation of pentameric molecules, failed to inhibit IgM rosette formation. This suggests that intact intrachain disulfide bridges may be required for IgM binding to the T-cell surface receptor (Ferrarini *et al.*, 1976).

Reports from several laboratories indicate that relatively low concentrations of IgM are required for saturation of the receptor and consequent inhibition of IgM rosette formation. This, together with the fact that IgM rosettes can be detected using indicator cells coated with relatively low amounts of rabbit IgM antibody, suggests that human T cells are equipped with a low number of relatively high avidity receptors.

Although receptors for IgG on human lymphocytes have been investigated in a variety of experimental situations, detailed studies of the specificity of the IgG receptors on isolated T cells have not yet been carried out. Some of the characteristics of this receptor are similar to those of the IgG receptors found on B cells and on the third incompletely characterized subset of lymphocytes, often called "null cells." This receptor recognizes molecules of the IgG class only, binds preferentially to IgG aggregated by antigens or other means, and has a low avidity for the substrate as shown by inhibition studies (Dickler, 1976). A common membrane molecular structure could therefore possibly serve as an IgG receptor of the various lymphocyte subsets. If this were the case, then by analogy with the receptors of other lymphocyte subpopulations, the IgG receptor on T cells would have affinity for the Fc portion of all human IgG subclasses (Dickler, 1976). It is interesting, however, that the different methods used to detect IgG receptors on human lymphocytes preferentially reveal these receptors on different cell subpopulations. For example, aggregated IgG seems to bind best to B cells (Dickler and Kunkel, 1972), while rosette formation by Rh⁺ human red cells coated with anti-Rh antibody detects IgG receptors on "null" and T cells only (Frøland and Natvig, 1973; van Oers *et al.*, 1977). In addition, fluoresceinated immune complexes bind to one or another cell subset, depending on the ratio of antigen and antibody used (Winfield *et al.*, 1977; R. J. Winchester, unpublished).

Very recently, two types of IgG receptors have been distinguished on mouse macrophages (reviewed by Silverstein *et al.*, 1977). One is a trypsin-sensitive Fc receptor that binds IgG antibodies uncomplexed with antigens, and the other a trypsin-resistant Fc receptor that binds aggregated IgG or IgG–antigen complexes. The Fc receptors for IgG on human $T._G$ cells appear to resemble the latter type (see Section II.E).

D. Receptors for IgM and IgG Discriminate between Distinct Subpopulations of T Cells

The use of rosette formation for the detection of cell-surface receptors for Ig affords an easy way to separate subpopulations of T cells according to the presence or absence of a given receptor. This experimental approach has been used to study whether receptors for IgG and IgM are carried by the same or different cells (Moretta *et al.*, 1976*a*). The protocol used for these experiments is shown in Fig. 2. T-cell suspensions were fractionated according to the presence or absence of IgG receptors. The two subpopulations of T cells so obtained were cultured overnight and then examined for the presence of receptors for IgM. Only the subpopulation of T cells which lacked receptors for IgG expressed receptors for IgM. When human T cells were fractionated according to the presence or absence of receptors for IgM, cells bearing receptors for IgG were found only in the fraction of cells lacking receptors for IgM. These results indicate that receptors for IgG and IgM represent useful markers for two different subsets of T cells, which, for simplicity, have been called $T._G$ and $T._M$ cells. The percentages of $T._M$ cells in the $T._G$-deprived subpopulation of T cells and of $T._G$ cells in the $T._M$-cell-depleted fraction were always below 100. This is consistent with the findings that in all of the lymphoid tissues examined (see Section IIF), the sum of the percentages of $T._G$ and $T._M$ cells was always below 100. The results suggest the existence of a third subpopulation of T cells ("T null cells"), lacking both receptors for IgG and IgM. Another possibility is that the identification of T null cells may represent an artifact which is due to the limitations of the technique. Other data, to be discussed in Section IIIA, favor the first possibility, i.e., the existence of a third subpopulation of T cells lacking IgM and IgG receptors.

E. Turnover of Receptors for IgM and IgG on T Cells

This has been investigated in experiments in which T cells were treated with proteolytic enzymes, and receptor reexpression *in vitro* was determined as a function of time (Moretta *et al.*, 1977*c*). Preliminary studies revealed that pronase exposure could eliminate receptors for both IgM and IgG, although a higher concentration of the enzyme (600 μg/ml) was needed for eliminating the binding capacity for IgG than for IgM (50 μg/ml). By contrast, trypsin treatment abolished IgM binding but not the IgG binding by T cells. Resistance to trypsin treatment of IgG receptors on B and "null" lymphocytes has been

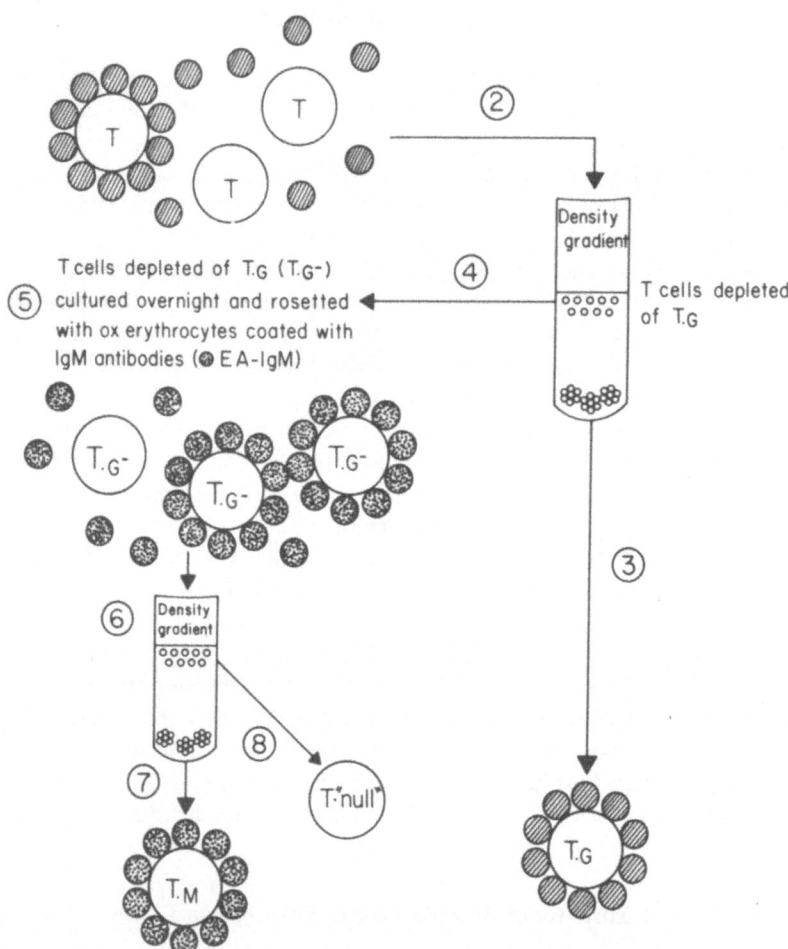

(1) Purified T-cell fraction rosetted with ox erythrocytes coated with IgG antibodies (● E A-IgG)

(2)

Density gradient

T cells depleted of T.G

T cells depleted of T.G (T.G-)
(5) cultured overnight and rosetted
with ox erythrocytes coated with
IgM antibodies (● E A-IgM)

(4)

(3)

(6) Density gradient

(7)

(8)

T.null

T.M

T.G

Figure 2. Schematic outline of the sequence of procedures used for separating purified T cells into three subpopulations: T cells with receptors for IgM (T.$_M$), T cells
with receptors for IgG (T.$_G$), and ones that fail to bind IgM- or IgG-coated red cells
(T.$_{null}$).

previously observed by others (Dickler, 1976). Following pronase digestion, IgM receptors reappeared within 4 hr and resynthesis appeared to be completed by 6 hr. IgG receptors were reexpressed by T cells after 6 hr, and resynthesis was completed by 8–12 hr (Moretta et $al.$, 1977c).

In another series of experiments (Mingari et $al.$, 1978; Moretta et $al.$, 1978), the effect of contact with IgG or IgM immune complexes on the turnover of the receptors was investigated. Purified T cells were rosetted with EA_G or EA_M and rosettes separated on Ficoll–Hypaque density gradients. Following removal of indicator red cells, $T._G$ or $T._M$ cells were treated with pronase, placed in culture, and examined at different intervals for the reappearance of the receptor on the cell surface. The time needed for the reexpression of IgM receptors by $T._M$ cells was unchanged as compared with cells which had been reacted with IgM immune complexes. By contrast, only a minority of the $T._G$ cells, which had been reacted with IgG immune complexes prior to pronase treatment, were able to reexpress IgG receptors. This suggests that contact with IgG immune complexes may act as a "switch-off" signal for synthesis and/or membrane insertion of the IgG receptor by $T._G$ cells. If this proves to be the case, it could have a significant effect on the modulation of the normal immune response and on the impaired immunological reactions which may be observed in the course of diseases with circulating immune complexes. Alternatively, although less likely in our view, contact with immune complexes may increase the rate of "shedding" of the IgG receptor from the cell surface, so that its presence could not be detected by the rosette method. It is of interest in this connection that a very rapid turnover rate has been detected for the IgG receptors of antigen-activated T cells and of certain lymphoblastoid T-cell lines (Fridman and Goldstein, 1974; Molenaar et $al.$, 1977).

F. Tissue Distribution of $T._M$ and $T._G$ Cells

The percentages of $T._G$ and $T._M$ cells detected in various lymphoid organs (Grossi et $al.$, 1977; Cooper et $al.$, 1977) are shown in Table I. $T._M$ cells were present in significant numbers in all of the lymphoid tissues with the remarkable exception of the thymus. $T._G$ cells outnumbered the $T._M$ cells in the spleen but were found in smaller proportions in other lymphoid tissues and were virtually lacking in the normal lymph node and thymus. Since thymocytes are largely immature T cells, our observations suggest that receptors for Ig molecules are expressed by T cells at later stages of the maturational process. Changes in the expression of membrane components during the process of maturation and differentiation of mouse T cells have been well documented (reviewed by Katz, 1977). T-cell precursors acquire most of the T-cell-specific antigens (G_{IX}, Ly, Thy, and TL) within the mouse thymus. During subsequent

Table I. Distribution of Total T, $T._M$, and $T._G$ Cells in Peripheral Blood and Lymphoid Organs

Tissues examined[a]	Total T[b] (%)	$T._M$[c] (%)	$T._G$[c] (%)
Thymus (4)	98 ± 1	3 ± 2	1.0 ± 1
Tonsils (5)	25 ± 5	59 ± 7	6 ± 3
Spleen (4)	37 ± 5	13 ± 3	45 ± 6
Peripheral blood (23)	70 ± 5	56 ± 9	11 ± 1
Cord blood (5)	–	51 ± 3	34 ± 2
Lymph nodes (3)	46 ± 3	56 ± 4	<1

[a]None of the tissues examined (number in parentheses) had disease manifestations. Except for the umbilical cord blood, all samples were obtained from immunologically mature individuals, most of whom were adults.
[b]Expressed as the mean percentage ±S.E. of mononuclear cells.
[c]Expressed as the mean percentages ± S.E. of the total T-cell population.

maturation within the thymus and in peripheral lymphoid organs, T cells lose their G_{IX} and TL markers and express a smaller amount of Thy 1 antigen. Furthermore, different subclasses of mouse T cells may show a selective loss of Ly antigenic specificities (see Cantor and Boyse, 1977). Since the relatively immature thymocytes apparently do not express receptors for Ig, it is possible that the T null cells found in other lymphoid organs may represent T cells at the early differentiation stages. This hypothesis should be testable by studying the capacity of such substances as thymosin or thymopoietin, which are known to promote T-cell maturation, to induce the expression of receptors for IgM and IgG.

G. Morphology of $T._M$ and $T._G$ Cells

Analysis of purified $T._M$ and $T._G$ cells by light and electron microscopy has revealed distinct morphological differences (Grossi *et al.*, 1977, 1978). Cytocentrifuged preparations of $T._M$ cells stained with the standard Giemsa dye mixture exhibit the characteristics of typical small lymphocytes, with dense accumulations of nuclear chromatin and a thin rim of basophilic cytoplasm. By contrast, $T._G$ lymphocytes are larger cells with a homogeneously stained nucleus and a much wider rim of weakly basophilic cytoplasm. Cytoplasmic vacuoles are often seen, and characteristic eosinophilic granules, which vary in number, size, and distribution, are a very distinctive feature of $T._G$ cells. Electron microscopy of $T._M$ lymphocytes reveals a smooth surface and a relative paucity of cytoplasmic organelles. $T._G$ cells have a rough surface, with many long microvilli; the cytoplasm is rich in mitochondria, single ribosomes, and scattered strands of rough endoplasmic reticulum; the Golgi apparatus is also well developed in piles of tubules and cisternae. The granules characteristic of the $T._G$ cells contain a dense matrix surrounded by a membrane unit, and they are often located mainly in the region between the Golgi apparatus and the overlying plasma membrane.

III. FUNCTIONAL ANALYSIS OF $T._M$ AND $T._G$ CELLS

A. Response to Mitogens and Allogeneic Cells

$T._M$ and $T._G$ cells have been examined for their patterns of responsiveness to two T-cell mitogens, concanavalin A (Con A) and phytohemagglutinin (PHA) (Moretta *et al.*, 1976*a*). This was done by culturing purified $T._G$ and $T._M$ cells and T cells depleted of $T._G$ cells ($T._G$-depleted) with different concentrations of Con A and PHA for 3 days. The proliferative response was determined by incorporation of ^{3}H-thymidine and compared with that of unfractionated T cells. Almost identical dose response curves to Con A were observed for all of the populations tested. On the contrary, consistent differences were detected in the PHA response. PHA elicited a response of $T._M$ cells only at concentrations higher than those capable of inducing stimulation in unfractionated T cells. Although $T._G$ cells responded at all of the PHA concentrations tested, their response was consistently lower than that of the unfractionated T cells. The responses of T-cell populations depleted of $T._G$ cells varied among different individuals, and the dose response curves observed were distributed between those of unfractionated T cells and those of the $T._M$ cells. In some individuals the curves were more like those observed with unfractionated T cells; i.e., a proliferative response was obtained even at low PHA concentrations. For others the response was more similar to that of $T._M$ cells; i.e., proliferative responses were observed only when high mitogen concentrations were present. Representative dose response curves are shown in Fig. 3. The differences in the PHA responses of purified $T._M$ cells and of T cells deprived of the $T._G$ subpopulation further suggest that these two fractions of T cells cannot be equated; the $T._G$-depleted fraction of T cells are likely to contain another T-cell subpopulation in addition to $T._M$ cells. Differences in the proportions of $T._M$ cells and a third subpopulation of T cells in the $T._G$-depleted cell fraction are probably responsible for the differences in the individual responses that we have observed.

Thus, these results are consistent with our notion that T null cells, lacking receptors for Ig, constitute one or more distinct T-cell subpopulations, at least some of which could mature into $T._M$ or $T._G$ cells under thymic influence

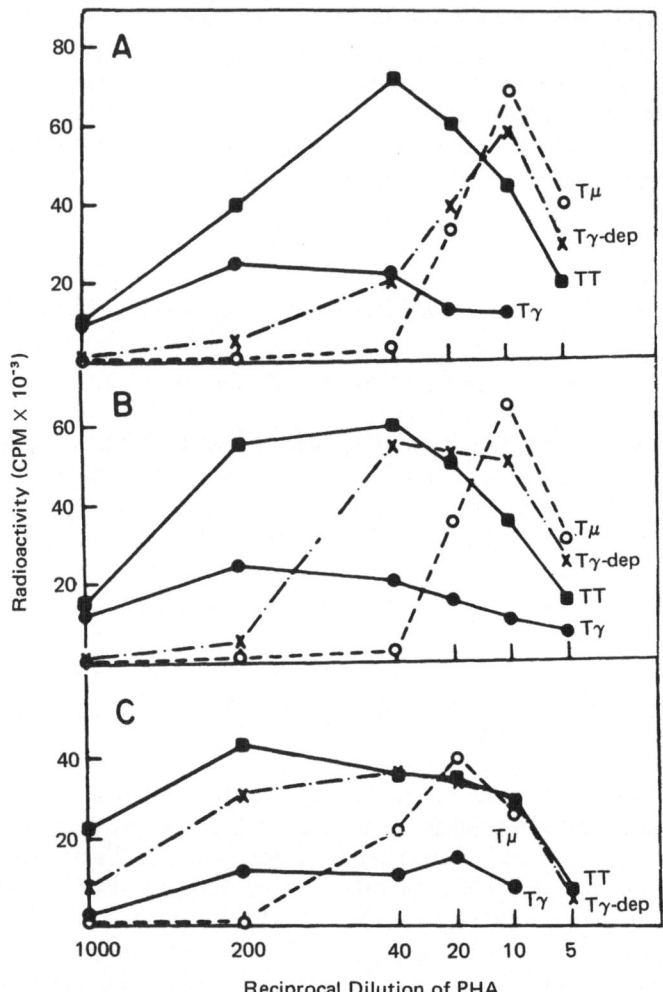

Figure 3. Proliferative response to phytohemagglutinin of different populations of T cells from three donors: ■, total T cells (TT); ×, T cells depleted of T_G cells (Tγ-dep); ●, T_G cells (Tγ); ○, T_M cells (Tμ). [Reproduced from Moretta *et al.* (1976*a*), with permission from The Williams & Wilkins Co., Baltimore.]

(Section IVA) or as a consequence of antigen stimulation (Yoshida and Andersson, 1972; Stout and Herzenberg, 1975*a*; van Boxel and Rosenstreich, 1974).

   The capacity of the various T-cell subpopulations to recognize and proliferate in response to alloantigens has been studied in one way mixed lymphocyte cultures (MLC) using allogeneic E_N-rosette-depleted peripheral blood lymphocytes as stimulator cells (Webb *et al.*, 1977, and manuscript in preparation). $T._M$ cells and $T._G$-depleted cells responded to allogeneic cells as well as unfractionated T cells. The response of $T._G$ cells, although different in the various individuals tested, was always lower than that of the other T-cell fractions. However the $T._G$-cell response to allogeneic cells, as detected by ^{3}H-thymidine uptake, was always significantly greater than the $T._G$ cell responses to autologous E_N-rosette-depleted stimulators (Kunz *et al.*, 1976). At the present it is not known whether the lower response of $T._G$ cells is an intrinsic property of this lymphocyte subclass or whether it is consequent to the fact that $T._G$ cells were reacted with IgG-coated erythrocytes during the isolation procedure. As will be discussed later (Section IIID), interaction with IgG immune complexes may play an essential role in the functional activation of $T._G$ cells. Nevertheless, the capacity of all of the T-cell subpopulations in human blood to respond in the MLC assay indicates that the specific recognition of allogeneic cells is not an exclusive property of one or another T-cell subpopulation, at least as defined by the presence or absence of receptors for IgM and IgG. It is interesting to note in this context that Evans *et al.* (1977), who fractionated human T cells according to the presence of surface heteroantigens, found differences in the capacity of their cell fractions to respond in the MLC assay. By contrast, in the mouse, MLC responsiveness has been shown for both FcR^+ and FcR^- subpopulations of T lymphocytes (Stout *et al.*, 1976) and for T cells having different Ly phenotypes (Cantor and Boyse, 1975*b*).

B. Response to Pokeweed Mitogen as an *in Vitro* Model for Human T- and B-Cell Interactions

It is now well documented that pokeweed mitogen (PWM) not only triggers proliferation of human lymphocytes, but also induces maturation of B cells. Following PWM stimulation, a certain proportion of cells with a well-developed endoplasmic reticulum and the appearance of plasmablasts or plasma cells can be observed by electron microscopy (Janossy and Greaves, 1975; Douglas, 1972). These cells contain all classes of Ig detectable in their cytoplasm by immunofluorescence on fixed cell preparations (Wu *et al.*, 1973; Keightley *et al.*, 1976) and secrete these immunoglobulins into the culture supernatants in amounts measurable by radioimmunoassays (Wu *et al.*, 1973; Waldmann *et al.*, 1974). PWM also induces the *in vitro* production of specific antibodies to different antigens measurable by plaque-forming cell (PFC) assays (Fauci and Pratt, 1976*a,b*; Friedman *et al.*, 1976). In this regard, PWM behaves as a polyclonal cell activator.

Studies of separated lymphocyte subpopulations have demonstrated that induction of B-lymphocyte proliferation and maturation is dependent upon the presence of T cells (Janossy and Greaves, 1975; Clot *et al.*, 1975; Cooper *et al.*, 1975; Keightley *et al.*, 1976). Similarly, the number of sheep erythrocyte PFCs is greatly reduced following removal of T cells prior to PWM stimulation (Friedman *et al.*, 1976; Fauci *et al.*, 1976; Insel and Merler, 1977). The helper activity of purified T cells in the B-cell response to PWM is resistant to γ irradiation in doses as high as 3000 rad (Keightley *et al.*, 1976; Fauci *et al.*, 1976; Insel and Merler, 1977; Kreth and Herzenberg, 1974; Moretta *et al.*, 1977a), and the magnitude of the plasma cell response obtained directly correlates with the number of T cells added (Fig. 4). The addition of supernatants of PWM-stimulated cells to B-cell cultures (Janossy and Greaves, 1975; Cooper *et al.*, 1975; Insel and Merler, 1977) or, under certain conditions, pretreatment of B cells with anti-Ig antisera can overcome the requirement for T-cell help (Fridman and Goldstein, 1974; Friedman *et al.*, 1976).

Recent studies have also demonstrated that proliferation of T cells in response to PWM depends on the presence of an accessory cell within the B-cell-enriched fraction obtained by removal of T cells and plastic adherent cells (Moretta *et al.*, 1977a). Although not completely characterized for surface

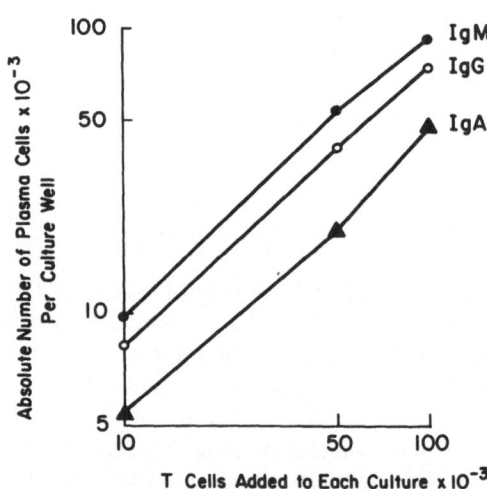

Specific Plasma Cells From B Cells Alone x 10^{-3}		
IgM	IgG	IgA
0	0.8	0.2

Figure 4. T-cell dependence of B-lymphocyte differentiation induced by pokeweed mitogen. Seven-day microcultures were harvested and plasma cells were enumerated after staining with fluorochrome-labeled antibodies specific for the major Ig classes. [Reproduced from Cooper *et al.* (1975), with permission from North-Holland Publishing Company, Amsterdam.]

markers, this auxiliary cell is likely to be a nonadherent, sIg-negative cell (Kreth and Herzenberg, 1974; Moretta *et al.*, 1977*a*).

The complex collaboration between cell subpopulations required for an *in vitro* response of human lymphocytes to PWM seems to mimic that occurring in the course of the response to T-dependent antigens. Therefore, the *in vitro* response to PWM would appear to be a suitable model system for studies on human T-cell interactions. In the following sections we shall review experiments intended to elucidate the regulatory role of T-cell subpopulations on PWM-induced B-cell differentiation.

C. Identification of $T._M$ Cells as "Helper" Cells

In order to identify the T-cell subpopulation(s) capable of promoting B-cell proliferation and differentiation, different numbers of "total T," $T._G$-enriched, or $T._G$-depleted cell fractions were mixed with a constant number of B cells from peripheral blood. Each cell combination was stimulated with PWM and help was assessed after 7 days in culture by measuring the proliferative response and the numbers of intracytoplasmic Ig-containing (cIg^+) cells. $T._G$-depleted cells provided help in a dose-dependent fashion that was not different from that provided by total T-cell population. In contrast, $T._G$ cells did not promote proliferation or differentiation of B cells. When $T._G$-depleted cells were separated further into $T._M$-enriched and -depleted cell fractions, it was found that the helper activity of $T._M$-enriched cells usually was even greater than that of total T cells. $T._M$-depleted cells, although capable of providing some help, were much less efficient than both $T._M$-enriched and total T cells. Figure 5 shows the results of a typical experiment carried out with various combinations of T cells and B cells. In evaluating these experiments, it should be noted that, owing to the relative instability of the IgM rosettes, the removal of $T._M$ cells was never complete. The helper activity observed in the $T._M$-depleted cell population, therefore, could have been associated with the presence of residual $T._M$ cells. However, the alternative possibility that T null cells may have some helper activity cannot be excluded.

D. Suppressor Capacity of $T._G$ Cells

Since $T._G$ cells were incapable of helper cell function, the possibility that this subpopulation contained cells with suppressor activity was considered. This hypothesis was tested as follows (Moretta *et al.*, 1977*a*). A combination of $T._M$ cells (1×10^4) and B cells (5×10^4) which provided for efficient B-cell responses to PWM, was mixed with different numbers of, alternatively, $T._M$, $T._G$, or total T cells. Addition of $T._G$ cells effectively suppressed B-cell differentiation, and the suppression observed directly correlated with the number of $T._G$ cells added. The suppressive effect of $T._G$ was completely abrogated by γ irradiation (3000 rad) of $T._G$ cells prior to culture. This result (see Fig. 6) and the similar observations of Siegal and Siegal (1977) suggest, but do not prove, that proliferation is required for $T._G$ cells to exert their suppressive function. It is worth noting that in mice suppressor activity, although radiosensitive, is not affected by mitomycin C (Basten *et al.*, 1975). Suppression of B-cell differentiation by $T._G$ cells was also obtained when higher ratios of helper $T._M$ cells to B cells (4:5) were used. When, instead of $T._G$ cells, $T._M$ or unseparated T cells were added, enhancement rather than suppression of B-cell differentiation was observed. Since isolation of purified $T._G$ cells required interaction with IgG-coated erythrocytes, it was possible that the lack of B-cell differentiation in the presence of $T._G$ cells might have been due to interaction of residual immune complexes with Fc receptors on the B cells. This possibility was excluded, however, by experiments in which B cells were rosetted with indicator bovine erythrocytes coated with IgG antibodies. Following lysis of the erythrocytes, B cells were mixed with appropriate numbers of $T._M$ cells and tested for their capacity to differentiate in response to PWM. These cells responded to PWM as well as control cell suspensions in which

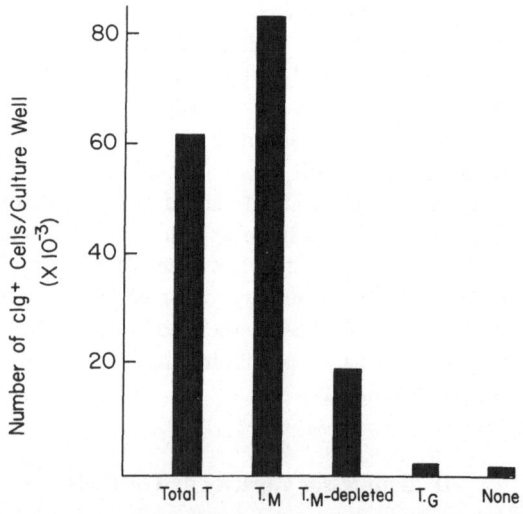

Figure 5. Plasma cell differentiation of human B lymphocytes induced by pokeweed mitogen in the presence of different T-cell populations. 5×10^4 cells of the B-enriched fraction were cultured alone or cocultured with different populations of T cells (5×10^4) in the presence of pokeweed mitogen. After 7 days in culture, cytoplasmic (c) Ig+ cells were enumerated by immunofluorescence.

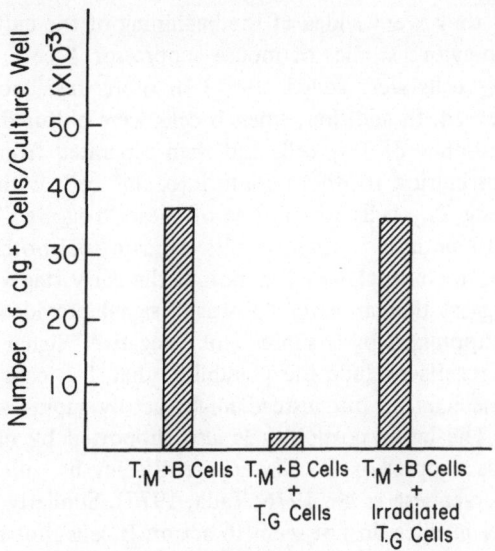

Figure 6. Radiosensitive $T._G$ cells are capable of suppressing the $T._M$-cell help of B-cell differentiation in response to pokeweed mitogen. See the text for further description of the experiments.

treatment with the immune complexes was omitted (Moretta *et al.*, 1977*a*). This experiment also indicates that suppressor capacity is restricted to $T._G$ cells; other cells with IgG receptors present among the "B-cell fraction," when reacted with IgG immune complexes, did not prevent B-cell differentiation.

Interaction with immune complexes was found to be necessary for the $T._G$ cells to suppress B-cell differentiation, as shown by the following experiments (Moretta *et al.*, 1977*a*). Enriched $T._G$-cell fractions were prepared by removing $T._M$ cells from purified T-cell populations. These suspensions contained 40–50% $T._G$ cells. Aliquots of these cells were reacted with IgG-antibody-coated erythrocytes and the red cells removed by hypotonic lysis. Both IgG-immune-complex-treated and -untreated $T._G$-enriched cells were then tested for their capacity to suppress B-cell differentiation. Suppressor activity was found exclusively in the cell suspension enriched for $T._G$ cells, which had been reacted with immune complexes prior to culture.

E. Mode of Suppression by $T._G$ Cells

The mechanisms whereby $T._G$ cells suppress B-cell differentiation have been investigated in a series of experiments employing the PWM model system (Moretta *et al.*, in preparation). $T._G$ cells were able to suppress B-cell differentiation only if they were added at the beginning of the cultures. In keeping with results of previous studies of mouse suppressor T cells (Dutton, 1975), when human $T._G$ cells were added after 1 or more days, no significant suppression was observed. In addition, when B cells were cultured for 2 days with an appropriate number of $T._M$ cells and then separated from helper T cells, they continued in culture to differentiate into cIg^+ cells without any further T-cell help. Adding $T._G$ cells to cultures of these "triggered" B cells did not suppress their differentiation. These results indicate that both helper and suppressor cells exert their regulatory function at the early stages of B-cell differentiation and suggest that an early "positive" signal provided by helper $T._M$ cells cannot be suppressed by a subsequent "negative" signal from suppressor $T._G$ cells. These results exclude the possibility that $T._G$ cells suppress B cells by a cytotoxic mechanism, but instead might act by suppressing the $T._M$-cell helper function. The latter possibility is also supported by observations indicating that mouse suppressor T cells apparently act by suppressing relevant helper T cells (Herzenberg *et al.*, 1976; Tada, 1977). Similarly, Con A-induced suppressor T cells in mice do not seem to act on B cells, but rather on T cells at very early stages of the immune response (Ekstedt *et al.*, 1977; Harwell *et al.*, 1977).

To test further the suggestion that human $T._G$ suppressor cells act by inhibiting $T._M$ helper activity, several different experimental approaches have been tried (Moretta *et al.*, in preparation). B cells were cultured together with either $T._M$ cells or a mixture of $T._M$ and $T._G$ cells in the presence of PWM. Following 2 or 3 days in culture, the T and B cells were reseparated and different combinations of T and B cells were cultured for an additional 4–5 days. B cells previously cultured with a mixture of $T._M$ and $T._G$ cells did not differentiate into cIg^+ cells when recultured with the same combination of helper and suppressor cells, but were capable of doing so when recultured with $T._M$ helper cells alone. This indicates that cells from a "suppressed" culture are still fully capable of differentiating into plasma cells and also supports the idea that suppression may not affect B cells directly. However, the alternative hypothesis that suppression of B cells is reversible was not excluded by these results. When B cells previously cultured with $T._M$ cells were isolated and cultured again with a mixture of $T._M$ and $T._G$ cells, no suppression of differentiation was observed, confirming the results reported above that $T._G$ cells cannot suppress differentiation of B cells which have already received an effective helper signal by $T._M$ cells.

In another series of experiments, B cells were stimulated with PWM in culture media supplemented with special batches of fetal calf serum (Moretta *et al.*, in preparation) selected for their capacity to promote PWM-induced proliferation and differentiation of B cells in the absence of helper T cells. When $T._G$ cells were added to these cultures, no suppression of B-cell differentiation was observed. This finding again suggests that $T._G$ cells do not directly suppress B-cell differentiation. However, in interpreting these data, the possibility should be considered that the B cells differentiating in the absence of T-cell help could be different from those requiring T-cell help, and that this special B-cell subpopulation might be insensitive to regulatory signals (help or suppression) provided by T cells. Another possibility is that the differentiation of B cells may be inducible by different mechanisms. In any case the findings above are compatible with, but do not provide final proof for, the hypothesis that human $T._G$ cells act by suppressing the helper function of $T._M$ cells. As mentioned above, factors in the supernatants of PWM-stimulated cultures, which have now been partially characterized (Insel and Merler, 1977), can effectively substitute for T cells in promoting PWM-induced differentiation of B cells. The use of this experimental approach is likely to be of great value in clarifying the mechanism of suppression by $T._G$ cells, and experiments along this line are being carried out.

IV. $T._M$ AND $T._G$ CELLS IN IMMUNODEFICIENCY DISEASES AND MALIGNANCIES

A. Immunodeficiencies

Since $T._M$ and $T._G$ cells may exert an important regulatory control over terminal B-cell differentiation, both numerical and functional imbalances in these T-cell subpopulations could conceivably be expected in immunodeficiencies. For example, in common variable hypogammaglobulinemia, an excess of suppressor activity of T cells has been demonstrated in vitro (Waldmann et al., 1974; Siegal et al., 1976) and offers one possible explanation for the pathogenesis of this syndrome in patients in whom intrinsic defects of B-cell maturation are not basic to the pathogenesis of the immunodeficiency (Wu et al., 1973; Geha et al., 1974; Cooper et al., 1975; De La Concha et al., 1977).

We found that abnormalities in the numbers of T cells or in the relative proportions of $T._G$ and $T._M$ cells were infrequently found in patients with primary immunoglobulin deficiencies (Moretta et al., 1976b; Cooper et al., 1977; Moretta et al., 1977d). These included patients with infantile agammaglobulinemia, selective IgA deficiency, and common variable hypogammaglobulinemia, a diagnostic category that includes a diverse group of syndromes. Although more correlative functional studies are needed, these results appear to be consistent with those of previous studies which implied that many if not most patients with immunoglobulin deficiency reflect inherent abnormalities of B cells or in the mechanisms involved in their triggering (Wu et al., 1973; Geha et al., 1974; Cooper et al., 1975; De La Concha et al., 1977).

On the other hand, imbalances in the proportions of $T._G$ and $T._M$ cells were consistently found in patients with severe combined immunodeficiencies, idiopathic defects of cell-mediated immunity, and both congenital and acquired abnormalities of the thymus. Of 15 such patients tested, 13 were deficient in $T._M$ cells, 9 had coexistent increases in the percentages of $T._G$ cells, and 10 had an expanded population of T null cells. Four of the patients were deficient in numbers of circulating T cells, and each had a coexisting relative decrease in the proportion of $T._M$ cells. Among other implications of these results, this study provided evidence that the thymus may play an important role in maintaining the normal balance of circulating T-cell subpopulations. Thus, two patients, who had undergone thymectomy because of mediastinal masses, which proved to be normal thymus, had normal numbers of circulating T cells and no immunodeficiencies, but the percentages of $T._M$ cells were abnormally low. By contrast, a patient with congenital thymic aplasia (Di George syndrome), who had received a thymus transplant, had normal T-cell numbers and normal proportions of $T._G$ and $T._M$ cells. In addition, Mingari *et al.* (1976, unpublished) have observed not only an increase in the number of circulating T cells, but also a raised proportion of $T._M$ cells in a patient with congenital thymus dysplasia (Nezelof's syndrome) following treatment with thymosin.

A further indication of the suppressive function of $T._G$ cells came from lymphocyte studies of a patient with thymoma, hypogammaglobulinemia, and an elevated proportion of circulating $T._G$ cells (Moretta *et al.*, 1977*d*). Purified, but unfractionated, T cells from this patient were found to inhibit PWM-induced differentiation of B cells from normal individuals. Removal of the $T._G$ cells completely eliminated the suppressive capacity of the patient's T cells. These observations also demonstrate that $T._G$ cells from this patient, in contrast to those from normal individuals, did not require *in vitro* activation with immune complexes to exert their suppressive function, indicating that his $T._G$ cells were already activated or primed *in vivo*. The *in vivo* mechanisms by which suppressor T cells from this immunodeficient patient were activated, as well as those from others for which *in vitro* suppressor activity has been demonstrated, remain unknown. One intriguing possibility is that $T._G$ cells may be activated *in vivo* as a consequence of the treatment of hypogammaglobulinemic patients with exogenous gamma globulin as replacement therapy. The gamma globulin preparations contain aggregates that could cause $T._G$ cell activation or priming for activation by a second signal, such as antigens. Similar mechanisms involving the IgG receptors of $T._G$ cells may also be involved in both normal physiological situations and in disease states in which an abundance of immune complexes are present. As one possible example, an unusually high number of naturally occurring activated $T._G$ cells can also be found in the newborn. These cells are capable of suppressing both mixed lymphocyte cultures and PWM induction of B-cell differentiation and could play a physiological role in inhibiting maternal immunocompetent cells from rejecting the fetus as an allograft (Olding and Oldstone, 1976; Hayward and Lawton, 1977; Oldstone *et al.*, 1977). In this regard, it is noteworthy that circulating immune complexes have been observed during normal human pregnancy (Masson *et al.*, 1977).

B. Leukemias

Use of lymphocyte surface markers for the analysis of lymphoproliferative disorders suggests that in the majority of cases the malignant cells belong to the B-cell lineage (reviewed by Cooper and Seligmann, 1977). Malignant proliferation of T cells appear to be less frequent but accounts for a significant proportion (20–30%) of acute lymphoblastic leukemias (ALL), some chronic lymphocytic leukemias, and occasional non-Hodgkin's lymphomas (see Seligmann *et al.*, 1973). In addition, the malignant cells of Sézary syndrome and mycosis fungoides have been found to be of T-cell origin (Brouet *et al.*, 1973; Zucker-Franklin *et al.*, 1976; Broome *et al.*, 1973).

Surface receptors for Ig have been analyzed on the neoplastic T cells from a few affected individuals. In a study of six patients with T-cell ALL, malignant T cells from four individuals expressed receptors for IgM only, whereas in the remaining two patients the leukemic T lymphoblasts had both IgG and IgM receptors (Moretta *et al.*, 1977b). The latter finding is in contrast with that observed for normal T cells, where receptors for IgM and IgG receptors are carried by different cells. The simultaneous expression of the two surface receptors may be a peculiar characteristic of certain malignant T cells. In this connection it may be worth noting that simultaneous expression of both T- and B-cell markers by neoplastic cells has been reported for an occasional lymphoproliferative disorder (Hsu *et al.*, 1975). More recent surveys of ALLs with T-cell characteristics have revealed instances in which the T lymphoblasts have no surface receptors for Ig molecules (T. Hoffman, personal communication).

Neoplastic T cells from some individuals with Sézary's disease have been found to have helper activity in the pokeweed model system of B-cell differentiation (Broder *et al.*, 1976). Unfortunately, correlative studies of both T-cell receptors for Ig and T-cell functions are lacking but should provide a rich source of further information on T-cell subpopulations in the future.

V. CONCLUDING REMARKS AND SPECULATIONS

The use of receptors for molecules of different Ig classes as surface markers has permitted the identification of two distinct T-cell subclasses, which we have named $T._G$ and $T._M$ cells, and tentative identification of a third T-cell subset referred to as T null cells. The first two of these T-cell subpopulations, although both capable of responding in MLC, differ in their mitogen responsiveness, morphology, and tissue distribution. In addition, *in vitro* analysis of the T-cell capacity for promoting the PWM induction of B-cell differentiation has demonstrated that helper cells reside in the $T_{.M}$-cell subpopulation, whereas $T_{.G}$ cells under appropriate conditions can exert a suppressive function. These results are in agreement with experiments involving analysis of specific antigenic responses in the mouse, which have demonstrated that helper and suppressor functions are mediated by different T-cell subpopulations distinguishable by membrane markers and physical properties (Cantor and Boyse, 1975*a,b*; Stout and Herzenberg, 1975*a*; Basten *et al.*, 1975; Jandinski *et al.*, 1976; Tse and Dutton, 1976; Okumura *et al.*, 1977). The complementary nature of these results reaffirms the value of polyclonal activators as probes in dissecting the diverse cell populations involved in the human immune response.

Animal studies have indicated the fundamental importance of the balance between helper and suppressor T cells in the regulation of the immune response (Gershon, 1974; Herzenberg *et al.*, 1976; Pierce and Kapp, 1976; Tada, 1977), and, more recently, suppressor capabilities have been demonstrated for human lymphocytes (Waldmann *et al.*, 1974; Sampson *et al.*, 1975; Shou *et al.*, 1976; reviewed by Waldmann and Broder, 1977). An excess of suppressor-T-cell activity has been tentatively associated with the pathogenesis of certain forms of primary immunodeficiencies (Waldmann *et al.*, 1974; Siegal *et al.*, 1976), and may be involved in the depressed immune status of patients with Hodgkin's disease, multiple myeloma, and fungal infections (Stobo *et al.*, 1976; Waldmann *et al.*, 1976; Twomey *et al.*, 1975). On the other hand, loss of T-cell suppressor activity has been implicated in the pathogenesis of the autoimmune disease of NZB mice (Dauphinee and Talal, 1975; Hardin *et al.*, 1973), and may be involved in the pathogenesis of systemic lupus erythematosus (Abdou *et al.*, 1976; Krakauer *et al.*, 1976; Bresnihan and Jasin, 1977; Horowitz *et al.*, 1977). The correlation between increased proportions of $T_{.G}$ cells and augmented suppressor activity in certain immunodeficient patients and in normal newborn babies' blood emphasizes the potential value of receptors for IgG as markers for further pathophysiologic studies on human suppressor T cells.

Although human suppressor T cells have been identified within the $T_{.G}$-cell population, it is not known whether all $T_{.G}$ cells are destined to serve a suppressor function. Cells with other functions, such as cytotoxic T lymphocytes and cells mediating antibody-dependent cell cytotoxicity (ADCC), have been detected in the $T_{.G}$-cell subpopulation (Stout *et al.*, 1976; West *et al.*, 1977; Lamon *et al.*, 1977; van Oers *et al.*, 1977; Saal *et al.*, 1977; Pape *et al.*, 1977). Although all the functions above could, in principle, be exerted by a single cell population, it appears more likely, as some recent data would suggest (Stout *et al.*, 1977), that $T_{.G}$ cells may be subdivided further into distinct subsets that have very specialized functional capabilities. An increased proportion of $T._G$ cells, therefore, may not necessarily give a precise indication of an excess of suppressor T-cell numbers or of suppressor activity.

The mechanism by which $T._G$ cells exert their suppressive function is not yet totally understood. However, some aspects of the problem deserve comment. Our studies with the PWM model system demonstrate that suppression may be achieved only when $T._G$ cells are primed for activation by contact with IgG immune complexes. The homeostatic role of antibody in general and of IgG antibody in particular on the immune response has been amply documented (Uhr and Möller, 1968). Antibody may suppress an ongoing immune response by masking antigenic determinants, and thereby compete with specific receptors of immunocompetent cells. However, evidence has also been obtained indicating the role of the Fc portion of IgG in potentiating the suppressive function of antibody (Sinclair, 1969). It has been suggested that the greater efficiency of intact IgG molecules over the corresponding $F(ab')_2$ fragments in inhibiting an immune response may be explained by the capacity of intact IgG to interact with IgG-Fc receptors on suppressor T cells (Playfair, 1974). In this connection, it is of interest that stimulation of idiotype-specific suppressor T cells of the mouse may require interaction with complexes formed by the relevant idiotype and the specific antigen (Eichmann, 1975; Owen *et al.*, 1977).

Fc receptors on $T._G$ cells bind strongly to IgG aggregated by antigen or other means, but poorly to native IgG molecules. This may be explained by the low avidity of the receptor for the Fc portion of the IgG and the consequent need for a multipoint attachment in order to stabilize the binding. Alternatively, the Fc portion of the IgG molecule may, upon contact with antigen, undergo conformational changes and expose new sites for which the receptor located on the cell surface could have preferential affinity. Whatever the fine molecular mechanism involved may be, binding of IgG molecules to Fc receptors and consequent $T._G$-cell activation could occur at certain antigen–antibody proportions obtainable *in vivo* only at particular stages of an ongoing immune response. Thus, we view the special requirements for interaction between Fc-IgG receptors and immune complexes acting as a safety device in promoting the activation of suppressor T cells only under specific conditions. Interaction between immune complexes and the receptor on the $T._G$ cell surface may also considerably slow down the turnover rate of the receptor itself, and consequently render these cells less susceptible to activation by immune complexes. This, too, may represent a safety device but in this case one that prevents an excess of suppression.

Having discussed potential advantages offered by interaction with immune complexes in order to activate $T._G$ cells, one has also to try to answer the following questions: (1) Is this interaction absolutely necessary in order to obtain a suppressive effect? (2) Is this interaction *per se* sufficient to determine a suppressive effect? Although binding of immune complexes by $T._G$ cells appears to play a role in activation of suppressor activity, it is not clear that this step is either invariably necessary or sufficient. For example, treatment of T cells with Con A induces suppressor activity which may block both antigen-specific and polyclonal mitogen-induced B-cell differentiation, with no apparent requirement for binding of immune complexes (Dutton, 1973; Rich and Pierce, 1973; Haynes and Fauci, 1977*a*). It is, however, possible that Con A-induced suppressor cells may belong to subpopulations other than T.$_G$ cells (Haynes and Fauci, 1977*b*; Lawton *et al.*, unpublished observations). More directly pertinent to this argument is the fact that suppressor activity is radiosensitive, suggesting the need for suppressor cell proliferation. Since contact of T.$_G$ cells with IgG immune complexes does not induce detectable proliferation but activation of T.$_G$ cell suppression *in vitro* normally appears to require prior contact with IgG immune complexes (Moretta *et al.*, 1976*a*), we suggest that a second signal may be required for T.$_G$-cell triggering. This second signal is likely provided, in the *in vitro* PWM model system, by the mitogen itself. A specific second signal may be delivered *in vivo* to T.$_G$ cells via interaction between the native antibody receptor and free antigenic determinants present on the antigen-IgG antibody complex. Via the antigen bridge, suppressor T.$_G$ cells of a specific clonotype may be activated in this way. Ample demonstration has been provided for the selective antigen specificity of mouse suppressor T cells (see Gershon, 1974; Pierce and Kapp, 1976), but for human suppressor T cells only limited evidence for antigen specificity is so far available (McMichael and Susazuki, 1977). This problem is amenable to further study as it is now possible to study the specific response of human lymphocytes to classical antigens *in vitro* (Fauci and Pratt, 1976*a*,*b*; Geha *et al.*, 1977).

Other ways in which two activating signals may be simultaneously delivered to specific T.$_G$ cells can be postulated within the context of a network theory of immune response regulation (Jerne, 1976). One straightforward possibility would be that an IgG antibody reacting with the idiotypic determinant of the native antigen receptor of a T.$_G$ cell may undergo conformational changes leading to secondary binding of the Fc portion to its receptor on the same cell (Eichmann, 1975). Among other theoretical possibilities of this nature, T.$_G$ cells with native antigen receptors specific for a given IgG allotype or idiotype could receive their second signal by reacting with one of these determinants after binding an appropriate IgG antibody-antigen complex via the Fc receptor. The common assumption for each of these hypotheses, which are not mutually exclusive, is that activation of T.$_G$ cells requires one specific (interaction between the native receptor for antigen and its specific target) and one less specific step (interaction between the Fc receptor and IgG immune complexes). The latter step could be envisaged as a device to restrict the function of suppressor T cells to certain stages of immune response only.

Unlike the comparable set of circumstances for T.$_G$ cells, interaction with IgM or IgM-antigen immune complexes was not a necessary prerequisite for the T.$_M$ cells to promote PWM induced B-cell differentiation. This could mean that receptors for IgM are not directly involved in the helper function of $T._M$ cells. Recent evidence has indicated that one potential function of IgM receptor is the "arming" of T cells; i.e., passively adsorbed IgM molecules may serve to direct T-cell cytotoxic activity against tumor cells or other cell types (Lamon et al., 1977; Wahlin et al., 1976; Fuson and Lamon, 1977). However, whether helper and cytotoxic $T._M$ cells belong to the same or to different lymphocyte subsets is presently unknown. Alternatively, IgM receptors may be involved in the activation of helper T cells under certain normal circumstances, but this role may have gone undetected in the PWM stimulation model system. Previous experiments have demonstrated an enhancing effect of passively administered IgM antibody on the immune response of experimental animals (Henry and Jerne, 1968) and a dependence of this effect on the presence of T cells (Dennert, 1971; McBride and Schierman, 1973). It is therefore possible that, as in the case of $T._G$ cells, antigen-specific activation of $T._M$ cells may involve both native antigen-specific receptors and passively acquired IgM molecules. In this connection it may be worth recalling (1) that $T._M$ cells have receptors with an apparent high avidity for the Fc portion of IgM, and (2) that binding of the molecule to the cell surface is not dependent upon prior aggregation by antigen–IgM. IgM antibody bound to the cell surface through its Fc portion may, therefore, bind antigen through its exposed free combining sites, thus passively arming T cells (Webb and Cooper, 1973) in the same manner as cytophilic antibody does for basophils, monocytes, and macrophages. This raises the possibility that physiological interactions between IgM molecules and antigen(s) may be initiated on the T-cell surface rather than by T-cell contact with preformed antigen–IgM complexes. Assuming random attachment of IgM antibodies on the T cell, this would require that minute numbers of IgM molecules of the appropriate specificity be able to deliver, upon contact with the antigen, an augmentary signal for activation of $T._M$ cells. On the other hand, it would seem more economical if the stability of the interaction between the $T._M$-cell receptors and IgM were favorably affected by preformed antigen–IgM complexes. One could then envision several ways in which triggering of the appropriate clone of helper $T._M$ cells could be enhanced by IgM antibody. Logically, IgM antibodies should be present at the outset in order to favorably influence the immune response via $T._M$ cells. These could be shed by virgin B lymphocytes, secreted by cells at an even earlier stage in differentiation (i.e., mammalian pre-B or avian bursal cells), or from IgM plasma cells. As for the latter cell source, there is clear evidence for the existence of T-independent B cells, which, interesting enough, may be stimulated to produce IgM antibody only (Playfair and Purves, 1971; Mitchell et al., 1972). The IgM antibodies from pre-B cells and B lymphocytes would be monomeric and present in smaller quantities than the pentameric IgM antibodies produced by stimulated plasmablasts and plasma cells. Clearly, this is a problem area that needs further study, especially at a biochemical level.

Thus, according to our view, the mechanism of activation of both helper and suppressor T cells may have a high degree of symmetry. Triggering of both T_G and T_M cells involve a specific and a nonspecific step, and for both cell types the Ig receptor is viewed as having a major regulatory role on the cell function. Such a regulatory role of antibody on T-cell functions has been previously proposed, although from perspectives differing somewhat from ours, by Playfair (1974) and by Gorczynski *et al.* (1976).

Let us now consider some of the implications of having antibody of two different Ig classes play a significant role in regulating the function of two distinct T-cell subclasses. First, it should be noted that T cells can be specifically triggered by antigen in the absence of antibodies produced by B cells; e.g., the immune responses directly attributable to T cells are intact in humans, chickens, and mice devoid of B cells and their products (see Good, 1973; Cooper *et al.*, 1966; Lawton and Cooper, 1974). However, T-cell helper activity might be expected to be deficient when the helper T cells have been derived from B-cell-deprived animals. This indeed appears to be the case when T-cell helper function has been carefully measured using carrier-primed T cells from mice depleted of B cells since birth by chronic treatment with anti-μ antibodies (Janeway *et al.*, 1977). Another implication of our view on the interaction of T and B cells via the receptors for IgM and IgG on T-cell subpopulations is that helper T_M cells should have the opportunity of being triggered before suppressor T_G cells. This would be the consequence of both the class of antibody needed in order to perceive what we have viewed as a "second signal," and the differential mode of binding of IgG and IgM to T_G or T_M cells, respectively. Thus the early stages of an immune response will be characterized by T-cell help but not suppression. Suppression will occur only when enough IgG antibody is produced to form immune complexes in sufficient quantities, and perhaps sufficient size, to bind to T_G cells. The third, and possibly most questionable implication, is that intervention of suppressor T cells occurs relatively early in the immune response when the amount of antigen available is sufficient to reach equilibrium with antibody and form stable immune complexes. Suppressor T cells, on the other hand, may not function efficiently in the closing stages of the immune responses when, owing to an excess of antibody production, formation of stable immune complexes would be much more difficult. Moreover, as discussed earlier, it is possible that interaction of immune complexes with surface receptors of T_G cells may slow down the turnover of the receptor itself with significant physiological effects. One final and rather appealing implication is that, according to this model, the single T lymphocyte, whether it belongs to the helper or suppressor subclass, will be able to recognize the antigen not as a single antigenic determinant, but as a complete antigenic molecular entity. Being clonally distributed, the single lymphocytes will recognize and bind a single determinant located on an antigen molecule through their native antigen-specific receptor. At this point activation may not take place in an efficient manner unless a second signal is delivered by passively adsorbed antibody molecules which, in all probability, would recognize different antigenic determinants on the same antigen molecule. The delivery, and possibly the intensity, of this second signal would then depend on whether other components of the immune system have previously recognized determinants present on the antigen molecule. As a consequence, help and suppression of the immune response would be exerted by T cells more at the level of antigenic molecular (or multimolecular) entities made of several antigenic determinants rather than at the level of a single antigenic determinant.

The hypothetical model that we have described represents an attempt to explain some of the functions of receptors for different Ig classes on T cells in providing specific signals that may be needed for triggering of helper and suppressor T cells and normal modulation of the antibody response. As we have already indicated, under certain circumstances these signals may be bypassed.

ACKNOWLEDGMENTS

We thank our colleagues who participated in these studies and who freely shared their ideas with us. Tina Chaffin, Martha Dagg, and Summer King provided invaluable assistance in preparing the manuscript.

This work was supported by a J. E. Fogarty Fellowship from the National Institutes of Health, Grants CA 16673 and CA 13148, awarded by the National Cancer Institute, DHEW; 5MO1-RR32, awarded by National Institutes of Health, DHEW; and 1-354, awarded by The National Foundation, March of Dimes.

VI. REFERENCES

Abdou, N. I., Sagawa, A., Pascual, E., Hebert, J., and Sadeghee, S., 1976, Suppressor T-cell abnormality in idiopathic systemic lupus erythematosus, *Clin. Immunol. Immunopathol.* 6:192.

Anderson, C. L., and Grey, H. M., 1974, Receptors for aggregated IgG on mouse lymphocytes. Their presence on thymocytes, thymus-derived and bone marrow derived lymphocytes, *J. Exp. Med.* 139:1175.

Balch, C. M., Dagg, M. K., and Cooper, M. D., 1976, Cross-reactive T-cell antigens among mammalian species, *J. Immunol.* 117:447.

Balch, C. M., Dougherty, P. A., Vogler, L., and Cresswell, P., 1977, Fluorescent detection of a human B-cell differentiation antigen (Ag) on normal and neoplastic lymphocytes, *Fed. Proc.* 36:1317A.

Basten, A., Miller, J. F. A. P., Sprent, J., and Pye, J., 1972, A receptor for antibody on B lymphocytes. I. Method for detection and functional significance, *J. Exp. Med.* 135:610.

Basten, A., Miller, J. F. A. P., and Johnson, P., 1975, T cell-dependent suppression of an anti-hapten antibody response, *Transplant Rev.* **26**:130.

Billing, R., Rafizadeh, B., Drew, I., Hartman, G., Gale, R., and Terasaki, P., 1976, Human B-lymphocyte antigens expressed by lymphocytic and myelocytic cells. I. Detection by rabbit antisera, *J. Exp. Med.* **144**:167.

Bresnihan, B., and Jasin, H. E., 1977, Suppressor function of peripheral blood mononuclear cells in normal individuals and in patients with systemic lupus erythematosus, *J. Clin. Invest.* **59**:106.

Broder, S., Edelson, R. L., Lutzner, M. A., Nelson, D. L., MacDermott, R. P., Durm, M. E., Goldman, C. K., Meade, B. D., and Waldmann, T. A., 1976, The Sézary syndrome. A malignant proliferation of helper T cells, *J. Clin. Invest.* **58**:1297.

Broome, J. D., Zucker-Franklin, D., Weiner, M. S., Bianco, C., and Nussenzweig, V., 1973, Leukemic cells with membrane properties of thymus-derived (T) lymphocytes in a case of Sézary's syndrome: Morphologic and immunologic studies, *Clin. Immunol. Immunopathol.* **1**:319.

Brouet, J. C., Flandrin, G., and Seligmann, M., 1973, Indications of the thymus-derived nature of the proliferating cells in six patients with Sézary's syndrome, *N. Engl. J. Med.* **289**:341.

Brown, G., and Greaves, M. F., 1974, Cell surface markers for human T and B lymphocytes, *Eur. J. Immunol.* **4**:302.

Cantor, H., and Boyse, E. A., 1975*a*, Functional subclasses of T lymphocytes bearing different Ly antigens. I. The generation of functionally distinct T-cell subclasses is a differentiation process independent of antigen, *J. Exp. Med.* **141**:1376.

Cantor, H., and Boyse, E. A., 1975*b*, Functional subclasses of T lymphocytes bearing different Ly antigens. II. Cooperation between subclasses of Ly^+ cells in the generation of killer activity, *J. Exp. Med.* **141**:1390.

Cantor, H., and Boyse, E., 1977, Regulation of the immune response by T-cell subclasses, in: *Contemporary Topics in Immunobiology*, Vol. 7 (O. Stutman, ed.), pp. 47–67, Plenum Press, New York.

Cantor, H., Simpson, E., Sato, V. L., Fathmann, C. G., and Herzenberg, L. A., 1975, Characterization of subpopulation of T lymphocytes. I. Separation and functional studies of peripheral T-cells binding different amounts of fluorescent anti-Thy 1.2 (theta) antibody using a fluorescence-activated cell sorter (FACS), *Cell. Immunol.* **15**:180.

Clot, J., Massip, H., and Mathieu, O., 1975, *In vitro* studies on human B and T cell purified populations. Stimulation by mitogens and allogeneic cells, and quantitative binding of phytomitogens, *Immunology* **29**:445.

Conradie, J. D., and Bubb, M. D., 1977, $C\mu 4$ domain of IgM has cytophilic activity for human lymphocytes, *Nature* **265**:160.

Cooper, M. D., and Seligmann, M., 1977, B and T lymphocytes in lymphoproliferative and immunodeficiency diseases, in: *B and T Cells in Immune Recognition* (F. Loor and G. E. Roelants, eds.), p. 377–406, John Wiley & Sons Ltd., London.

Cooper, M. D., Peterson, R. D. A., South, M. A., and Good, R. A., 1966, The functions of the thymus system and the bursa system in the chicken, *J. Exp. Med.* **123**:75.

Cooper, M. D., Keightley, R. G., and Lawton, A. R., 1975, Defective T and B cells in primary immunodeficiencies, in: *Membrane Receptors of Lymphocytes* (M. Seligmann, J. L. Preud'homme, and F. M. Kourilsky, eds.), p. 431, North-Holland, Amsterdam.

Cooper, M. D., Moretta, L., Webb, S. R., Pearl, E. R., Okos, A. J., and Lawton, A. R., 1977, Diversity of defects in human B-cell differentiation, in: *Immunopathology*, Vol. VII (P. A. Miescher, ed.), pp. 343–354, Schwabe & Co., Basel/Stuttgart.

Dauphinee, M. J., and Talal, N., 1975, Reversible restoration by thymosin of antigen-induced depression of spleen DNA synthesis in NZB mice, *J. Immunol.* 114:1713.

De La Concha, E. G., Oldham, G., Webster, A. D. B., Asherson, G. L., and Platts-Mills, T. A. E., 1977, Quantitative measurements of T- and B-cell function in "variable" primary hypogammaglobulinemia: Evidence for a consistent B-cell defect, *Clin. Exp. Immunol.* 27:208.

Dennert, G., 1971, The mechanism of antibody-induced stimulation and inhibition of the immune response, *J. Immunol.* 106:951.

Dickler, H. B., 1976, Lymphocyte receptor for immunoglobulin, in: *Advances in Immunology* (F. J. Dixon and H. G. Kinkel, eds.), p. 167, Academic Press, New York.

Dickler, H. B., and Kunkel, H. G., 1972, Interaction of aggregated γ-globulin with B lymphocytes, *J. Exp. Med.* 136:191.

Douglas, S. D., 1972, Electron microscopic and functional aspects of human lymphocyte response to mitogens, *Transplant. Rev.* 11:39.

Dutton, R. W., 1973, Inhibitory and stimulatory effects of concanavalin A on the response of mouse spleen cell suspensions to antigen. II. Evidence for separate stimulatory and inhibitory cells, *J. Exp. Med.* 138:1496.

Dutton, R. W., 1975, Suppressor T cells, *Transplant. Rev.* 26:39.

Eichmann, K., 1975, Idiotype suppression. II. Amplification of a suppressor T cell with anti-idiotypic activity, *Eur. J. Immunol.* 5:511.

Ekstedt, R. D., Waterfield, J. D., Nespoli, L., and Möller, G., 1977, Mechanism of action of suppressor cells. *In vivo* concanavalin-A-activated suppressor cells do not directly affect B cells, *Scand. J. Immunol.* 6:247.

Evans, R. L., Breard, J. M., Lazarus, H., Schlossman, S. F., and Chess, L., 1977, Detection, isolation, and functional characterization of two human T-cell subclasses bearing unique differentiation antigens, *J. Exp. Med.* 145:221.

Fathman, C. G., Cone, J. L., Sharrow, S. O., Tyrer, H., and Sachs, D. H., 1975, *Ia* alloantigen(s) detected on thymocytes by use of a fluorescence-activated cell sorter, *J. Immunol.* 115:584.

Fauci, A. S., and Pratt, K. R., 1976a, Polyclonal activation of bone-marrow-derived lymphocytes from human peripheral blood measured by a direct plaque-forming cell assay, *Proc. Natl. Acad. Sci. U.S.* 73:3676.

Fauci, A. S., and Pratt, K. R., 1976b, Activation of human B lymphocytes. I. Direct plaque-forming cell assay for the measurement of polyclonal activation and antigenic stimulation of human B lymphocytes, *J. Exp. Med.* 144:674.

Fauci, A. S., Pratt, K. R., and Whalen, G., 1976, Activation of human B lymphocytes. II. Cellular interactions in the PFC response of human tonsillar and peripheral blood B lymphocytes to polyclonal activation by pokeweed mitogen, *J. Immunol.* 117:2100.

Felsburg, P. J., and Edelman, R., 1977, The active E-rosette test: A sensitive *in vitro* correlate for human delayed-type hypersensitivity, *J. Immunol.* 118:62.

Ferrarini, M., Moretta, L., Abrile, R., and Durante, M. L., 1975a, Receptors for IgG molecules on human lymphocytes forming spontaneous rosettes with sheep red cells, *Eur. J. Immunol.* 5:70.

Ferrarini, M., Tonda, G. P., Risso, A., and Viale, G., 1975b, Lymphocyte membrane receptors in human lymphoid leukemias, *Eur. J. Immunol.* 5:89.

Ferrarini, M., Moretta, L., Mingari, M. C., Tonda, P., and Pernis, B., 1976, Human T cell receptor for IgM: Specificity for the pentameric Fc fragment, *Eur. J. Immunol.* 6:520.

Ferrarini, M., Hoffman, T., Fu, S. M., Winchester, R. J., and Kunkel, H. G., 1977, Receptors for IgM on certain human B lymphocytes, *J. Immunol.* 119:1525.

Fridman, W. H., and Goldstein, P., 1974, Immunoglobulin-binding factor present on and produced by thymus-processed lymphocytes (T cells), *Cell. Immunol.* **11**:442.

Friedman, S. M., Breard, J. M., and Chess, L., 1976, Triggering of human peripheral blood B cells: Polyclonal induction and modulation of an *in vitro* PFC response, *J. Immunol.* **117**:2021.

Frøland, S. S., and Natvig, J. B., 1973, Identification of three different human lymphocyte populations by surface markers, *Transplant. Rev.* **16**:114.

Fuson, E. W., and Lamon, E. W., 1977, IgM-induced cell-mediated cytotoxicity with antibody and effector cells of human origin, *J. Immunol.* **118**:1907.

Geha, R. S., Schneeberger, E., Merler, E., and Rosen, F. S., 1974, Heterogeneity of "acquired" or common variable agammaglobulinemia, *N. Engl. J. Med.* **291**:1.

Geha, R. S., Mudawwar, F., and Scheeberger, E., 1977, The specificity of T-cell helper factor in man, *J. Exp. Med.* **145**:1436.

Gershon, R. K., 1974, T cell control of antibody production, in: *Contemporary Topics in Immunobiology*, Vol. 3 (M. D. Cooper and N. L. Warner, eds.), p. 1–40, Plenum Press, New York.

Gmelig-Meyling, F., van der Ham, M., and Ballieux, R. E., 1976, Binding of IgM by human T lymphocytes, *Scand. J. Immunol.* **5**:487.

Gonzales-Molina, A., and Spiegelberg, H. L., 1977, A subpopulation of normal human peripheral B lymphocytes that bind IgE, *J. Clin. Invest.* **59**:616.

Good, R. A., 1973, Immunodeficiency in developmental perspective, *Harvey Lect.* **67**:1.

Gorczynski, R., Kontiainen, S., Mitchison, N. A., and Tigelaar, R. E., 1976, Antigen–antibody complexes as blocking factors on the T lymphocyte surface, in: *Cellular Selection and Regulation in the Immune Response* (E. M. Edelman, ed.), p. 143, Raven Press, New York.

Grossi, C. E., Moretta, L., Webb, S. R., Mingari, M. C., Moretta, A., Lydyard, P. M., Licca, A., and Cooper, M. D., 1977, Analysis of surface properties, fine structure and surface distribution of two distinct T-cell subpopulations: Tμ and Tγ, in: *Regulatory Mechanisms in Lymphocyte Activation: Proceedings of the Eleventh Leukocyte Culture Conference* (David O. Lucas, ed.), pp. 509–511, Academic Press, New York.

Grossi, C. E., Webb, S. R., Zicca, A., Lydyard, P. M., Moretta, L., Mingari, M. C., and Cooper, M. D., 1978, Morphological and histochemical analyses of two human T-cell subpopulations bearing receptors for IgM (T.$_M$) or IgG (T.$_G$), *J. Exp. Med.* (in press).

Hallberg, T., Gurner, B. W., and Coombs, R. R. A., 1973, Opsonic adherence of sensitized ox red cells to human lymphocytes as measured by rosette formation, *Int. Arch. Allergy Appl. Immunol.* **44**:500.

Hardin, J. A., Chused, T. M., and Steinberg, A. D., 1973, Suppressor cells in the graft vs. host reaction, *J. Immunol.* **111**:650.

Harwell, L., Marrack, P., and Kappler, J. W., 1977, Suppressor T-cell inactivation of a helper T-cell factor, *Nature* **265**:57.

Haynes, B. F., and Fauci, A. S., 1977*a*, Activation of human B lymphocytes. III. Concanavalin A-induced generation of suppressor cells of the plaque-forming cell response of normal human B lymphocytes, *J. Immunol.* **118**:2281.

Haynes, B. F., and Fauci, A. S., 1977*b*, Characterization of concanavalin A generated suppressor cells of the plaque forming cell response of human peripheral blood lymphocytes, *Clin. Res.* **25**:359A.

Hayward, A. R., and Lawton, A. R., 1977, Induction of plasma cell differentiation of human fetal lymphocytes: Evidence for functional immaturity of T and B cells, *J. Immunol.* **119**:1213.

Hellström, U., Dillner, M-L., Hammerström, S., and Perlmann, P., 1976, Fractionation of human T lymphocytes on wheat germ agglutinin-Sepharose, *J. Exp. Med.* **144**:1381.

Henry, C., and Jerne, N. K., 1968, Competition of 19S and 7S antigen receptors in the regulation of the primary immune response, *J. Exp. Med.* **128**:133.

Herzenberg, L. A., Okumura, K., Cantor, H., Sato, V. L., Shen, F. W., Boyse, E. A., and Herzenberg, L. A., 1976, T-cell regulation of antibody responses: Demonstration of allotype-specific helper T cells and their specific removal by suppressor T cells, *J. Exp. Med.* **144**:330.

Hoffman, T., and Kunkel, H. G., 1976, The E-rosette test in *in vitro* methods, in: *Cell Mediated and Tumor Immunity* (B. R. Bloom and J. R. David, eds.), p. 71, Academic Press, New York.

Hoffman, T., Wang, C. Y., Winchester, R. J., Ferrarini, M., and Kunkel, H. G., 1977, Human lymphocytes bearing "Ia-like" antigens; absence in patients with infantile agammaglobulinemia, *J. Immunol.* **119**:1520.

Horowitz, S., Borcherding, W., Moorthy, A. V., Chesney, R., Schulte-Wissermann, H., Hong, R., and Goldstein, A., 1977, Induction of suppressor T cells in systemic lupus erythematosus by thymosin and cultured thymic epithelium, *Science* **197**:999.

Horwitz, D. A., and Garrett, M. A., 1977, Distinctive functional properties of human blood lymphocytes: A comparison with T lymphocytes, B lymphocytes and monocytes, *J. Immunol.* **118**:1712.

Hsu, C. C. S., Marti, G. E., Schreck, R., and Williams, R. C., 1975, Lymphocytes bearing B- and T-cell markers in patient with lymphosarcoma cell leukemia, *Clin. Immunol. Immunopathol.* **3**:385.

Huber, B., Devinsky, O., Gershon, R. K., and Cantor, H., 1976, Cell-mediated immunity: Delayed-type hypersensitivity and cytotoxic responses are mediated by different T-cell subclasses, *J. Exp. Med.* **143**:1534.

Humphreys, R. E., McCune, J. M., Chess, L., Herrman, H. C., Malenka, D. J., Mann, D. L., Parham, P., Schlossman, S. F., and Strominger, J. L., 1976, Isolation and immunologic characterization of a human, B lymphocyte-specific, cell surface antigen, *J. Exp. Med.* **144**:98.

Insel, R. A., and Merler, E., 1977, The necessity for T cell help for human tonsil B cell responses to pokeweed mitogen: Induction of DNA synthesis, immunoglobulin, and specific antibody production with a T cell helper factor produced with pokeweed mitogen, *J. Immunol.* **118**:2009.

Jandinski, J., Cantor, H., Tadakuma, T., Peavy, D. L., and Pierce, C. W., 1976, Separation of helper T cells from suppressor T cells expressing different Ly components. I. Polyclonal activation: Suppressor and helper activities are inherent properties of distinct T-cell subclasses, *J. Exp. Med.* **143**:1382.

Janeway, C. A., Jr., Murgita, R. A., Weinbaum, F. I., Asofsky, R., and Wigzell, H., 1977, Evidence for a primed T cell that increases helper T cell activity, *Proc. Natl. Acad. Sci. U.S.* **74**:4582.

Janossy, G., and Greaves, M., 1975, Functional analysis of murine and human B lymphocyte subsets, *Transplant. Rev.* **24**:177.

Jerne, N. K., 1976, Clonal selection in a lymphocyte network, in: *Cellular Selection and Regulation in the Immune Response* (G. M. Edelman, ed.), p. 39, Raven Press, New York.

Katz, D. H., 1977, *Lymphocyte Differentiation, Recognition and Regulation*, p. 124, Academic Press, New York.

Keightley, R. G., Cooper, M. D., and Lawton, A. R., 1976, The T cell dependence of B cell differentiation induced by pokeweed mitogen, *J. Immunol.* **117**:1538.

Krakauer, R. S., Strober, W., Rippeon, D. L., and Waldmann, T. A., 1976, Prevention of autoimmunity in experimental lupus erythematosus by soluble immune response suppressor, *Science* **196**:56.

Kreth, H. W., and Herzenberg, L. A., 1974, Fluorescence-activated cell sorting of human T and B lymphocytes. I. Direct evidence that lymphocytes with a high density of membrane-bound immunoglobulin are precursors of plasmacytes, *Cell. Immunol.* **12**:396.

Kunz, M. M., Innes, J. B., and Weksler, M. E., 1976, Lymphocyte transformation induced by autologous cells. IV. Human T lymphocyte proliferation induced by autologous or allogeneic non-T lymphocytes, *J. Exp. Med.* **143**:1043.

Kurnick, J. T., and Grey, H. M., 1975, Relationship between immunoglobulin-bearing lymphocytes and cells reactive with sensitized human erythrocytes, *J. Immunol.* **115**: 305.

Lamon, E. W., Shaw, M. W., Goodson, S., Lidin, B., Walia, A. S., and Fuson, E. W., 1977, Antibody-dependent cell-mediated cytotoxicity in the Maloney sarcoma virus system: Differential activity of IgG and IgM with different subpopulations of lymphocytes, *J. Exp. Med.* **145**:302.

Lawton, A. R., and Cooper, M. D., 1974, Modification of B lymphocyte differentiation by anti-immunoglobulins, in: *Contemporary Topics in Immunobiology*, Vol. 3 (M. D. Cooper and N. L. Warner, eds.), pp. 193–225, Plenum Press, New York.

Lee, S. -T., and Paraskevas, F., 1972, Cell surface-associated gamma globulins in lymphocytes. IV. Lack of detection of surface γ globulin on B-cells and acquisition of surface γG globulin by T-cells during primary response, *J. Immunol.* **109**:1262.

Masson, P. L., Delire, M., and Cambiaso, C. L., 1977, Circulating immune complexes in normal human pregnancy, *Nature* **266**:542.

McBride, R. A., and Schierman, L. W., 1973, Thymus dependency of antibody-mediated helper effect, *J. Immunol.* **110**:1710.

McConnell, I., and Hurd, C. M., 1976, Lymphocyte receptors. II. Receptors for rabbit IgM on human T lymphocytes, *Immunology* **30**:835.

McMichael, A. J., and Susazuki, T., 1977, A suppressor T cell in the human mixed lymphocyte reaction, *J. Exp. Med.* **146**:368.

Mingari, M. C., Moretta, L., Moretta, A., Ferrarini, M., and Preud'homme, J. L., 1978, Fc-receptors for IgG and IgM immunoglobulins on human T lymphocytes: Mode of reexpression following proteolysis or interaction with immune complexes, *J. Immunol.* (in press).

Mitchell, G. F., Grumet, F. C., and McDevitt, H. O., 1972, Genetic control of the immune response. The effect of thymectomy on the primary and secondary antibody response of mice to poly-L(tyr, glu)-poly-D, L-ala-poly-1-lys, *J. Exp. Med.* **135**:126.

Molenaar, J. L., van Galen, M., Hannema, A. J., Ziejlemaker, W., and Pondman, K. W., 1977, Spontaneous release of Fc receptor-like material from human lymphoblastoid cell lines, *Eur. J. Immunol.* **7**:230.

Moretta, L., Ferrarini, M., Durante, M. L., and Mingari, M. C., 1975, Expression of a receptor for IgM by human T cells *in vitro*, *Eur. J. Immunol.* **5**:565.

Moretta, L., Ferrarini, M., Mingari, M. C., Moretta, A., and Webb, S. R., 1976*a*, Subpopulations of human T cells identified by receptors for immunoglobulins and mitogen responsiveness, *J. Immunol.* **117**:2171.

Moretta, L., Webb, S. R., Grossi, C. E., Lydyard, P. M., and Cooper, M. D., 1976*b*, Functional analysis of two subpopulations of human T cells and their distribution in immunodeficient patients, *Clin. Res.* **24**:448A.

Moretta, L., Webb, S. R., Grossi, C. E., Lydyard, P. M., and Cooper, M. D., 1977*a*, Functional analysis of two human T-cell subpopulations: Help and suppression of B cell responses by T cells bearing receptors for IgM ($T._M$) or IgG ($T._G$), *J. Exp. Med.* **146**:184.

Moretta, L., Mingari, M. C., Moretta, A., and Lydyard, P. M., 1977*b*, Receptors for IgM are expressed on acute lymphoblastic leukemia cells having T-cell characteristics, *Clin. Immunol. Immunopathol.* **7**:405.

Moretta, L., Mingari, M. C., and Moretta, A., 1977*c*, Characterization of receptors for IgG and IgM on human T lymphocytes, *Fed. Proc.* **36**:1314.

Moretta, L., Mingari, M. C., Webb, S. R., Pearl, E. R., Lydyard, P. M., Grossi, C. E., Lawton, A. R., and Cooper, M. D., 1977d, Imbalance in T-cell subpopulations associated with immunodeficiency and autoimmune syndromes, *Eur. J. Immunol.* 7:696.

Moretta, L., Mingari, M. C., and Romanzi, C. A., 1978, Loss of Fc receptors for IgG from human T lymphocytes exposed to IgG immune complexes, *Nature* (in press).

Okumura, K., Takemori, T., and Tada, T., 1977, Specific enrichment of suppressor T cells bearing the product of *I-J* subregion, in: *ICN-UCLA Symposium Proceedings, Immune System II: Regulation and Genetics,* Vol. 8 (E. Sercarz, A. Herzenberg, and C. Fox, eds.), Academic Press, New York.

Olding, L. B., and Oldstone, M. B. A., 1976, Thymus-derived peripheral lymphocytes from human newborns inhibit division of the mothers' lymphocytes, *J. Immunol.* 116:682.

Oldstone, M. B. A., Tishon, A., and Moretta, L., 1977, Active thymus derived suppressor lymphocytes in human cord blood, *Nature* 269:333.

Owen, F. L., Ju, S.-T., and Nisonoff, A., 1977, Presence on idiotype-specific suppressor T cells of receptors that interact with molecules bearing the idiotype, *J. Exp. Med.* 145: 1559.

Pape, G. R., Troye, M., and Perlmann, P., 1977, Characterization of cytolytic effector cells in peripheral blood of healthy individuals and cancer patients. II. Cytotoxicity to allogeneic or autochthonous tumor cells in tissue culture, *J. Immunol.* 118:1925.

Pichler, W. J., and Knapp, W., 1977, Receptors for IgM-coated erythrocytes on chronic lymphatic leukemia cells, *J. Immunol.* 118:1010.

Pierce, C. W., and Kapp, J. A., 1976, Regulation of immune responses by suppressor T cells, in: *Contemporary Topics in Immunobiology,* Vol. 5 (W. O. Weigle, ed.), pp. 91–143, Plenum Press, New York.

Playfair, J. H. L., 1974, The role of antibody in T-cell responses, *Clin. Exp. Immunol.* 17:1.

Playfair, J. H. L., and Purves, E. C., 1971, Separate thymus dependent and thymus independent antibody forming cell precursors, *Nature New Biol.* 231:149.

Preud'homme, J. L., Gonnot, M., Tsapis, A., Brouet, J. C., and Mihaesco, C., 1977, Human T lymphocyte receptors for IgM: reactivity with monomeric 8S subunits, *J. Immunol.* 119:2206.

Rich, R. R., and Pierce, C. W., 1973, Biological expressions of lymphocyte activation. II. Generation of a population of thymus-derived suppressor lymphocytes, *J. Exp. Med.* 137:649.

Saal, J. G., Rieber, E. P., Hadam, M., and Riethmuller, G., 1977, Lymphocytes with T-cell markers cooperate with IgG antibodies in the lysis of human tumour cells, *Nature* 265:158.

Samarut, C., Brochier, J., and Revillard, J. P., 1976, Distribution of cells binding erythrocyte-antibody (EA) complexes in human lymphoid populations, *Scand. J. Immunol.* 5:221.

Sampson, D., Grotelueschen, C., and Kauffman, H. M., 1975, The human splenic suppressor cell, *Transplantation* 20:362.

Seligmann, M., Preud'homme, J. L., and Brouet, J. C., 1973, B and T cell markers in human proliferative blood diseases and primary immunodeficiencies, with special reference to membrane bound immunoglobulins, *Transplant. Rev.* 16:85.

Shou, L., Schwartz, S. A., and Good, R. A., 1976, Suppressor cell activity after concanavalin A treatment of lymphocytes from normal donors, *J. Exp. Med.* 143:1100.

Siegal, F. P., and Siegal, M., 1977, Enhancement by irradiated T cells of human plasma cell production: Dissection of helper and suppressor functions *in vitro, J. Immunol.* 118:642.

Siegal, F. P., Siegal, M., and Good, R. A., 1976, Suppression of B-cell differentiation by leukocytes from hypogammaglobulinemic patients, *J. Clin. Invest.* 58:109.

Silverstein, S. C., Steinman, R. M., and Cohn, Z. A., 1977, Endocytosis, *Annu. Rev. Biochem.* 46:669.

Sinclair, N. R. S., 1969, Regulation of the immune response. I. Reduction in ability of specific antibody to inhibit long-lasting IgG immunological priming after removal of the Fc fragment, *J. Exp. Med.* 129:1183.

Soteriades-Vlachos, C., Gyöngyössy, M. I. C., and Playfair, J. H. L., 1974, Rosette formation by mouse lymphocytes. III. Receptors for immunoglobulin on normal and activated T cells, *Clin. Exp. Immunol.* 18:187.

Stobo, J. D., 1972, Phytohemagglutinin and concanavalin A: Probes for murine "T" cell activation and differentiation, *Transplant. Rev.* 11:60.

Stobo, J. D., Paul, S., van Scoy, R. E., and Hermans, P. E., 1976, Suppressor thymus-derived lymphocytes in fungal infection, *J. Clin. Invest.* 57:319.

Stout, R. D., and Herzenberg, L. A., 1975*a*, The Fc receptor on thymus-derived lymphocytes. I. Detection of a subpopulation of murine T lymphocytes bearing the Fc receptor, *J. Exp. Med.* 142:611.

Stout, R. D., and Herzenberg, L. A., 1975*b*, The Fc receptor on thymus-derived lymphocytes. II. Mitogen responsiveness of T lymphocytes bearing the Fc receptor, *J. Exp. Med.* 142:1041.

Stout, R. D., Waksal, S. D., and Herzenberg, L. A., 1976, The Fc receptor on thymus-derived lymphocytes. III. Mixed lymphocyte reactivity and cell-mediated lympholytic activity of Fc^- and Fc^+ T lymphocytes, *J. Exp. Med.* 144:54.

Stout, R. D., Murphy, D. B., McDevitt, H. O., and Herzenberg, L. A., 1977, The Fc receptor on thymus-derived lymphocytes. IV. Inhibition of binding of antigen–antibody complexes to Fc receptor-positive T cells by anti-*Ia* sera, *J. Exp. Med.* 145:187.

Tada, T., 1977, Regulation of the antibody response by T cell products determined by different I subregions, in: *ICN-UCLA Symposium Proceedings, Immune System II: Regulation and Genetics*, Vol. 8 (E. Sercarz, L. A. Herzenberg, and C. F. Fox, eds.), Academic Press, New York.

Tse, H., and Dutton, R. W., 1976, Separation of helper and suppressor T lymphocytes on a Ficoll velocity sedimentation gradient, *J. Exp. Med.* 143:1199.

Twomey, J. J., Laughter, A. H., Farrow, S., and Douglass, C. C., 1975, Hodgkin's disease. An immunodepleting and immunosuppressive disorder, *J. Clin. Invest.* 56:467.

Uhlenbruck, G., Seaman, G. V. F., and Coombs, R. R. A., 1967, Factors influencing the agglutinability of red cells. III. Physico-chemical studies on ox red cells of different classes of agglutinability, *Vox Sanguinis* 12:420.

Uhr, J. W., and Möller, G., 1968, Regulatory effect of antibody on the immune response, *Adv. Immunol.* 8:81.

van Boxel, J. A., and Rosenstreich, D. L., 1974, Binding of aggregated γ-globulin to activated T lymphocytes in the guinea pig, *J. Exp. Med.* 139:1002.

van Oers, M. H. J., Zeijlemaker, W. P., and Schellekens, P. Th. A., 1977, Separation and properties of EA-rosette-forming lymphocytes in humans, *Eur. J. Immunol.* 7:143.

Wahlin, B., Perlmann, H., and Perlmann, P., 1976, Analysis by a plaque assay of IgG- or IgM-dependent cytolytic lymphocytes in human blood, *J. Exp. Med.* 144:1375.

Waldmann, T. A., and Broder, S., 1977, Suppressor cells in the regulation of the immune response, *Progr. Clin. Immunol.* 3:155.

Waldmann, T. A., Durm, M., Broder, S., Blackman, M., Blaese, R. M., and Strober, W. S., 1974, Role of suppressor T cells in pathogenesis of common variable hypogammaglobulinemia, *Lancet* 2:609.

Waldmann, T. A., Broder, S., Krakauer, R., MacDErmott, R. P., Durm, M., Goldman, C., and Meade, B., 1976, The role of suppressor cells in the pathogenesis of common variable hypogammaglobulinemia and the immunodeficiency associated with myeloma, *Fed. Proc.* 35:2067.

Webb, S. R., and Cooper, M. D., 1973, T cells can bind antigen via cytophilic IgM antibody made by B cells, *J. Immunol.* **111**:275.

Webb, S. R., Lydyard, P. M., Moretta, L., Ferrarini, M., Mingari, M. C., Moretta, A., and Cooper, M. D., 1977, Proliferative responsiveness of two distinct human T-cell subpopulations to Con A, PHA and alloantigens, in: *Regulatory Mechanisms in Lymphocyte Activation: Proceedings of the Eleventh Leukocyte Culture Conference* (David O. Lucas, ed.), pp. 512–514, Academic Press, New York.

Weiner, M. S., Bianco, C., and Nussenzweig, V., 1973, Enhanced binding of neuraminidase-treated sheep erythrocytes to human T lymphocytes, *Blood* **42**:939.

West, W. H., Cannon, G. B., Kay, H. D., Bonnard, G. D., and Herberman, R. B., 1977, Natural cytotoxic reactivity of human lymphocytes against a myeloid cell line: Characterization of effector cells, *J. Immunol.* **118**:355.

Winchester, R. J., Fu, S. M., Hoffman, T., and Kunkel, H. G., 1975, IgG on lymphocyte surfaces; technical problems and the significance of a third cell population, *J. Immunol.* **114**:1210.

Winchester, R. J., Wang, C. Y., Halper, J., and Hoffmann, T., 1976, Studies with B-cell allo- and hetero-antisera: Parallel reactivity and special properties, *Scand. J. Immunol.* **5**:745.

Winfield, J. B., Lobo, P. I., and Hamilton, M. E., 1977, Fc receptor heterogeneity. Immunofluorescent studies of B, T and third population lymphocytes in human blood using rabbit IgG b_4-anti b_4 complexes, *J. Immunol.* **119**:1778.

Wu, L. Y. F., Lawton, A. R., and Cooper, M. D., 1973, Differentiation capacity of cultured B lymphocytes from immunodeficient patients, *J. Clin. Invest.* **52**:3180.

Yoshida, T. O., and Andersson, B., 1972, Evidence for a receptor recognizing antigen complexed immunoglobulin on the surface of activated mouse thymus lymphocytes, *Scand. J. Immunol.* **1**:401.

Zucker-Franklin, D., Melton, J. W., III, and Quagliata, F., 1976, Ultrastructural, immunologic, and functional studies on Sézary cells: A neoplastic variant of thymus-derived (T) lymphocytes, *Proc. Natl. Acad. Sci. U.S.* **71**:1877.

Chapter 3

Metazoan and Protozoan Parasitic Infections in Nude Mice

Graham F. Mitchell

Laboratory of Immunoparasitology
The Walter and Eliza Hall Institute of Medical Research
Royal Melbourne Hospital P.O.
Melbourne, Victoria 3050, Australia

I. INTRODUCTION*

Congenitally hypothymic, *nu/nu* (nude) mice have virtually displaced all other types of T-cell-deficient mice in studies on the consequences of T-cell deficiency, the dissection of T-cell functions, and analyses of T-cell-dependent and T-cell-independent immunological phenomena *in vivo*. Nude mice are severely hypothymic if not totally athymic (Loor and Roelants, 1974); the same cannot be said for the other types of T-cell-deficient mice (e.g., Mitchell, 1974). Large numbers of SPF-derived nude[†] and intact, heterozygous *nu/+* littermates are now available from several centers. Their usefulness has been increased further by the availability of inbred nude mice of various genotypes (e.g., BALB/c.*nu/nu*, CBA/H.*nu/nu*, C57BL/6.*nu/nu*, etc.).

Comparisons and dissection of the susceptibility and resistance of nude, *nu/+*, and selectively reconstituted nude mice to various metazoan and protozoan

---

*Abbreviations: T cell, thymus-influenced cell; B cell, non-thymus-derived precursor of antibody-secreting cells; SPF, specific-pathogen-free; PFC, Jerne plaque-forming cell; Ig, immunoglobulin; BCG, *Mycobacterium* bacillus Calmette–Guérin; DNP, dinitrophenol hapten; DTH, delayed-type hypersensitivity.

†Raising nude mice in an SPF facility not only reduces the mortality rate but, theoretically at least, obviates any selection for the more immunocompetent individuals in the breeding program. Against this being an important consideration is the fact that in most breeding programs, thymus-grafted nude males are mated to intact *nu/+* females.

parasites are likely to provide important new information on the immunological and paraimmunological responses of hosts to parasites. Equally important information will be obtained on the reactions of parasites to potentially host-protective immune responses. Moreover, such mice will certainly provide new insights on concomitant immunity (see below). This article aims to illustrate just how valuable the nude mouse is becoming in this regard, the text being divided into sections dealing with nematode (roundworms), cestode (tapeworms), trematode (flatworms), and protozoal infections. Data obtained using other types of T-cell-deficient mice have been reviewed by Targett (1973).

A common observation in parasitic disease (metazoan parasitic disease in particular) is what has been broadly termed concomitant immunity (Clegg, 1974; Smithers et al., 1969). This type of immunity (i.e., resistance to *reinfection* of an individual which is already parasitized by that particular parasite) is to be expected in a balanced "adaptation tolerance" situation (Sprent, 1959). Without this immunity, hosts would be susceptible to superinfection and death, such a consequence militating against the evolutionary survival of the parasite. The existence of concomitant immunity in numerous host-parasite relationships augurs well for the development of vaccines capable of preventing first infection. Clearly, the challenge facing the immunoparasitologist is twofold: (1) to identify the antigens responsible for concomitant immunity (i.e., induction of resistance to reinfection), and (2) to identify and exploit the mechanisms whereby *established* parasites are resistant to an immune response which is fully effective in eliminating *establishing* parasites.

Mechanisms which have been proposed to account for the resistance of parasites to host protective immunities are (1) antigenic variation, especially in the case of chronic protozoal infections; (2) lability of antigens at the parasite-host interface; (3) uptake of host "blindfolding" molecules; (4) production of immunosuppressive, anticomplementary, or antiinflammatory molecules; (5) induction of immune responses which suppress host-protective immunities; and (6) location in sequestered (e.g., intracellular) sites and resistance to degradative enzymes when the parasitized cell is a phagocyte (Brown, 1971; Cohen and Sadun, 1976; Ogilvie and Wilson, 1976; Porter and Knight, 1974; Trager, 1974). While not a mechanism of the type mentioned above, transmission to the next generation is ensured in the case of some nematodes by a periparturient relaxation in resistance and the commencement of further development of arrested parasites in pregnant and lactating females (reviewed on Ogilvie and Jones, 1973).

Most of the available reports on susceptibility and resistance (or immune reponses) to parasites in nude mice are contained in brief communications. Comprehensive analyses have only recently begun. Obviously, data on parasite numbers in nude mice are easy to generate, and several cautionary comments regarding interpretation are warranted. No statement can be made on T-cell dependence of susceptibility and resistance, or T-cell dependence of a particular response, unless at least three groups of mice are examined: nude, littermate *nu/+*, and T-cell-reconstituted nude. Moreover, observations in at least certain types of T-cell reconstituted nudes must closely resemble those in intact heterozygotes, and interpretations are simplified by the use of highly inbred nude mice in reconstitution studies. No statement on *specifically reactive* T cells can be made until properties such as specific immunological memory or tolerance have been demonstrated in the reconstitutive T-cell inoculum (Miller and Mitchell, 1969). In general, it must be shown whether or not T cells from either immune or tolerant mice are more and less efficient in reconstitution of nudes, respectively. Results of this type of study, plus direct assays of T-cell reactivity to parasite antigens, are required before the conclusion is warranted that T cells with reactivity to parasite antigens are required in a reconstitutive inoculum. The point here is that one must discount the possibility that an inoculum of T cells, simply by improving the general health of the recipient nude mouse, enables another totally T-cell-independent mechanism to mediate parasite rejection or resistance to infection.

Finally, it must be emphasized that the demonstration of a host-protective effect with serum antibodies is relatively easy to interpret.* However, the contribution of cell-mediated (or cellular) immunity in host protection is extremely difficult to assess. A positive transfer of protection with one injection of cells, and a negative with one injection of serum, does not exclude a major contribution of antibodies (of any, or all, Ig classes) produced by the transferred lymphoid cells. Moreover, ablation of an otherwise positive cellular transfer by treatment of the cells with anti-T serum, or a positive transfer with enriched populations of T cells, simply demonstrates that the positive event is T-cell-dependent and does not implicate T cells as the *direct* mediators of antiparasite immunity.

II. NEMATODES

The rejection of those intestinal nematode worms which are rejected by intact mice is impaired in nude mice. Although based on fewer observations, the susceptibility of nudes to tissue-migrating forms of nematodes may not be very different from that of intact mice.

A circulating eosinophilia and an intestinal mast cell response are prominent features of the response of intact mice and rats to certain nematodes (Basten and Beeson, 1970; Dobson, 1972; Miller and Jarrett, 1971; Walls *et al.*, 1971). Both

---

*The existence of host-protective antibodies also provides the investigator with a very powerful tool with which to isolate antigens of relevance in the induction of host-protective immune responses. With antibodies, solid-phase immunoabsorbents or coprecipitation techniques can be used to separate the antigens responsible for induction of these particular antibodies.

responses are absent in nematode-parasitized nude mice (Mitchell *et al.*, 1976*a*; Nielsen *et al.*, 1974; Ruitenberg and Elgersma, 1976). In the case of the mast cell response, one of several possibilities to account for the absence of mast cell accumulation in the intestinal wall of nude mice is that these particular mast cells [but not others located elsewhere (Keller *et al.*, 1976; Ruitenberg and Elgersma, 1976; Vicklicky *et al.*, 1973)] are derived from T cells (Burnet, 1978).

A. *Nippostrongylus brasiliensis*

Nippostrongylus brasiliensis is a direct-infection nematode or rats and mice and has been used extensively in rats in studies on the host components required for worm rejection (e.g., Dineen *et al.*, 1973). After subcutaneous injection of infective third-stage larvae (L3) and migration via the blood, lungs, trachea, and esophagus, adults appear in the intestines and are rejected by day 8-10 from intact mice. Rejection times are slightly longer in the case of rats, and the rat is likely to be the more natural host. Elimination of the intestinal adults of this parasite is achieved most efficiently by a combination of cellular and humoral immunity (Dineen *et al.*, 1973; Jacobson and Reed, 1977; Ogilvie and Love, 1974), although in mice, limited quantities of antibody may suffice (Jacobson *et al.*, 1977; Mitchell *et al.*, 1976*b*; Reed *et al.*, 1978). Nude mice are highly defective in their ability to reject *N. brasiliensis* and parasite burdens are maintained long after normal mice have rejected the parasite (Jacobson and Reed, 1974*a*; Mitchell *et al.*, 1976*b*). In the case of normal mice, resistance to reinfection is striking, but in nude mice, the second infection appears to superimpose itself on the first (Mitchell *et al.*, 1976*b*). An injection of T cells either before or several days after injection of L3 restores the capacity to reject the worms from the intestines (Mitchell *et al.*, 1976*b*). Treatment of the reconstitutive T cells with well-characterized anti-Ly sera, for example, should provide useful information on the type of T cell required for worm rejection.

B. *Ascaris suum*

Ascaris suum is a direct-infection nematode of pigs, the larval migration stages of which occur in various mammals, including mice (Sprent, 1952), Embryonated eggs, administered orally, hatch in the intestines and larvae migrate to the liver and lungs, reaching peak numbers in these organs at days 3-5 and 7-8, respectively. In terms of the number of lung larvae recovered, various strains of mice differ in susceptibility; C57BL/6 mice are particularly susceptible. Nude mice of either susceptible (e.g., C57BL/6.*nu/nu*) or relatively resistant (i.e., BALB/c.*nu/nu* or CBA/H.*nu/nu*) genotypes are not more susceptible than their respective *nu*/+ littermates to first infection. In fact, day-7 lung larvae numbers are often lower, although numbers at later points are comparable (Mitchell *et al.*, 1976a). Intact mice are highly resistant to reinfection, but an answer to the question of whether nude, in particular C57BL/6.*nu/nu*, mice are resistant to second infection has not been resolved satisfactorily. Nude mice lose condition very rapidly after second oral administration of eggs, and results obtained with surviving mice are thus unreliable.

C. Other Nematodes

After oral administration of infective larvae of *Trichinella spiralis*, adults develop in the intestines and are rejected from intact mice more rapidly than from nude mice (Ruitenberg and Elgersma, 1976). No reports on numbers of *T. spiralis* tissue larvae in nude versus intact mice are yet available, although numbers in other T-cell-deficient mice are increased 2–5 times over those in controls (Walls *et al.*, 1973). Nude mice are more susceptible than intact or T-cell-reconstituted mice to the intestinal pinworms *Aspicularis tetraptera* and *Syphacia obvelata* (Jacobson and Reed, 1974b). No published data are yet available on the susceptibility of nude mice to *Nematospiroides dubius* larvae and intestinal worms, the migrating larvae of *Toxocara canis*, and *Trichuris muris* intestinal worms, although it is likely that nudes will be very susceptible to the latter (Wakelin and Selby, 1974).

III. CESTODES

Nude mice are markedly more susceptible than intact mice to either adult intestinal tapeworms or the tissue larval forms of cestodes.

A. *Hymenolepis* Species

Experiments by Bland (1976) and, in particular, the Montana group (Isaak *et al.*, 1975; Reed *et al.*, 1978) have demonstrated that expulsion of *Hymenolepis nana* and *H. diminuta* intestinal tapeworms is deficient in nude mice and that the time course of infection in T-cell-reconstituted nudes is similar to that in intact mice. *Hymenolepis nana* is capable of autoinfection and intestinal tapeworm, and villus cysticercoid numbers may reach very high levels in nude mice. As in the case of intestinal *N. brasiliensis* and *T. spiralis* nematode worms, all the data on intestinal tapeworms in nude mice are compatible with the hypothesis that expulsion of worms and the development of reinfection immunity are T-cell-dependent phenomena.

B. *Taenia taeniaeformis*

Taenia taeniaeformis is a common, nonproliferating, cystic larval cestode of mice and rats, the adult tapeworms being found in the intestines of cats. Infection of mice is achieved readily by oral administration of oncospheres (eggs). Recent studies have established that *T. taeniaeformis* liver cysts grow more rapidly in nude mice (Mitchell *et al.*, 1977a). Moreover, strains of mice differ markedly in susceptibility and nude mice of relatively resistant genotype (e.g., BALB/c. *nu/nu*) contain as many liver cysts as normal mice of susceptible genotype (e.g., C3H/He and A/J). There is substantial evidence that concomitant immunity to *T. taeniaeformis* in rats (Lloyd and Soulsby, 1974; Musoke and Williams, 1975) and mice (Mitchell *et al.*, 1977a) is mediated partly, if not wholly, by circulating complement-fixing IgG antibodies. Such antibodies are not produced in BALB/c. *nu/nu* mice, and these mice can be protected, absolutely, by injection of IgG antibodies from infected mice given at the time of oral egg administration. Injections of the anticomplementary material, cobra venom factor, to nude mice inhibits the protective activity of immune serum. Interestingly, there is evidence that established cysts have complement-altering activities (Hammerberg *et al.*, 1976; Mitchell *et al.*, 1977a).

C. *Mesocestoides corti*

Mesocestoides corti is a noncystic larval cestode of mice and rats which proliferates in the liver and spills over into the peritoneal cavity. Infection of mice is accomplished by either oral or i.p. administration of peritoneal larvae. In nude mice, *M. corti* liver larvae increase much more rapidly in number than in intact mice, and it is clear that T cells recognize *M. corti* antigens since intact but not nude mice respond to DNP-*M. corti* larvae by production of anti-DNP antibodies (Mitchell *et al.*, 1977b). The established noncystic larvae of *M. corti*, like the established cystic larvae of *T. taeniaeformis*, are relatively resistant to immunological effector mechanisms and larvae are not rejected; rather their rate of accumulation (proliferation?) appears to be reduced by some T-cell-dependent influence. Recent work by W. L. Nicholas and colleagues (personal communication) suggests that collagen deposition in the liver is defective in nude mice, and this defective inflammatory response may facilitate parasite proliferation. Moreover, an eosinophil response is very prominent in the peritoneal cavity of infected normal mice but is absent in infected nude mice (G. Johnson, D. Metcalf, S. Pollacco, W. L. Nicholas, and G. F. Mitchell, unpublished observations). We do not yet know whether these cells reduce parasite numbers in intact versus nude mice; on this point it is clear that eosinophils are at least one cell type capable of initiating schistosomule and *Schistosoma mansoni* egg destruction (Butterworth *et al.*, 1977; James and Colley, 1977).

Peritoneal *M. corti* larvae in normal mice are coated with large amounts of IgG_1 antibodies and levels of IgG_1 in the serum of infected intact mice increase 10 times. IgG_1 antibodies are absent on the larvae harvested from nude mice. Such antibodies do not appear to be in any way host-protective and they may well be parasite-protective (Mitchell *et al.*, 1977*b*).

IV. TREMATODES

A. *Schistosoma mansoni* and *Fasciola hepatica*

Nude mice are not more susceptible than intact littermates to the blood fluke, *S. mansoni* (Phillips *et al.*, 1977), and pathological consequences of infection such as granuloma formation around eggs (Warren, 1972) are less intense (Hsu *et al.*, 1976; Phillips *et al.*, 1977). T cells recognize *S. mansoni* antigens as evidenced by the observations that anti-TNP responses to TNP-schistosomules are lower in nude mice than in intact mice (Ramalho-Pinto *et al.*, 1976). Studies with *S. mansoni* in nude mice (Hsu *et al.*, 1976; Phillips *et al.*, 1977; A. Sher, personal communication) have confirmed that the eosinophilia associated with schistosomiasis is defective in T-cell-depleted mice (Fine *et al.*, 1973).* In the case of the liver fluke *F. hepatica*, initial findings are that nudes (BALB/c.*nu*/*nu* mice) are not obviously more susceptible to infection than intact littermates (G. F. Mitchell, G. S. Rajasakariah, and R. S. Hogarth-Scott, unpublished observations). It is not yet known whether infected nude and infected intact mice differ in their susceptibility to reinfection with *F. hepatica* and whether liver larvae differ in surface antigen composition or host antibody content when harvested from normal and nude mice (cf. *M. corti*, described above).

V. PROTOZOA

A. *Giardia muris* and *Hexamita muris*

Boorman *et al.* (1973) have reported that conventionally raised nude mice contain high numbers of *G. muris* and *H. muris* protozoa in the intestines and that thymus grafting reduces the parasite burden. Nudes infected with *H. muris* at 4 weeks of age excreted cysts throughout life, whereas intact *nu*/+ mice

---

*From *all* the studies on eosinophils in parasitic infections it is clear that T-cell-deficient mice, including nude mice, have eosinophils but that they are defective in their ability to mount a response in terms of increased numbers in the circulation or in localized sites.

eliminated the infection within 4–5 weeks (Kunstyr *et al.*, 1978). Similar observations have been made using *G. muris* in nudes, additional observations being that the alteration in the intestinal villus:crypt ratio (Roberts-Thomson *et al.*, 1976) may be less intense in infected nudes, and that cells from previously infected intact mice are more efficient in reconstitution than cells from normal intact mice (Roberts-Thomson and Mitchell, 1978).

B. *Plasmodium* and *Babesia* Species

Intact mice eliminate *Plasmodium yoelii*, an intraerythrocytic murine malaria parasite, within 2–3 weeks after injection of parasitized blood, but the infection in nude mice progresses slowly until the mice die with high parasitemias (Clark and Allison, 1974; G. F. Mitchell, unpublished observations). Weinbaum *et al.* (1976) have demonstrated that both nude and anti-μ-injected (i.e., B-cell-deficient) mice die of *P. yoelii* infection, whereas controls are fully resistant. In our laboratory, BALB/c.*nu/nu* and intact mice have comparable mortality curves after infection with the lethal murine malaria parasite *P. berghei* (Mitchell, 1977), although Waki and Suzuki (1978) have reported that *nu/nu* mice survive longer. This latter observation may be related to that of Sheagren and Monaco (1969), who observed a decreased rate of mortality in mice given antilymphocyte serum before infection with *P. berghei*. A similar observation in *Babesia rodhaini*-infected nude mice will be discussed below. BCG protects mice (and nude mice) against various intraerythrocytic protozoa, including *P. berghei* (Clark *et al.*, 1976). We have confirmed some of these observations, although in our studies the effect has been highly variable, largely confined to CBA/H mice, and protection cannot be induced in CBA/H.*nu/nu* mice (G.F.Mitchell, unpublished observations). T cells recognize *P. berghei* antigens since a DTH response to infected blood is demonstrable in intact and T-cell-reconstituted nude mice but not in nudes themselves (Whitelaw *et al.*, 1977).

Clark and Allison (1974) reported that nude mice differed from intact mice in that they were unable to eliminate the intraerythrocytic parasite *Babesia microti*. Interestingly, the parasitaemia in *B. microti*-infected nude mice stayed at approximately 50% throughout the course of the infection. The reasons for this stable parasite count in nude mice are not known. *Babesia rodhaini* is a lethal intraerythrocytic parasite of mice, intact mice dying within 1–2 weeks of injection of infected blood. Nude mice (BALB/c.*nu/nu*) are more resistant to *B. rodhaini* (in that the mean survival time is longer), although the difference between nude and *nu/+* mice is not marked with *B. rodhaini* isolates which are very rapidly lethal in intact mice. Moreover, the antibabesial drug Amicarbalide protects most *nu/+* mice but not nude mice (Mitchell, 1977).

We have tested whether the difference in susceptibility of BALB/c.*nu/nu* and BALB/c.*nu/+* mice to *B. rodhaini* is due to the presence of T-cell-dependent antierythrocytic autoantibodies in *nu*/+ mice. It has been proposed that autoanti-bodies exacerbate the anaemia in malaria and babesiosis (e.g., Zuckerman, 1970; Ristic, 1970; Porter and Knight, 1974). *Babesia rodhaini*-infected BALB/c.*nu*/+, but not infected BALB/c.*nu*/*nu* mice contain increased numbers of antibody-secreting cells (PFC) directed against enzyme-modified mouse erythrocytes. The contribution of the autoantibodies to the pathogenesis of babesiosis is unknown, but it is noteworthy that only small numbers of PFC are detected and enzyme modification of erythrocytes is obligatory for detection of PFC (discussed in Cox *et al.*, 1977).

C. Other Protozoa

Yet to be reported are studies on the susceptibility of nude mice to protozoa such as *Toxoplasma gondii, Leishmania tropica, Leishmania donovani, Trypanosoma brucei,* and *Trypanosoma duttoni (musculi).* Nude mice, after irradiation, have been used to grow *Theileria parva*-infected bovine lymphoid cells (Irvin *et al.*, 1975).

VI. CONCLUDING REMARKS

The value of nude mice in the study of the immunological aspects of host-parasite relationships is illustrated by the following: (1) nude mice are markedly compromised in their ability to reject intestinal cestodes, nematodes, and protozoa. The consequences of selective additions of cells and/or antibodies to nude mice enable conclusions to be drawn about the involvement of certain immunological components in parasite rejection or inhibition of parasite establishment; (2) at least one parasite, the larval cestode *Mesocestoides corti,* has been shown to be very different when harvested from nude versus intact mice; and (3) in several situations, nude mice are slightly more resistant to lethal in-traeythrocytic protozoa, and a lack of T-cell-dependent autoantibodies in such mice may be related to their increased resistance.

In the next several years we can expect to see a proliferation in the number of strains of mice in which the *nu* gene has been incorporated. This will be an important development since in many model systems, mouse strain variation in susceptibility is very obvious. The existence of resistant and susceptible mouse strains makes the task of the immunoparasitologist easier in that, in some instances, particular immune responses can be implicated at being host (or parasite)-pro-tective. Inbred nude mice of these various genotypes will be of great assistance in the dissection of the immunological consequences of metazoan and protozoan parasitism.

ACKNOWLEDGMENTS

The studies on various parasites conducted in this laboratory were funded by NIH grant AI-12677, The Bushell Trust, and the Australian National Health and Medical Research Council. I thank Dr. Norman Reed for numerous reprints and preprints on the subject of susceptibility of nude mice to nematodes and cestodes. In addition, I wish to take this opportunity to acknowledge the enormous contribution of others within and outside the Hall Institute who continue to be indispensable in the immunoparasitology program. Dr. Margaret Holmes and her team, including Alison Parsons, Joan Evans, and Jenny West, provide all inbred and nude mice and are developing new inbred *nu/nu* strains. Colleagues in the veterinary, medical, and zoology fields in Melbourne, Canberra, and Adelaide have, without exception, been particularly willing to perform collaborative experiments with various parasites and to share information on these parasites. In this regard I am indebted to R. S. Hogarth-Scott, M. D. Rickard, W. L. Nicholas, I. C. Roberts-Thomson, R. P. Herd, R. D. Edwards, K. O. Cox, I. J. O'Donnell, M. C. Howell, G. R. Rajasakariah, C. R. Jenkins, and P. Ey.

VII. REFERENCES

Basten, A., and Beeson, P. B., 1970, Mechanism of eosinophilia. I. Factors affecting the eosinophil response of rats to *Trichinella spiralis, J. Exp. Med.* 131:1271.

Bland, P. W., 1976, Immunity to *Hymenolepis diminuta*: unresponsiveness of the athymic nude mouse to infection, *Parasitology* 72:93.

Boorman, G. A., Lina, P. H. C., Zurcher, C., and Nieuwerkerk, H. T. M., 1973, *Hexamita* and *Giardia* as a cause of mortality in congenitally thymus-less (nude) mice, *Clin. Exp. Immunol.* 15:623.

Brown, K. N., 1971, Protective immunity to malaria provides a model for the survival of cells in an immunologically hostile environment, *Nature* 230:163.

Burnet, F. M., 1978, The probable relationship of some or all mast cells to the T cell system, *Cell. Immunol.* (in press).

Butterworth, A. E., David, J. R., Franks, D., Mahmoud, A. A. F., David, P. H., Sturrock, R. F., and Houba, V., 1977, Antibody-dependent eosinophil-mediated damage to ^{51}Cr-labelled *Schistosoma mansoni.* Damage by purified eosinophils, *J. Exp. Med.* 145:136.

Clark, I. A., and Allison, A. C., 1974, *Babesia microti* and *Plasmodium berghei yoelii* infections in nude mice, *Nature* 252:328.

Clark, I. A., Allison, A. C., and Cox, F. E., 1976, Protection of mice against *Babesia* and *Plasmodium* with BCG, *Nature* 259:309.

Clegg, J. A., 1974, Host antigens and the immune response in schistosomiasis, in: *Parasites in the Immunized Host: Mechanisms of Survival* (R. Porter and J. Knight, eds.), p. 161, Associated Scientific, Amsterdam.

Cohen, S., and Sadun, E. H. (eds.), 1976, *Immunology of Parasitic Infections*, Blackwell Scientific, Oxford.

Cox, K. O., Howard, R. J., and Mitchell, G. F., 1977, Studies on immune responses to parasite antigens in mice. VII. Cells secreting antibodies to modified mouse erythrocytes in *Babesia rodhaini* infected mice, *Cell. Immunol.* **32**:223.

Dineen, J. K., Ogilvie, B. M., and Kelly, J. D., 1973, Expulsion of *Nippostrongylus brasiliensis* from the intestine of rats. Collaboration between humoral and cellular components of the immune response, *Immunology* **24**:467.

Dobson, D., 1972, Immune response to gastrointestinal helminths, in: *Immunity to Animal Parasites* (E. J. L. Soulsby, ed.), p. 191, Academic Press, New York.

Fine, D. P., Buchanan, R. D., and Colley, D. G., 1973, *Schistosoma mansoni* infection in mice depleted of thymus-dependent lymphocytes, *Amer. J. Pathol.* **71**:193.

Hammerberg, B., Musoke, A. J., Hustead, S. T., and Williams, J. F.,1976, Anticomplementary substances associated with Taeniid metacestodes, in: *Pathophysiology of Parasitic Infections* (E. J. L. Soulsby, ed.), p. 233, Academic Press, New York.

Hsu, C.-K., Hsu, S. H., Whitney, R. A., and Hansen, C. T., 1976, Immunopathology of schistosomiasis in athymic mice, *Nature* **262**:397.

Irvin, A. D., Stagg, D. A., Kanhai, G. K., and Brown, C. G., 1975, Heterotransplantation of *Theileria parva*-infected cells to athymic mice, *Nature* **253**:549.

Isaak, D. D., Jacobson, R. H., and Reed, N. D., 1975, Thymus dependence of tapeworm *(Hymenolepis diminuta)* elimination from mice, *Infect. Immun.* **12**:1478.

Jacobson, R. H., and Reed, N. D., 1974*a*, The immune response of congenitally athymic (nude) mice to the intestinal nematode *Nippostrongylus brasiliensis*, *Proc. Soc. Exp. Biol. Med.* **147**:667.

Jacobson, R. H., and Reed, N. D., 1974*b*, The thymus dependency of resistance to pinworm infection in mice, *J. Parasitol.* **60**:976.

Jacobson, R. H., and Reed, N. D., 1977, The requirement of thymus competence for both humoral and cell mediated steps in expulsion of *Nippostrongylus brasiliensis* from mice, *Int. Arch. Allergy Appl. Immunol.* **52**:160.

Jacobson, R. H., Reed, N. D., and Manning, D. D., 1977, Expulsion of *Nippostrongylus brasiliensis* from mice lacking antibody production potential, *Immunology* **32**:867.

James, S. L., and Colley, D. G., 1977, Eosinophil-mediated destruction of *Schistosoma mansoni* eggs, *J. Retic. Soc.* **20**:359.

Keller, R., Hess, M. W., and Riley, J. F., 1976, Mast cells in the skin of normal, hairless and athymic mice, *Experientia* **32**:171.

Kunstyr, I., Ammerpohl, E., and Meyer, B., 1978, Hexamitiasis in nude mice: an animal model for immunoparasitologic studies, in: *Proc. 2nd Int. Workshop on Nude Mice*, Tokyo (in press).

Lloyd, S., and Soulsby, E. J. L., 1974, The passive transfer of immunity to the metacestodes of *Taenia taeniaeformis* and *Taenia saginata*, in: *Parasitic Zoonoses, Clinical and Experimental Studies* (E. J. L. Soulsby, ed.), p. 231, Academic Press, New York.

Loor, F., and Roelants, G. E., 1974, High frequency of T lineage lymphocytes in nude mouse spleen, *Nature* **251**:229.

Miller, H. R. P., and Jarrett, W. F. H., 1971, Immune reactions in mucous membranes. Intestinal mast cell response during helminth expulsion in the rat, *Immunology* **20**:277.

Miller, J. F. A. P., and Mitchell, G. F., 1969, Thymus and antigen-reactive cells, *Transplant. Rev.* **1**:3.

Mitchell, G. F., 1974, T cell modification of B cell responses to antigen in mice, *Contemporary Topics in Immunobiology*, Vol. 3 (M. D. Cooper, ed.), p. 97, Plenum Press, New York.

Mitchell, G. F., 1977, Studies on immune responses to parasite antigens in mice V. Different susceptibilities of hypothymic and intact mice to *Babesia rodhaini*, *Int. Arch. Allergy Appl. Immunol.* **53**:385.

Mitchell, G. F., Hogarth-Scott, R. S., Lewers, H. M., Edwards, R. D., Cousins, G., and Moore,

T., 1976a, Studies on immune responses to parasite antigens in mice. I. *Ascaris suum* larvae numbers and antiphosphorylcholine responses in infected mice of various strains and hypothymic nu/nu mice, *Int. Arch. Allergy Appl. Immunol.* 52:64.

Mitchell, G. F., Hograth-Scott, R. S., and Edwards, R. D., 1976b, Studies on immune responses to parasite antigens in mice. III. *Nippostrongylus brasiliensis* infection in hypothymic *nu/nu* mice, *Int. Arch. Allergy Appl. Immunol.* 52:95.

Mitchell, G. F., Goding, J. W., and Rickard, M. D., 1977a, Studies on immune responses to larval cestodes in mice. I. Increased susceptibility of certain mouse strains and hypothymic mice to *Taenia taeniaeformis* and analysis of passive transfer of resistance with serum, *Aust. J. Exp. Biol. Med. Sci.* 55:165.

Mitchell, G. F., Marchalonis, J. J., Smith, P. M., Nicholas, W. L., and Warner, N. L., 1977b, Studies on immune responses to larval cestodes in mice. II. Immunoglobulins associated with the larvae of *Mesocestoides corti*, *Aust. J. Exp. Biol. Med. Sci.* 55:187.

Musoke, A. J., and Williams, J. F., 1975, The immunological response of the rat to infection with *Taenia taeniaeformis*. II. Sequence of appearance of protective immunoglobulins and the mechanism of action of $7S\gamma2a$ antibodies, *Immunology* 29:855.

Nielsen, K., Fogh, L., and Andersen, S., 1974, Eosinophil response to migrating *Ascaris suum* larvae in normal and congenitally thymusless mice, *Acta Pathol. Microbiol. Scand. B.* 82:919.

Ogilvie, B. M., and Jones, V. E., 1973, Immunity in the parasitic relationship between helminths and hosts, *Progr. Allergy* 17:93.

Ogilvie, B. M., and Love, R. J., 1974, Co-operation between antibodies and cells in immunity to a nematode parasite, *Transplant. Rev.* 19:147.

Ogilvie, B. M., and Wilson, R. J. M., 1976, Evasion of the immune response by parasites, *Brit. Med. Bull.* 32:177.

Phillips, S. M., Diconza, J. J., Gold, J. A., and Reid, W. A., 1977, Schistosomiasis in the congenitally athymic (nude) mouse. I. Thymic dependency of eosinophil granuloma formation and host morbidity, *J. Immunol.* 118:594.

Porter, R., and Knight, J. (eds.), 1974, *Parasites in the Immunized Host: Mechanisms of Survival*, Associated Scientific, Amsterdam.

Ramalho-Pinto, F. J., deSouza, J. M., and Playfair, J. H. L., 1976, Stimulation and suppression of response of mouse T cells to the schistosomules of *Schistosoma mansoni* during infection, *Nature* 259:603.

Reed, N. D., Isaak, D. D., and Jacobson, R. H., 1978, The use of nude mice in model systems for studies on acquired immunity to parasite helminths, in: *Proc. 2nd Int. Workshop on Nude Mice*, Tokyo (in press).

Ristic, M., 1970, Babesiosis and theileriosis, in: *Immunity to Parasitic Animals*, Vol. 2 (G. J. Jackson, R. Herman, and I. Singer, eds.), p. 793, Appleton-Century-Crofts, New York.

Roberts-Thomson, I. C., and Mitchell, G. F., 1978, Giardiasis in mice. I. Prolonged infections in certain mouse strains and hypothymic (nude) mice, *Gastroenterology* (in press).

Roberts-Thomson, I. C., Stevens, D. P., Mahmoud, A. A. F., and Warren, K. S., 1976, Giardiasis in the mouse: An animal model, *Gastroenterology* 71:57.

Ruitenberg, E. J., and Elgersma, A., 1976, Absence of intestinal mast cell response in congenitally athymic mice during *Trichinella spiralis* infection, *Nature* 264:258.

Sheagren, J. N., and Monaco, A. P., 1969, Protective effect of antilymphocyte serum on mice infected with *Plasmodium berghei*, *Science* 164:1423.

Smithers, S. R., Terry, R. J., and Hockley, D. J., 1969, Host antigens in schistosomiasis, *Proc. Roy. Soc. London B.* 171:483.

Sprent, J. F. A., 1952, On the migratory behaviour of the larvae of various ascaris species in white mice. I. Distribution of larvae in tissues, *J. Infect. Dis.* 90:165.

Sprent, J. F. A., 1959, Parasitism, immunity and evolution, in: *The Evolution of Living Organisms* (G. S. Leeper, ed.), p. 149, Melbourne University Press, Melbourne.

Targett, G. A. T., 1973, Thymus dependency and chronic antigenic stimulation: Immunity to parasitic protozoans and helminths, in: *Contemporary Topics in Immunobiology*, Vol. 2 (A. J. S. Davies and R. L. Carter, eds.), p. 217, Plenum Press, New York.

Trager, W., 1974, Some aspects of intracellular parasitism, *Science* 183:269.

Vicklicky, V., Sima, P., and Pritchard, H., 1973, On the origin of mast cells in adult life, *Folia Biol.* 19:247.

Wakelin, D., and Selby, G. R., 1974, Thymus-dependency of the immune response of mice to a primary infection with the nematode *Trichuris muris, Int. J. Parasitol.* 4:657.

Waki, S., and Suzuki, M., 1978, Studies on malaria immunobiology using nude mice, in: *Proc. 2nd Int. Workshop on Nude Mice*, Tokyo (in press).

Walls, R. S., Basten, A., Leuchars, E., and Davies, A. J. S., 1971, Mechanism for eosinophilic and neutrophilic leucocytoses, *Brit. Med. J.* 3:157.

Walls, R. S., Carter, R. L., Leuchars, E., and Davies, A. J. S., 1973, The immunopathology of trichiniasis in T-cell deficient mice, *Clin. Exp. Immunol.* 13:231.

Warren, K. S., 1972, The immunopathogenesis of schistosomiasis: a multidisciplinary approach, *Trans. Roy. Soc. Trop. Med. Hyg.* 66:417.

Weinbaum, F. I., Evans, C. B., and Tigelaar, R. E., 1976, Immunity to *Plasmodium berghei yoelii* in mice. I. The course of infection in T cell and B cell deficient mice, *J. Immunol.* 117:1999.

Whitelaw, A., Miller, J. F. A. P., and Mitchell, G. F., 1977, Studies on immune responses to parasite antigens in mice. VI. Delayed type hypersensitivity to blood cells from *Plasmodium berghei* infected mice, *Cell. Immunol.* 32:216.

Zuckermann, A., 1970, Malaria in lower mammals, in: *Immunity to Parasitic Animals*, Vol. 2 (G. J. Jackson, R. Herman, and I. Singer, eds.), p. 793, Appleton-Century-Crofts, New York.

Chapter 4

In Vitro Induction and Expression of T-Cell Immunity to Tumor-Associated Antigens

Robert C. Burton

Transplantation Unit
Massachusetts General Hospital
Harvard University
Boston, Massachusetts 02114

Stanley E. Chism

Division of Radiation Oncology
University of California
San Francisco, California 94122

and

Noel L. Warner

Immunobiology Laboratories
Departments of Pathology and Medicine
University of New Mexico School of Medicine
Albuquerque, New Mexico 87131.

I. INTRODUCTION

The development of *in vitro* assays of cell-mediated cytotoxicity has provided a means both of quantitating cell-mediated immunity (CMI) induced *in vivo*, and also of identifying the cytotoxic effector cells (CL) involved. Studies with the ^{51}Cr release assay have clearly shown that a specific subpopulation of T lymphocytes (termed T_C-cytotoxic T lymphocytes) are responsible for mediating cytotoxicity *in vitro*, when cell preparations from animals undergoing allograft rejection or graft-versus-host reactions are assayed *in vitro* (Cerottini *et al.*, 1970; Miller *et al.*, 1971; Cerottini and Brunner, 1974). The T_C subpopulation has been further characterized in terms of cell-surface markers and is a distinct T-cell lineage of phenotype Ly-1 negative, Ly-2 positive, Ly-3 positive (Cantor and Boyse, 1976). Since cytotoxic T cells are, however, to be found in both Fc receptor-positive *and* -negative lymphocyte groups, some heterogeneity may still exist within the T_C population (Stout *et al.*, 1976). The results of *in vitro* assays of lymphoid cells from animals immunized with tumor cells have, however, been much less clear-cut, and the number of different effector cell types and the mechanisms of cytotoxicity have proliferated rapidly since the introduction of techniques for identifying different subpopulations of lymphocytes and mononuclear cells (Table I).

The *in vitro* investigation of CMI induced *in vivo* to tumor-associated antigens (TAA) has thus been complicated by a wealth of mechanisms and effector cell types. Furthermore, the relevance of results obtained from *in vitro* assays to *in vivo* mechanisms of tumor immunity is not fully defined, although T lymphocytes from animals immunized against TAA have been shown to protect nonimmune animals from the growth of the relevant tumor, both in Winn assays (Winn, 1961) when admixed with the tumor cells prior to transfer (Rollinghoff and Warner, 1973), and also when administered separately intravenously to animals inoculated with the tumor cells (Brunner *et al.*, 1975). These types of observations are, however, only correlative in nature, and do not prove that the T_C population identified *in vitro* is the same cell population effective *in vivo*.

The development of *in vitro* methods for immunizing T_C against TAA has provided tumor immunologists with a new tool with which to investigate CMI to tumors. The genesis of this technique lay in the discovery that phytohema-

Table I. Cell-Mediated *in Vitro* Lysis of Tumor Cell Lines

Cell type	Mechanism	Specificity	Reference
Macrophage	SMAF[a]	Ag-specific[b]	Evans *et al.* (1973)
	Direct lysis	"Nonspecific"	Meltzer (1976)
B cell	Ab-dependent[c]	Ag-specific	Lamon *et al.* (1975)
Polymorph	Ab-dependent	Ag-specific	Gale and Zighelboim (1975)
	Chemical mediator	Nonspecific	Takasugi *et al.* (1975)
Null cell (k)	Ab-dependent	Ag-specific	Pollack *et al.* (1975)
Natural killer	?	"Specific"	Kiessling *et al.* (1975)
T cell	Direct lysis	Ag-specific	Glaser *et al.* (1976*a*)
	Ab-dependent	Ag-specific	Lamon *et al.* (1975)
	Lectin-dependent	"Nonspecific"	Dennert (1976)

[a]SMAF, specific macrophage arming factor.
[b]Ag, antigen.
[c]Ab, antibody.

glutinin could induce blast transformation when added to *in vitro* cultures of lymphocytes (Nowell, 1960). A similar phenomenon was observed when lymphocytes from unrelated donors were cultured together *in vitro* (Schrek and Donnelly, 1961), in the mixed lymphocyte culture (MLC) technique. The subsequent investigation of the MLC, which was facilitated by treating one lymphocyte population (Stimulator cells) with irradiation (Kasakura and Lowerstein, 1965) or mitomycin C (Bach and Voynow, 1966) to prevent their proliferation, has revealed that the cellular proliferation in the other lymphocyte population (Responder cells) is restricted to T lymphocytes (Johnston and Wilson, 1970; Mosier and Cantor, 1971; Hayry *et al.*, 1972). The importance of the MLC as a means of investigating cell-mediated immunity *in vitro* was further enhanced with the recognition in 1970 that the reaction also resulted in the induction of CL with specificity for antigens expressed on the Stimulator cell population (Hayry and Defendi, 1970; Solliday and Bach, 1970; Wunderlich and Canty, 1970). MLCs which lead to the generation of CL with specificity for target cells bearing the stimulating alloantigens have been termed *in vitro* allograft reactions, and all of the cytotoxicity involved is T_C-mediated (Wagner *et al.*, 1972, 1973; Hayry *et al.*, 1972). It is important to note that a considerable amount of investigation of the *in vitro* allograft reaction has been directed toward an understanding of the relationship between the initial proliferative responses and the emergence of the T_C population. Current views on this aspect indicate that two separate cell lineages are involved, in that an Ly-1 positive T helper (T_H) population initially proliferates and collaborates with the Ly-2,3 positive T_C population to promote its differentiation to the effector T_C (Cantor and Boyse, 1975).

The first successful experimental *in vitro* induction of CMI to TAA was performed by McKhann and Jagarlamoody (1971), who cocultured spleen cells from C3H mice *in vitro* with tumor cells from a 3-methylcholanthrene (MCA)-induced C3H sarcoma, and then assayed them for specific antitumor immunity in a Winn assay. The results demonstrated that lymphocytes cocultured with stimulating tumor cells could protect mice against the growth of the particular stimulating tumor, but not of another MCA-induced C3H sarcoma. It was concluded, therefore, that *in vitro* immunization had occurred, and that the TAA involved were "unique" to the stimulating tumor.

Successful *in vitro* assays of CL induced *in vitro* to TAA were reported in 1973 employing the ^{51}Cr release assay to test CL induced *in vitro* to syngeneic plasmacytomas (Wagner and Rollinghoff, 1973) and a syngeneic mastocytoma (Lundak and Raidt, 1973). The following year Rollinghoff (1974) demonstrated that spleen cells from mice preimmunized to a syngeneic plasmacytoma (PCT) were significantly more cytotoxic following *in vitro* stimulation with the same tumor (secondary cytotoxic *in vitro* reaction) than were spleen cells from nonimmune

mice. It was also shown that the cytotoxicity induced in both the primary and
secondary *in vitro* reactions to TAA was mediated solely by T_C (Rollinghoff
and Wagner, 1973; Rollinghoff, 1974). These results have been confirmed in a
variety of *in vitro* systems which have employed a range of tumor cell types
(Table II). Therefore, the *in vitro* induction of CMI to TAA allows the study of
T_C responses to these antigens in the absence of any of the other cytotoxic

Table II. *In Vitro* Induction of Primary and Secondary Cytotoxic
CMI to TAA and OFA

Tissue type	Etiology	Strain(s)[a]	References
Sarcoma	3-Methyl-cholanthrene	C3H, C57B1	McKhann and Jagarlamoody (1971)
		BALB/c	Warnatz and Scheiffarth (1974); Nomoto *et al.* (1974); Kall and Hellstrom (1975); Kall *et al.* (1976); Burton and Warner (1978*a*)
Fibrosarcoma	Spontaneous	BALB/c	Burton and Warner (1978*a*)
Plasmacytoma	Mineral-oil-induced	BALB/c $\longrightarrow$ C57B1[b]	Wagner and Rollinghoff (1973)
		NZB	Rollinghoff (1974)
		BALB/c, C3H, NZB	Burton and Warner (1977*a*)
Mastocytoma	7,12-Dimethyl benzanthracene	DBA/2	Lundak and Raidt (1973); Takei *et al.* (1976)
Carcinoma	Spontaneous	C57B1	Ilfeld *et al.* (1973); Carnaud *et al.* (1973)
Carcinoma	7,12-Dimethyl benzanthracene	Fischer 344 rat	Kuperman *et al.* (1975*a,b*)
Sarcoma	Moloney (murine) sarcoma virus	C57B1	Plata *et al.* (1975); Senik *et al.* (1975); Kirchner *et al.* (1976)
Lymphoma	Radiation-induced	BALB/c	Burton and Warner (1978*b*)
Lymphoma	Spontaneous	DBA/2	Manson and Palmer (1975); Manson *et al.* (1975)
Lymphoma	Gross virus	W/Fu rats	Glaser *et al.* (1976*b*); Bernstein *et al.* (1976); Bruce *et al.* (1976)
Leukemia	Friend virus	C57B1	Ting and Bonnard (1976)
Fetal liver	—	BALB/c	Chism *et al.* (1976); Friend *et al.* (1976)
		(C57B1 × CBA)F$_1$ hybrid	Burton *et al.* (1977)

[a]Mouse strain: rats where indicated.
[b]Allophenic (tetra parental chimeric) mouse.

mechanisms which appear to operate when *in vivo* immunized cells are used as the CL source.

The aims of this review are to examine the techniques used to induce and assay tumor-specific immunity *in vitro* in the light of our own experience, and to consider three particular aspects of the phenomenon:

1. The distinction between this phenomenon and the *in vitro* induction of CL by culture of spleen cells in the absence of added stimulating cells.

2. The role of the major histocompatibility complex (MHC) at the inductive phase.

3. The role of the MHC in restricting lysis at the effector phase, and the implications of this for our current concept of the nature of TAA.

II. METHODOLOGY

A. *In Vitro* Induction of Tumor-Specific Immunity

A variety of culture conditions have been successfully employed to induce tumor-specific immunity *in vitro*. The culture vessels have included Marbrook flasks (Wagner and Rollinghoff, 1973), Mishell–Dutton cultures (Lundak and Raidt, 1973), petri dishes (Carnaud *et al.*, 1973), tissue culture flasks (Kall and Hellstrom, 1975), and plastic tubes (Takei *et al.*, 1976). Various tissue culture media supplemented with mammalian sera have been used, including Eagle's minimal essential medium (Wagner and Rollinghoff, 1973), Mishell–Dutton cocktail (Warnatz and Scheiffarth, 1974), Dulbecco's modified Eagle's medium (Carnaud *et al.*, 1973), medium 199 (Nomoto *et al.*, 1974), and RPMI 1640 (Kall and Hellstrom, 1975). In some cases 2-mercaptoethanol (2ME) was added (Kuperman *et al.*, 1975a,b); the use of 2ME is considered in more detail in Section IIC.

Since none of these techniques was optimal for an extensive analysis of the specificity of tumor immunity induced *in vitro*, a micro system was developed for this purpose. A 25-compartment plastic tissue culture tray (Sterilin Ltd., Richmond, Surrey, England, Cat. No. 3063) was used, and the cells were cultured in Eagle's minimal essential medium with nonessential amino acids (Grand Island Biological Co., New York, N.Y., Cat. No. F/15), supplemented with 10% fetal calf serum (FCS-Commonwealth Serum Laboratories, Melbourne, Australia), penicillin, and streptomycin, and buffered with sodium bicarbonate (MEMF). The medium was prepared fresh each day and 2ME was added to a final concentration of 5×10^{-5} M. The optimal number of irradiated stimulator tumor cells, in a volume of 0.1 ml, were placed into the compartments of the tray and 3.6 ml of MEMF was added. Then 15×10^{6} syngeneic or semisyngeneic responder viable nucleated spleen cells, in 0.2 ml, were added to each compartment and the trays placed in a humidified CO_2 incubator for 5-6 days, these conditions being optimal for induction of tumor-specific immunity (Burton *et al.*, 1975). At the end of the culture period the CL were harvested, identical compartments pooled, the viability determined by eosin dye exclusion, and then the CL adjusted to the concentration required for the assay.

B. *In Vitro* Assay of Tumor-Specific Immunity: [51]Cr Release

The ^{51}Cr release assay developed by Brunner *et al.* (1968) and the micro cytotoxicity assay of Takasugi and Klein (1970) are the two most popular *in vitro* assays for the quantitation of target cell lysis by CL. The ^{51}Cr release assay has been shown to reflect target cell lysis (Wigzell, 1965; Sanderson, 1976a,b), while the micro cytotoxicity assay, by comparison, has a number of disadvantages. It measures loss of adherence of target cells to plastic, and this may not accurately reflect the lysis of target cells (Takasugi and Terasaki, 1973). The technique usually involves long incubation times, 24-48 hr, and there is evidence that in this period *in vitro* sensitization may occur (Ginsberg, 1968), that memory cells may be activated (Forman and Britton, 1973; Trostmann *et al.*, 1976), that nonspecifically sensitized cells may be recruited (Perlmann, 1972), and that B cells and antibody can also be involved (Kiessling and Klein, 1973). Therefore, the short-term (less than 6 hr) ^{51}Cr release assay, which measures mainly T_C activity when used as an assay of CMI (Canty and Wunderlich, 1971; Cerottini and Brunner, 1974; Trostmann *et al.*, 1976), was the method of choice for the studies.

The assay of CMI *in vitro* by ^{51}Cr release has been considerably facilitated by the recent development of micro ^{51}Cr release assays (Thorn *et al.*, 1974), particularly when a short period of hyperthermia, which increases the rate of ^{51}Cr release from damaged cells, is also employed (Dunkley *et al.*, 1974). The micro assay used in our studies was performed in microtiter trays (Microtest II tissue culture plate, Falcon Plastics, Oxnard, California) in a total volume of 0.2 ml of Dulbecco's modified Eagle's medium supplemented with 10% FCS (DMEF). The assays were set up in quadruplicate over a range of CL to target (CL/T) ratios, with a constant number (2.5×10^4) of ^{51}Cr-labeled tumor target cells. The micro trays were then incubated for 4 hr at 37°C, followed by 1 hr at 45°C, before 100 microliters of the supernatant was removed from each well and counted in a Beckman biogamma scintillation counter. The results were expressed as

$$\text{percent specific lysis} = \frac{\text{test count} - \text{background count}}{\text{maximal count} - \text{background count}} \times 100$$

The background count was the ^{51}Cr released when target cells were incubated in the absence of CL, and the maximal release obtained by incubating target cells in detergent and distilled water.

C. Important Parameters of Induction and Assay

A number of factors which operated at either the inductive or effector (assay) stages of this *in vitro* system were important in determining the levels of specific lysis detected. Although both MEMF and DMEF were equivalent media for use at the inductive phase, the batch and concentration of fetal calf serum used was critical, and there was no cytotoxicity detected when 2ME was omitted, or added in excess (Burton *et al.*, 1975). The addition of 2ME to tissue culture media has been shown to enhance the induction of both humoral and cell-mediated immunity *in vitro* (Click *et al.*, 1972; Bevan *et al.*, 1974), to promote the growth of murine lymphoid tumor cells *in vitro* (Broome and Jeng, 1973), and to substitute for the requirement for a small number of macrophages at the inductive phase of the *in vitro* allograft reaction (Bevan *et al.*, 1974). Although these properties are shared with other thiols (Fanger *et al.*, 1970; Broome and Jeng, 1973), the mechanism of action of 2ME is not known, although it has been suggested that thiols stimulate induction of CLs by an intracellular process involving free sulfhydryl groups (Harris *et al.*, 1976).

The responder/stimulator cell (R/S) ratio was a *crucial* parameter of *in vitro* induction for all tumor types tested, and also for the *in vitro* induction of CL to oncofetal antigens (OFA) (Burton *et al.*, 1975, 1977; Chism *et al.*, 1976; Burton and Warner, 1977, 1978a). This is illustrated in Table III, and also by the R/S ratio curve for BALB/c CL induced *in vitro* to the BALB/c fibrosarcoma (FSA) WEHI-164. The CL were then assayed *in vitro* on two ^{51}Cr-labeled BALB/c FSA, WEHI-164 and WEHI-11 (Fig. 1). Since the optimal R/S ratio varies markedly with the tumor used to stimulate the induction of CL (Table III), it must be determined in each case. Our results with the PCT (Burton *et al.*, 1975; Burton and Warner, 1977a) were in general agreement with those of Wagner and Rollinghoff (1973), with a peak R/S ratio between 50 and 100 : 1. The method of stimulator cell inactivation did not appear to be a significant factor, and 5000 rad of X irradiation was as effective as treating the tumor cells with mitomycin C or glutaraldehyde.

The optimal period of *in vitro* culture proved to be 5 days when an additional day of incubation in fresh medium was employed, and 6 days when it was not. These findings are in agreement with those of others for both the *in vitro* allograft reaction (Wagner *et al.*, 1972), and also for the induction of tumor specific immunity (Rollinghoff and Wagner, 1973; Warnatz and Scheiffarth, 1974). It was found that an additional 18–21 hr of incubation in fresh culture medium at the end of the 5-day culture period considerably augmented the cytotoxicity

Table III. *In Vitro* Induction of Tumor-Specific Immunity:
Effect of Responder/Stimulator Ratio

Responder spleen cells	Stimulator tumor cell type	Optimal R/S[a]	Reference
Nonimmune	MCA sarcoma	2000:1	Burton and Warner (1978a)
Nonimmune	MCA sarcoma	100:1	Warnatz and Scheiffarth (1974)
Nonimmune	MCA sarcoma	12:1	Kall and Hellstrom (1975)
Nonimmune	Spontaneous sarcoma	10000:1	Burton and Warner (1978a)
Nonimmune	Plasmacytoma	30:1	Wagner and Rollinghoff (1973)
Nonimmune	Plasmacytoma	100:1	Burton *et al.* (1975)
Immune	Plasmacytoma	100:1	Rollinghoff (1974)
Immune	Plasmacytoma	10:1	Burton and Warner (1977a)
Nonimmune	Mastocytoma	350:1	Lundak and Raidt (1973)
Immune	Mastocytoma	10:1	Takei *et al.* (1976)
Nonimmune	Carcinoma	6:1	Carnaud *et al.* (1973)
Nonimmune	Carcinoma	30:1	Kuperman *et al.* (1975a)
Immune	Carcinoma	30:1	Kuperman *et al.* (1975b)
Nonimmune	Rauscher lymphoma	25:1	Plata *et al.* (1975)
Immune	Rauscher lymphoma	25:1	Plata *et al.* (1975)
Immune	Rauscher lymphoma	128:1	Kirchner *et al.* (1976)
Nonimmune	MSV sarcoma	300:1	Plata *et al.* (1975)
Nonimmune	Friend leukemia	150:1	Ting and Bonnard (1976a)
Immune	Friend leukemia	450:1	Ting and Bonnard (1976b)
Nonimmune	Gross leukemia	16:1	Glaser *et al.* (1976)
Immune	Gross leukemia	64:1	Glaser *et al.* (1976)
Immune	Gross leukemia	30:1	Bernstein *et al.* (1976)

[a]Responder/stimulator cell ratio.

detected. Although there was a loss of 20–40% of the CLs during this incubation, there was usually a two- to threefold increase in the levels of specific lysis detected, on a per cell basis (Burton *et al.*, 1975). The use of this additional incubation step was based on reports that such a procedure considerably enhanced the cytotoxicity of *in vivo*-derived CL harvested from tumor-immune animals (Ortiz de Landazuri and Herberman, 1972a; Vasudevan *et al.*, 1973; Laux and Lausch, 1974). The mechanism involved is not known, but the possibilities include an adherent cell-dependent differentiation (Ortiz de Landazuri and Herberman, 1972b), and release from tumor inhibitory factors (Laux and Lausch, 1974). This overnight incubation, however, was only effective when tumor cells were used as stimulators, and this step actually decreased the cytotoxicity observed when CL were induced *in vitro* to OFA (Chism *et al.*, 1976).

At the assay stage the most important parameter was the CL/T ratio (Fig. 2). The plot of specific lysis against CL/T on a semilog scale was always linear in the range of CL/T between 25:1 and 100:1, but plateaued or declined at higher ratios. This plateau effect has been attributed both to crowding in the microassay (Dunkley *et al.*, 1974), and also to a suppressor cell type present at low

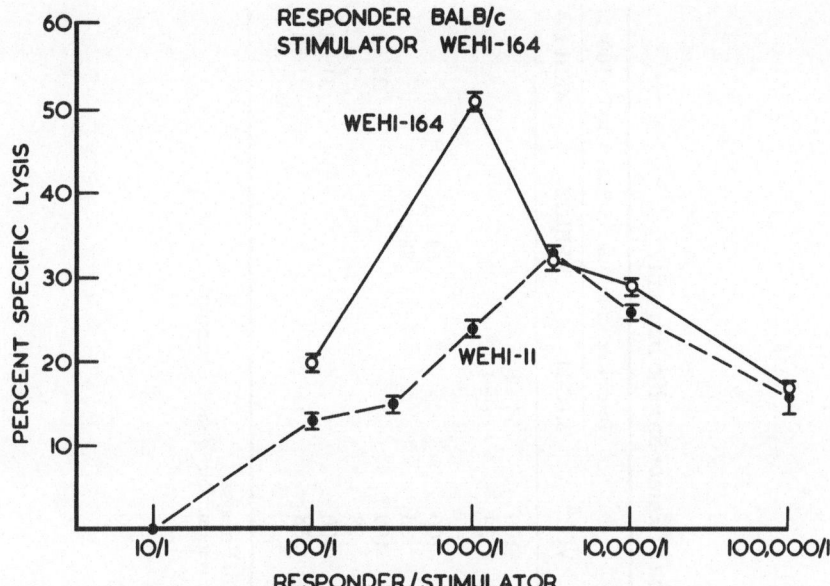

Figure 1. Dependence of cytotoxicity on R/S ratio. BALB/c responder spleen cells were cultured with irradiated WEHI-164 stimulator tumor cells over the range of R/S ratios shown, and the CL induced were then assayed on ^{51}Cr-labeled WEHI-164 (o———o) and WEHI-11 (•-----•) (CL/T = 100:1). [Reproduced with permission from-*Brit. J. Cancer* (1978, in press).]

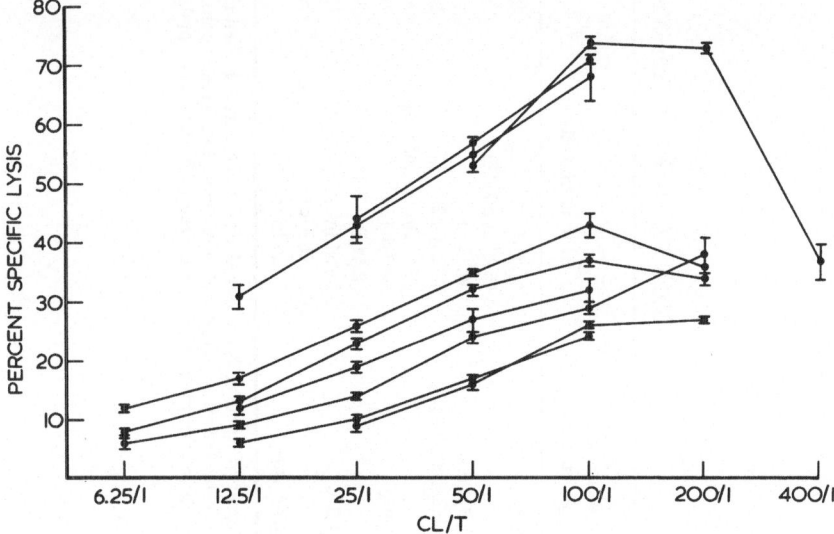

Figure 2. Effect of CL/T ratio on specific lysis. BALB/c T_C induced *in vitro* against the BALB/c PCT MPC-11 were assayed on ^{51}Cr MPC-11 (nine separate experiments).

Table IV. Role of T Cells in the *in Vitro* Induction of Tumor-Specific Immunity

Responder spleen cells	Stimulator cells	Treatment of CL	% VCC[a]	Percent specific lysis ± S.E.M. (CL/T = 100:1)		
				MPC-11	WEHI-22	WEHI-164
BALB/c	MPC-11 (BALB/c PCT)	NIL[b]	100	64 ± 2		
		Anti-Thy-1,2 + C'	33	1 ± 1		
BALB/c.nu (BALB/c × C57)F$_1$[c]	MPC-11	—	—	0		
BALB/c	WEHI-22 (BALB/c lymphoma)	NIL	100		64 ± 1	
		Anti-Thy-1,2 + C'	33		28 ± 1	
BALB/c	WEHI-164[a] (BALB/c-FSA)	NIL	100			22 ± 1
		Anti-Thy-1,2 + C'	28			3 ± 2
BALB/c	Fetal liver (BALB/c)	NIL	100			31 ± 1
		Anti-Thy-1,2 + C'	38			1 ± 1
BALB/c.nu	Fetal liver	—	—			0

[a] Percent of viable cells recovered after treatment; CL then made up for CL/T = 100:1 in assay.
[b] Anti-Thy-1,2 serum alone and complement (C') alone controls were included and were similar to the Nil control.
[c] Spleen cells from mice preimmunized to WEHI-22 (secondary *in vitro* induction).

frequency (Clark *et al.*, 1976). Whatever the mechanism, comparisons of specific lysis should not be made at CL/T ratios which are not on the linear part of the plot. When one CL/T ratio only is shown, the highest was usually chosen, i.e., CL/T = 100 : 1.

The crucial role of the T cell at both the inductive and assay stages of this *in vitro* phenomenon is illustrated in Table IV, where it can be seen that T cells were both mandatory for *in vitro* induction to occur, and were also the mediators of cytotoxicity. No cytotoxicity was detected when spleen cells from nude (athymic) mice were used as responders, and treatment of the CL with anti-Thy-1,2 antiserum and complement largely abolished target-cell lysis. This is shown for three different tumor types, and also for fetal cells as stimulators. One secondary *in vitro* induction is also shown; that of spleen cells from (BALB/c × C57BL)F_1 mice immunized to the BALB/c thymic (T) lymphoma WEHI-22.

D. Cellular Competitive Inhibition *in Vitro* Assay

The direct ^{51}Cr release assay does have a number of drawbacks in terms of its application to all tumor immunity systems:

1. Certain tumors do not grow well in tissue culture and since, with the exception of ascites tumors (Goodman, 1961), *in vivo* derived tumor cell suspensions generally label poorly with ^{51}Cr, many tumors cannot be tested in a ^{51}Cr release cytotoxicity assay.

2. Certain tumor cell lines do not tolerate the labeling or assay conditions well, and have unacceptable levels of background ^{51}Cr release. Since the labeling procedure requires a number of washing steps to remove the ^{51}Cr it has been suggested that the repeated dilutions may damage newly adapted tissue culture cells, which, in general, grow well only at high cell concentrations (A. W. Harris, personal communication).

3. One major problem with the ^{51}Cr release assay is related to the rate of ^{51}Cr release from a damaged target cell consequent upon T_C injury. The rate of ^{51}Cr release is considerably slower than the time taken for the lethal T-cell injury (Miller and Dunkley, 1974; Sanderson, 1976*b*); therefore, the number of interactions of T_C with target cells as estimated by ^{51}Cr release is probably considerably less than the actual number that have occurred. Furthermore, it has been shown that different cell lines may release ^{51}Cr at different rates following damage by T_C (Sanderson, 1976*b*). Therefore, comparisons of the number of T_C and target-cell interactions between *different* targets are very difficult.

The limitations of the ^{51}Cr release assay have led to the development of the cellular competitive inhibition assay (Ortiz de Landazuri and Herberman, 1972*b*; Herberman *et al.*, 1974). In such an assay the CL/T ratio, CL type, and the target-cell identity remain constant, and unlabeled viable (blocker) cells of various types are added at various blocker/target (B/T) ratios in an attempt to

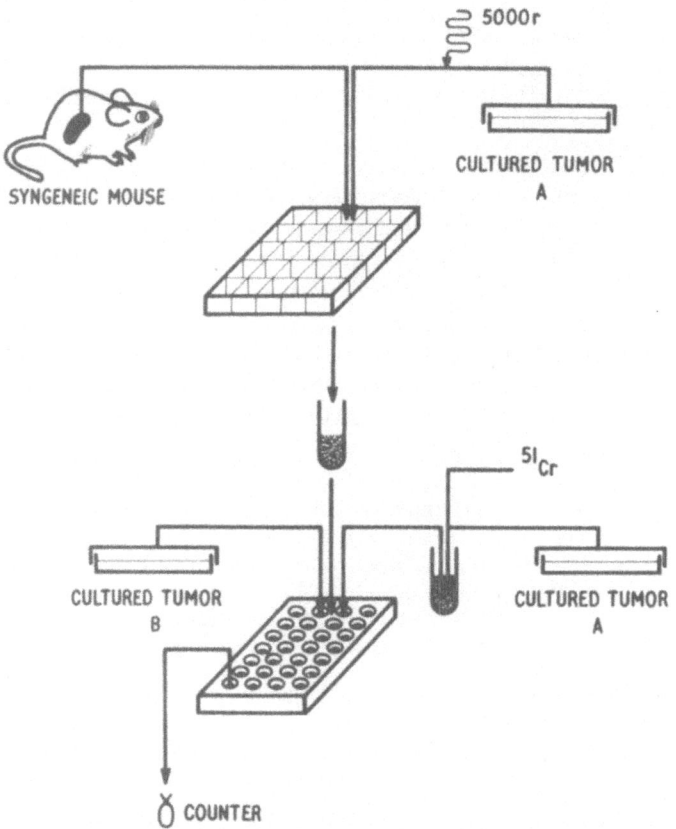

Figure 3. *In vitro* micro system for induction and assay of CL. As depicted, T_C are induced *in vitro* to TAA of tumor A. The ^{51}Cr release assay is accomplished by omitting the addition of blocker tumor cells B. The cellular competitive inhibition assay is performed by adding blocker cells as shown.

inhibit lysis of the ^{51}Cr-labeled target. If the blocker and target cells share antigens against which the CL are directed, then competition for lysis will occur, and there will be reduction in ^{51}Cr release which is proportional to the B/T ratio. A microcellular competitive inhibition assay was developed using the micro ^{51}Cr release assay (Chism *et al.*, 1977). It was found that for optimal sensitivity the CL/T ratio and assay times had to be adjusted to produce modest levels of specific lysis, between 20 and 50%. It was, however, found that nonspecific blocking could occur with certain tumor-cell lines, and that this was related to the volume of the blocker cells added at high B/T ratios. Accordingly, certain limits were set which usually distinguished the nonspecific effects. When tumor cells were used as blockers, levels of inhibition of lysis of up to 20% at B/T ratios of 30:1 or more were considered nonspecific. However, when fetal liver or adult spleen cells were used, nonspecific blocking of this order was not observed until B/T ratios of 90:1 or higher were reached. The micro *in vitro* techniques for induction and assay of CL are illustrated in Fig. 3. For the inhibition assay the results were calculated as

percent inhibition of cytotoxicity (lysis)

$$= \frac{\text{mean percent direct lysis control} - \text{mean percent test lysis}}{\text{mean percent direct lysis control}} \times 100$$

The direct control lysis was determined by omitting blockers from one group of four micro wells.

The reproducibility of the technique is illustrated in Fig. 4, where the mean percent inhibition of lysis curves for 11 experiments have been plotted for BALB/c spleen T_C induced *in vitro* to OFA by coculture with BALB/c 14-day fetal liver cells and assayed on the ^{51}Cr-labeled BALB/c FSA WEHI-164 (CL/T = 100:1, percent specific lysis = 30 ± 3%). BALB/c 14-day fetal liver cells, unlabeled WEHI-164 FSA cells, and MPC-11 BALB/c PCT cells all inhibited lysis of the labeled FSA cells, but adult BALB/c spleen cells did not.

Nonspecific blocking, which is the major limitation of this technique, is shown in Fig. 5, where B10.D2 T_C (H-2^d) induced *in vitro* to H-2^b alloantigens

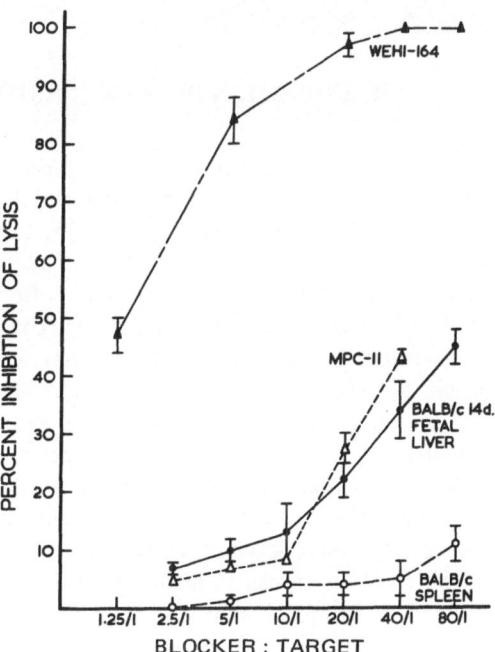

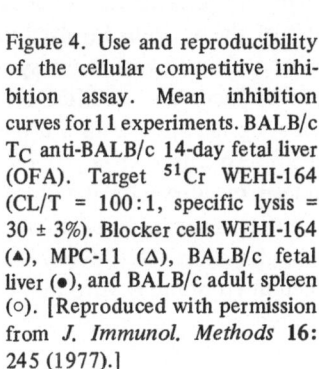

Figure 4. Use and reproducibility of the cellular competitive inhibition assay. Mean inhibition curves for 11 experiments. BALB/c T_C anti-BALB/c 14-day fetal liver (OFA). Target ^{51}Cr WEHI-164 (CL/T = 100:1, specific lysis = 30 ± 3%). Blocker cells WEHI-164 (▲), MPC-11 (Δ), BALB/c fetal liver (●), and BALB/c adult spleen (○). [Reproduced with permission from *J. Immunol. Methods* **16:** 245 (1977).]

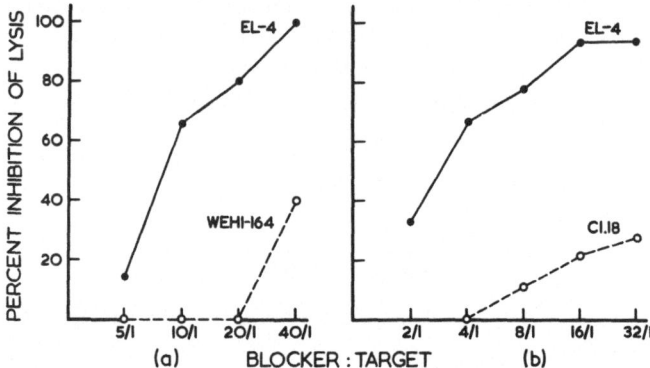

Figure 5. Tumor cells as specific and nonspecific inhibitors in an allogeneic system. B10.D2 anti-C57Bl CL, (a) CL/T = 20:1, assay time 2 hours, % specific lysis ^{51}Cr EL-4 = 15 ± 1%. Blocker cells EL-4 (●), WEHI-164, (○). (b) CL/T = 6:1, assay time 4 hr, specific lysis ^{51}Cr EL-4 = 18 ± 2%. Blocker cells EL-4 (●), C1.18 (○). [Reproduced with permission from *J. Immunol. Methods* **16**:245 (1977).]

on C57Bl spleen cells were assayed on ^{51}Cr-labeled EL-4, a C57Bl (H-2^b) lymphoma. Specific inhibition was produced by unlabeled EL-4 cells, but both WEHI-164 (H-2^d) and C1.18, a C3H (H-2^k) PCT, produced some nonspecific blocking at high B/T ratios.

III. INDUCTION OF CL IN "UNSTIMULATED" CULTURES

T_C can be induced *in vitro* by culturing rat or mouse spleen cells together with irradiated syngeneic normal tissue cells (Cohen *et al.*, 1971; Cohen and Wekerle, 1973; Ilfeld *et al.*, 1973, 1975; Carnaud *et al.*, 1974; Warnatz *et al.*, 1975). This phenomenon has been termed "autosensitization" *in vitro*, and is postulated to represent an *in vitro* escape from the *in vivo*-tolerant state (Cohen *et al.*, 1971; Cohen and Wekerle, 1973). The nature of the antigens involved in this phenomenon is not known; however, it has been claimed that when syngeneic fibroblasts are used as stimulator cells, the antigens are modified self *H-2* gene products (Ilfeld *et al.*, 1975), and when syngeneic liver cells are the stimulators, that the antigens are tissue-type-specific (Warnatz *et al.*, 1975). These specificities contrast with those of T_C induced *in vitro* with the T-cell mitogen in concanavalin A, where the major target antigens appear to be nonself H-2 determinants (Bevan *et al.*, 1976).

Since it was crucial to distinguish this phenomenon from the *in vitro* induction of T_C to TAA, controls of spleen cells cultured alone or together with syngeneic irradiated spleen cells were routinely included in all of our *in vitro* experiments. When spleen cells were cultured *in vitro*, either alone or with syngeneic irradiated spleen cells, CL were induced which could lyse tumor targets *in vitro*, and a peak of cytotoxicity was observed on day 6 of culture. However, the levels of lysis obtained were significantly lower than those mediated by CL from the same spleen cell pools induced *in vitro* to OFA (Fig. 6). Similar levels of cytotoxicity were observed whether or not syngeneic irradiated adult spleen cells were added as stimulators, which contrasted with the clear dependence on the R/S ratio of the *in vitro* induction of T_C to OFA or TAA. This would indicate that no additional effect was exerted by the presence of the irradiated spleen cells. All the tumor target cell lines tested *in vitro* were susceptible to lysis by CL induced in this way, and there was no apparent restriction by the MHC on the lysis of target cells (Table V).

Clear-cut quantitative and qualitative (specificity) differences were demonstrated between this phenomenon and the *in vitro* induction of tumor-specific immunity. As is shown in Fig. 7, the levels of lysis of ^{51}Cr-labeled MPC-11 mediated by CL from control cultures (spleen cells alone or plus irradiated spleen cells) were significantly lower than those of CL induced from the same spleen cell pools by *in vitro* culture with irradiated MPC-11 [$p < 0.001$, Mann–Whitney U-test for nonparametric data, probability (p) for group sizes over 20; Armitage, 1971]. There was, however, no statistically significant difference in the levels of lysis observed between the two control groups using the same

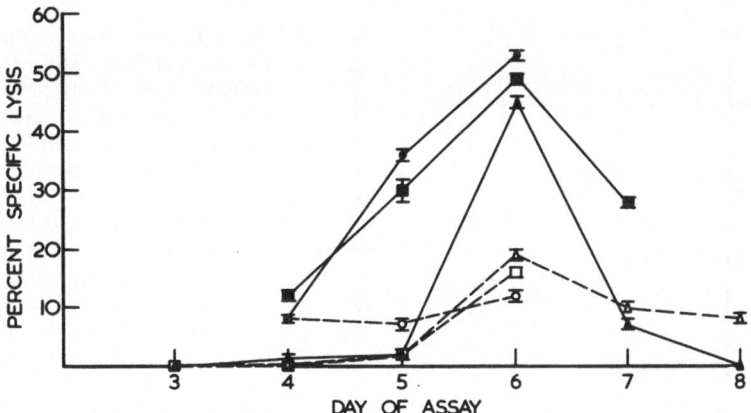

Figure 6. Kinetics of "autosensitization" compared to kinetics of induction of T_C to OFA. The lines ●———●, ▲———▲, and ■———■ are the kinetics curves of three separate experiments in which BALB/c CL were induced *in vitro* to irradiated 14-day BALB/c fetal liver for 3–8 days and then assayed on ^{51}Cr WEHI-164 at a CL/T = 100:1. The lines ○———○, △– – –△, and □– – –□ are the corresponding curves from the same experiments in which the BALB/c CL were induced *in vitro* to irradiated adult BALB/c spleen cells and assayed in the same way. [Reproduced with permission from *J. Immunol.* **119**:1329 (1977).]

Table V. Lysis of Tumor Cell Lines *in Vitro* by "Autosensitized" CL

[51]Cr-labeled tumor line (CL/T = 100:1)	Strain of origin	H-2	Percent specific lysis (mean ± S.E.M.)[a]		
			Strain of 6-day cultured spleen cells		
			BALB/c (H-2[d])	CBA (H-2[k])	C57B1 (H-2[b])
WEHI-164 (FSA)	BALB/c	d	20 ± 2 (38)	12 ± 3 (3)	18 ± 4 (3)
P815 (mastocytoma)	DBA/2	d	14 ± 4 (6)	14 ± 2 (4)	29 ± 5 (4)
EL.4 (T lymphoma)	C57B1	b	22 ± 2 (16)	20 ± 6 (7)	18 ± 2 (5)
HPC-10 (PCT)	NZB	d	8 ± 3 (6)	8 ± 3 (6)	9 ± 3 (5)
MPC-11 (PCT)	BALB/c	d	9 ± 1 (24)	14 ± 1 (1)	16 ± 1 (1)
C1.18 (PCT)	C3H	k	15 ± 3 (6)	5 ± 2 (2)	8 ± 1 (3)

[a]Mean ± S.E.M. of the total number of experiments noted in parentheses.

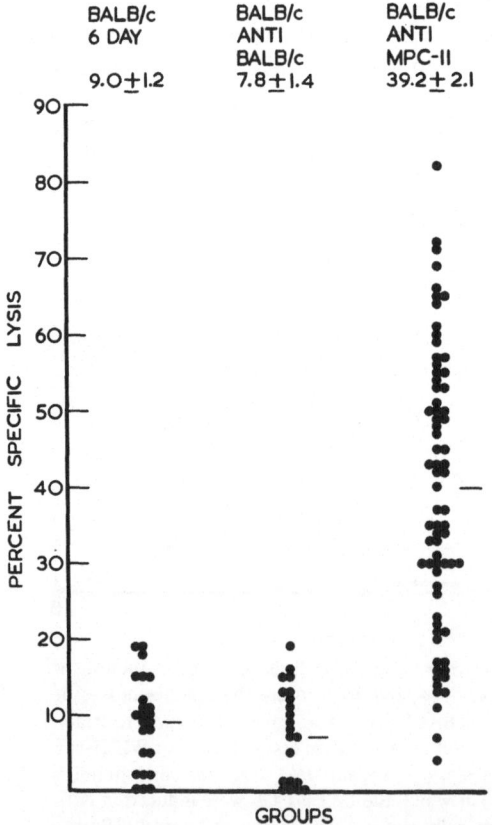

Figure 7. Comparison of tumor-immune and "autosensitized" CL-mediated lysis of MPC-11. This figure summarizes the results of all experiments in which BALB/c CL, induced *in vitro* by 6-day culture alone, or with irradiated BALB/c spleen or MPC-11 cells, were assayed on ^{51}Cr MPC-11 at a CL/T = 100:1. The mean percent specific lysis (●) is shown for each experiment, as is the median (———) of all the experiments in each group. The groups are labeled appropriately and the mean ± S.E. of each group is reported. These first two groups were the "autosensitized" CL controls for the third tumor-immune CL group. [Reproduced with permission from *J. Immunol.* **119**:1329 (1977).]

mode of analysis ($p = 0.26$). Statistically significant quantitative differences in lysis were also shown between control CL and CL induced *in vitro* to fetal liver and FSA cells (Burton and Warner, 1978*a*; Burton *et al.*, 1977*b*).

Experiments were performed to elucidate the identity of the responding cells, and the results indicated that both T and non-T cells were important (Table VI). At the inductive phase T cells were absolutely necessary, and no cytotoxicity was detected in cultures of nude spleen cells. However, at the effector stage, treatment of the CL with anti-Thy-1,2 serum and complement produced evidence that both T and non-T cells were involved. In the case of C1.18, all cytotoxicity was abolished by this treatment, but with the CL populations mediating lysis of WEHI-164 and EL-4, there was no reduction in the level of lysis detected at a CL/T of 100:1. These experiments were performed at least three times in parallel with experiments in which the cytotoxicity of CL induced *in vitro* by culture of spleen cells from the same pools with tumor or fetal cells was totally abolished by treatment with the same dilution of the same anti-Thy-1,2 antiserum and complement.

Subsequent investigation of this phenomenon did not indicate that self- or H-2-type antigens were involved, but rather that if the phenomenon was antigenically specific, the antigens involved were probably derived from the FCS used in the tissue culture media (Burton *et al.*, 1977*b*). The acquisition of antigens by cells grown in media containing mammalian serum was first reported for human melanoma cells grown in FCS by Irie *et al.* (1974), and has been confirmed by other workers (Sulit *et al.*, 1976; Forni and Green, 1976). Since FCS has also been reported to act as a mitogen (Golub and Zielske, 1975), the effect observed could be one of a general polyclonal stimulation of T_C,

Table VI. Role of T Cells in the Induction of CL in Unstimulated Cultures

CL source	Treatment	WEHI-164 (5)[a]		EL-4 (4)		C1.18 (2)	
		%[b] VCC	% Specific lysis	% VCC	% Specific lysis	% VCC	% Specific lysis
BALB/c spleen,	NIL	100	19 ± 3	100	14 ± 4	100	9 ± 1
6-day culture	Complement (C')	97	21 ± 3	97	16 ± 3	95	12 ± 1
	Anti-Thy-1,2	91	16 ± 3	83	20 ± 4	75	8 ± 1
	Anti-Thy-1,2 + C'	43	17 ± 6	41	19 ± 4	27	0
BALB/c. *nu* spleen, 6- day culture				0			

[a]% specific lysis shown is mean ± S.E. of the number of experiments in parentheses.
[b]% of viable cells recovered after treatment; CL then made up for CL/T = 100:1 in assay.

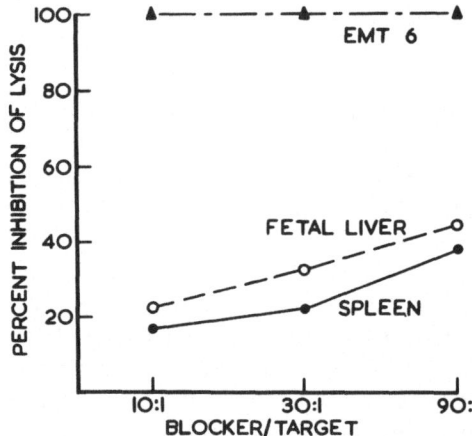

Figure 8. Failure to inhibit "auto-sensitized" CL with fetal liver cells. The lines ▲——————▲ (EMT-6), ●———● (BALB/c spleen), and ○----○ (BALB/c 14-day fetal liver) were the inhibition curves produced when the viable unlabeled cells indicated were added at the B/T ratios shown to the assay of "autosensitized" BALB/c CL (induced by culture of spleen cells for 6 days) and ^{51}Cr EMT-6 (specific lysis = 18 ± 1%, CL/T = 100:1). [Reproduced with permission from *J. Immunol.* 119:1329 (1977).]

although the studies listed above are more compatible with an antigen-specific nature for the phenomenon.

Another explanation for the phenomenon has been suggested by Gorczynski (1976*a*). On the basis of experiments which demonstrated that CL which developed in cultures of spleen cells were more effective in lysing syngeneic embryonic fibroblasts than syngeneic adult fibroblasts or allogeneic embryonic fibroblasts, and that this lysis could be inhibited by a heterologous rabbit antimurine embryo antiserum, he proposed that the antigens involved were OFA, which were induced on the spleens cells by *in vitro* culture. However, we have performed studies in a fully syngeneic system with the cellular competitive inhibition assay which have shown that the lysis of a ^{51}Cr-labeled tumor cell line by CL generated in unstimulated cultures could be inhibited by tumor cells, but not by adult spleen or fetal liver cells (Fig. 8). Furthermore, it has been shown both by ourselves (Table VI) and by Shustik *et al.* (1976) that both syngeneic and allogeneic targets are readily lysed by the CL which develop in cultures of "unstimulated" murine spleen cells.

There are a number of other conflicts between the observations of the various groups working in this field. In the studies of the "autosensitization" *in vitro* phenomenon (Cohen and Wekerle, 1973; Carnaud *et al.*, 1974), all the cytotoxicity was apparently T-cell-mediated. However, both in our studies (Table VI) and those of Gorczynski (1976*b*), it appeared that both T and non-T cells were involved. In another recent report, in which the phenomenon was termed T lymphocytes with promiscuous cytotoxicity (Sulit *et al.*, 1976), again only T cells were involved at the effector stage. It has also been claimed for the "autosensitization"-*in-vitro* phenomenon that CL do not develop if irradiated syngeneic spleen cells are substituted for fibroblasts (Cohen and Wekerle, 1973).

These contrasting observations and conclusions are illustrative of the current state of this field. Further work in carefully defined *in vitro* systems is obviously necessary to completely characterize the phenomenon. Regardless of the nature of the phenomenon, what is crucial to the whole field of *in vitro* induction of CMI is the definition of the part this phenomenon plays in any given system. In this regard we have shown that the phenomenon is both quantatively and qualitatively distinct from the *in vitro* induction of T_C to TAA and OFA, for in these latter two systems the levels of cytotoxicity are significantly higher, the CL themselves are all T_C, and the antigens involved show a different and distinct distribution.

The practical problem with this phenomenon is that in any particular T_C population stimulated by a specific TAA there may also be present a proportion of CLs of this "autosensitization" type. Thus, in assessing the specificity of the particular anti-TAA T_C population, some confusion may be introduced by the more general reactivity of the "autosensitized" CLs. Thus before these general cytotoxicity and inhibition assays can be fully exploited to resolve the nature and distribution of TAA, it will be necessary to develop means to either prevent the induction of these "autosensitized" CLs, or to negate their expression at the effector stage. Unfortunately, no universal substitute for FCS has yet been found.

IV. ROLE OF THE MHC AT THE INDUCTIVE PHASE OF T-CELL IMMUNITY *IN VITRO* TO TAA

The susceptibility to C-type oncogenic viral tumor induction has long been known to have a genetic basis. Of special interest, however, is the more recent demonstration that genes linked to the MHC play a role in the susceptibility to these tumors and/or in the immune response to TAA expressed by them. Lilly (1970, 1971) has demonstrated an *H-2*-linked susceptibility to some forms of Friend and Gross virus infection, and, more recently, it was reported that the *in vivo* immune response to TAA of a XI-VEA$^+$-virus-induced BALB/c leukemia was under *H-2*-linked genetic control (Sato *et al.*, 1973). These findings, and the discovery of the immune response (*Ir*) genes which are part of the MHC (Benacerraf and McDevitt, 1972; Shreffler and David, 1975; Green, 1974), stimulated a series of investigations in this laboratory into the possible role of *H-2*-linked *Ir* genes in the control of the *in vitro* T_C response to PCT TAA. Experiments were conducted using two NZB PCT cell lines, HPC-6 and HPC-10, as stimulators, and spleen cells from NZB, (NZB X C57B1)F_1, (NZB X B10.D2)-F_1, and (NZB X B10.Br)F_1 hybrid mice as responders.

Preliminary experiments were conducted which demonstrated that the optimal R/S ratio for the *in vitro* induction of T_C to NZB PCT TAA was 100:1 for the NZB parental strain and 10:1 for the various NZB F_1 *H-2* congenic hybrid

Table VII. F$_1$ *H-2* Congenic Hybrid—Immunity to HPC-6 *in Vitro*

Responder spleen cells	Stimulator cells (5000 rad)	R/S	Percent specific lysis[a]	
			^{51}Cr HPC-6	^{51}Cr MPC-11
NZB	HPC-6	10:1	29 ± 5	16 ± 4
(NZB × C57B1)F$_1$	HPC-6	10:1	62 ± 5	44 ± 3
(NZB × B10.D2)F$_1$	HPC-6	10:1	49 ± 5	23 ± 2
(NZB × B10.Br)F$_1$	HPC-6	10:1	37 ± 5	21 ± 1
NZB	HPC-6	100:1	16 ± 3	17 ± 2
(NZB × C57B1)F$_1$	HPC-6	100:1	37 ± 4	17 ± 4
(NZB × B10.D2)F$_1$	HPC-6	100:1	16 ± 2	14 ± 3
(NZB × B10.Br)F$_1$	HPC-6	100:1	22 ± 3	3 ± 1
CL	Treatment	% VCC[b]		
(NZB × C57BL)F$_1$	Nil	100	66 ± 1	56 ± 1
Anti-HPC-6	C'	100	53 ± 2	48 ± 2
R/S = 10/1	Anti-Thy1.2	100	42 ± 1	35 ± 1
	Anti-Thy1.2 + C'	18	12 ± 1	5 ± 1

[a]Mean ± S.E.M. for all experiments, CL/T = 100:1.
[b]Percentage of pretreatment CL viable after treatment.

mice. Therefore, all subsequent experiments were performed at these two ratios using the conditions described previously, including the overnight incubation step in fresh medium, and the results shown are expressed in terms of the percent lysis per 2.5×10^6 CL (CL/T = 100:1). Since the viable cell recoveries from the cultures of the various responder strains were all within the range 23 ± 3% of the original responding spleen cell number, and since the CL/T ratio chosen was on the linear part of the curve, the levels of lysis observed probably directly reflect the frequency of clones of T cells directed against NZB PCT TAA in the responding spleen cell populations.

The pooled results of a number of experiments employing HPC-6 at R/S ratios of both 10:1 and 100:1, and both HPC-6 and MPC-11 as targets, are shown in Table VII. In one particular experiment (NZB × C57B1)F$_1$ hybrid CL were treated with anti-Thy-1,2 antiserum and complement to demonstrate the T$_C$ nature of the response.

The results with HPC-6 as the target show that the (NZB × C57B1)F$_1$ hybrid response at the R/S ratio of 100:1 was significantly higher than that of any of the other strains ($p < 0.01$, Student's *t* test; Armitage, 1971), indicating that there is an *H-2*^{b}-linked gene controlling the *in vitro* high response to TAA on the NZB plasmacytoma. At the R/S ratio of 10:1, the response of the (NZB × C57B1)F$_1$ hybrid was again greater than that of the other hybrids but was not significantly greater than that of the $(NZB \times B10.D2)F_1$ hybrid ($p > 0.05$, Student's t test). When the various T_C were also assayed on MPC-11, the results suggested that most of the *in vitro* response had been to TAA shared between the two tumors. At the optimal R/S ratio (10:1) the $H\text{-}2^b$-linked high response was again quite evident, although at the R/S ratio of 100:1, the pattern of results was different, and the T_C from all the strains, except for the (NZB $\times$ B10.Br)F_1 hybrid, mediated essentially the same rather low level of lysis of this target.

The somewhat complex pattern of responses observed here might have been expected, as there are at least four classes of TAA of murine PCT: (1) "unique" TAA, (2) TAA shared to other PCT, (3) TAA shared to lymphomas and other tumor types, and (4) OFA (Chism *et al.*, 1976; Burton and Warner, 1977*a*, 1978*b,c*). The results of the direct ^{51}Cr release assay were confirmed in the competitive inhibition assay, in which it was shown that the lysis of HPC-6 or HPC-10 by (NZB $\times$ C57B1)F_1 hybrid T_C induced *in vitro* to either tumor was best inhibited by the two NZB PCT, to a lesser extent by the BALB PCT MPC 11, and to a small but significant extent by a BALB/c or a NZB lymphoma (Burton and Warner, 1978*c*).

These inhibition assay results had also suggested that there might be TAA restricted in distribution to NZB PCT and therefore not expressed on BALB/c-derived PCT. Therefore, the technique of induction of secondary T_C responses *in vitro* (Rollingoff, 1974) was employed to test this thesis. In a number of experiments, spleen cells from both nonimmune and immune (NZB $\times$ C57B1)F_1 hybrid mice, which had been immunized to HPC-6 by the technique of surgical tumor removal (Burton and Warner, 1977*a*), were used as Responder cells, with HPC-6 as the Stimulator. The pooled results of all the experiments that were performed (a minimum of 2 at each R/S ratio) are presented in Table VIII. It can be seen that spleen cells from preimmunized mice could be induced to yield considerably more active populations on a per-cell basis (secondary response) than those from nonimmunized mice (primary response). The most striking aspect of these results, however, is the restriction of the secondary cytotoxic response to the NZB PCT. It was subsequently confirmed by the cellular competitive inhibition assay, in which a variety of BALB/c and NZB tumors were used as blockers, that the specificity of T_C induced in the secondary cytotoxic response *in vitro* to NZB PCT was restricted to NZB plasmacytomas, thereby identifying a tumor and strain-specific TAA (Burton and Warner, 1977*c*).

$H\text{-}2$-linked genetic control of the *in vivo* immune response has been demonstrated for the TAA of polyoma (Oth *et al.*, 1976) and murine-leukemia-virus (MuLV)-induced tumors (Sato *et al.*, 1973). Virion and viral self surface antigens of the MuLV group are readily detectable on murine PCT (Aoki and Takahashi, 1972; Hyman *et al.*, 1972; Aoki *et al.*, 1973), and since most of the *in vitro* T_C responses were to *shared* TAA of PCT, it is likely that they were in part directed

Table VIII. Primary and Secondary *in Vitro* Responses of
(NZB × C57Bl)F$_1$ Hybrid Spleen Cells to HPC-6

$T_C{}^a$	Mean percent specific lysis (all experiments) ± S.E.M. (CL/T = 100:1)		
	HPC-6	HPC-10	MPC-11
(NZB × C57Bl)F$_1$ (R/S = 10:1) Anti-HPC-6 *Primary*	33 ± 2	45 ± 2	16 ± 1
(NZB × C57Bl)F$_1$ (R/S = 10:1) Anti-HPC-6 *Secondary*	70 ± 2	80 ± 2	22 ± 2
(NZB × C57Bl)F$_1$ (R/S = 100:1) Anti-HPC-6 *Primary*	7 ± 1	14 ± 1	0
(NZB × C57Bl)F$_1$ (R/S = 100:1) Anti-HPC-6 *Secondary*	27 ± 1	38 ± 3	0

^{a}T_C induced by coculturing (NZB × C57Bl)F$_1$ hybrid spleen cells from nonimmune (primary) or HPC-6 immune (secondary) mice with irradiated HPC-6 cells at the R/S ratios shown.

against antigens of this type. The NZB strain-specific PCT TAA might also be of this type and perhaps be related to the NZB xenotropic virus recently described by Levy *et al.* (1975).

V. ROLE OF THE MHC AT THE EFFECTOR PHASE OF T_C IMMUNITY *IN VITRO* TO TAA

In a number of recent *in vivo* and *in vitro* studies, it was found that T_C could only lyse target cells *in vitro* if they shared MHC determinants with the target. Thus lymphocytes from Rous-sarcoma-bearing chickens were cytotoxic for autochthonous but not allogeneic tumor cells (Wainberg *et al.*, 1974), and mouse cells infected with lymphocytic choriomeningitis (Zinkernagel and Doherty, 1975), ectromelia (Gardner *et al.*, 1975), vaccinia (Koszinowski and Ertl, 1975), and paramyxo (Doherty and Zinkernagel, 1976) viruses were only lysed by syngeneic or semiallogeneic T_C from virus-immunized animals. Furthermore, it has been shown *in vivo* that the transfer of cell-mediated immunity to *Listeria monocytogenes* is also restricted by the *H-2* gene complex (Zinkernagel, 1974). This *in vitro* restriction on the lysis of target cells by T_C also applies when the effectors are induced *in vitro* to haptenated cells (Shearer, 1974), the male specific (*H-Y*) antigen (Gordon *et al.*, 1975), minor histocompatibility antigens (Bevan, 1975), and "self" antigens (Ilfeld *et al.*, 1975).

A number of studies have indicated that the same kind of restriction may apply to CMI induced *in vivo* or *in vitro* to TAA. It has been shown that the *in vitro* lysis of Friend-virus-induced tumors of BALB/c *H-2* congenic mice, which express the Friend-virus-induced FMR cell surface antigen and viral envelope antigens, occurs only when the T_C are obtained from Friend-virus-immune mice that share MHC determinants with the target (Blank *et al.*, 1976). Similar findings were recorded for MSV-induced tumors with T_C which had been obtained from BALB/c and C57B1 *H-2* congenic mice which had been immunized with the virus (Gomard *et al.*, 1976). Furthermore, CMI to SV40-specific TAA is also restricted by the MHC (Trinchieri *et al.*, 1976). Less direct evidence indicating that T_C reactive to TAA must share *H-2* determinants with the target cells has come from studies in which the lysis of such target cells was blocked by anti-H-2 alloantisera (Germain *et al.*, 1975; Schrader and Edelman, 1976).

Many studies have demonstrated, however, that it is possible to alloimmunize T_C both *in vivo* and *in vitro*, that the immunization is specific to private H-2 alloantigens, and that allogeneic targets bearing those antigens are lysed *in vitro* (Wagner *et al.*, 1973; Cerottini and Brunner, 1974; Brondz *et al.*, 1975). In order to account for both sets of findings, two models for the biological role of the MHC have been developed (Zinkernagel and Doherty, 1974; Doherty and Zinkernagel, 1975). The first, the "physiological interaction" model, proposes that the T_C antigen receptor recognizes the relevant antigen on the target-cell surface, but that a second interaction between *H-2*-coded structures on the T cell and target cell are necessary for lysis to occur, and physiological interaction occurs only with MHC-determined self-complementary molecules. The second proposes that T lymphocytes can recognize only modified or unmodified H-2 antigens, and has been called the "altered-self" hypothesis. A number of studies with F_1 hybrid mice (Zinkernagel and Doherty, 1974, 1975; Shearer *et al.*, 1975; Bevan, 1975), and with T_C from a secondary *in vitro* induction with ectromelia-virus-infected cells (Davidson *et al.*, 1976), have strongly suggested that the physiological interaction model is untenable, and current interest has therefore been focused on the altered-self hypothesis.

Since this is a general hypothesis which carries profound implications for both basic and tumor immunology, studies were undertaken to determine whether the MHC restricted the *in vitro* lysis of tumor targets by T_C induced *in vitro* to OFA or PCT TAA. In the first instance T_C were induced under the conditions described above to syngeneic 14- or 15-day fetal liver cells at the optimal R/S ratio (10:1). These OFA-immune T_C could mediate lysis of a wide variety of syngeneic and allogenic tumor cell lines (Table IX). Additional studies with the cellular competitive inhibition assay indicated that both syngeneic and allogeneic tumor cells could inhibit the lysis of a BALB/c tumor by BALB/c T_C induced *in vitro* to BALB/c fetal liver (Burton *et al.*, 1977).

When BALB/c T_C induced *in vitro* against MPC-11 were assayed on both the syngeneic PCT MPC-11 and the allogeneic C3H PCT C1.18, they readily lysed both tumor lines (Burton *et al.*, 1977). *In vitro* studies with the cellular inhibition assay supported the results of the direct lysis experiments. The lysis of ^{51}Cr-labeled MPC-11 by BALB/c T_C induced *in vitro* to MPC-11 was inhibited by two BALB/c (H-2d) PCT, MPC-11 (Fig. 9A and B) and MOPC-315 (Fig. 9B), and also by the allogeneic C3H (H-2k) PCT C1.18 (Fig. 9A and B). BALB/c spleen or lymphoma (WEHI-22) cells did not inhibit lysis (Fig. 9A). The level of inhibition mediated by MPC-11 blocker cells was two to three times greater than that seen with MOPC-315 or C1.18 blocker cells, whether the responder was of the strain of origin of the tumor (Fig. 9A) or the F_1 hybrid (Fig. 9B). Since the *in vitro* induction was performed with MPC-11 as the stimulator cell, the unlabeled MPC-11 should compete best with the ^{51}Cr-labeled MPC-11 for BALB/c T_C. What is of *crucial* importance here, however, is that C1.18, the H-2-incompatible PCT, produced the *same* levels of inhibition of lysis as the H-2-compatible PCT MOPC-315.

A second series of experiments was performed in which both allogeneic and syngeneic ^{51}Cr-labeled PCT cells were pretreated with well-characterized H-2 alloantisera prior to being employed as targets for the assay of T_C induced *in vitro* to PCT TAA. No reduction in the levels of specific lysis of alloantiserum-treated target cells was observed in a total of four experiments, although the

Table IX. Lysis of Allogeneic and Syngeneic Tumor Target Cells
by T_C Induced *in Vitro* to OFA

Responder spleen cells	Stimulator fetal liver cells (5000 rad)	Lysis of tumor target cells (CL/T = 100:1)	
		Tumor line (*H-2* type)	% Specific lysis (Mean ± S. E.)
BALB/c	BALB/c	WEHI-164 (d)	36 ± 2
BALB/c	BALB/c	EMT-6 (d)	50 ± 3
BALB/c	BALB/c	MPC-11 (d)	28 ± 2
BALB/c	BALB/c	HPC-10 (d)	26 ± 5
BALB/c	BALB/c	EL-4 (b)	32 ± 2
BALB/c	BALB/c	RILQ (k)	20 ± 2

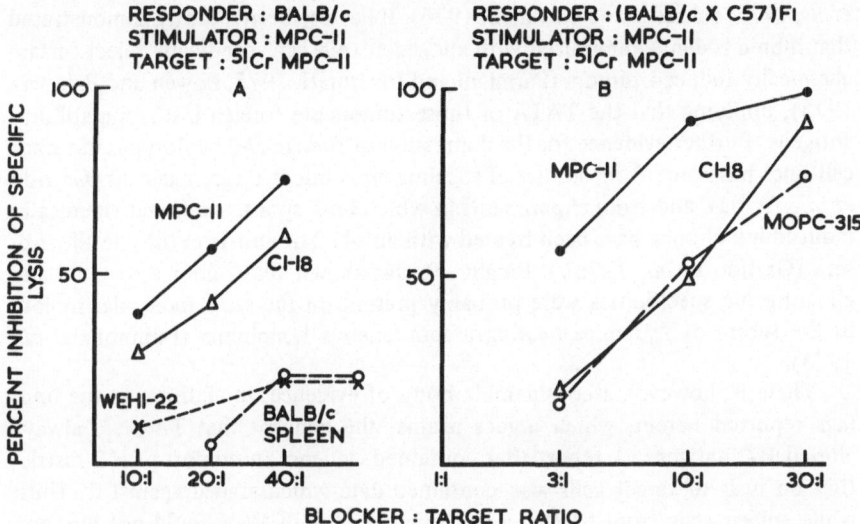

Figure 9. PCT inhibition studies: lack of *H-2* restriction. (A) The lines ●——● (MPC-11), △——△ (C1.18), x---x (WEHI-22), and ○---○ (BALB/c spleen) show the results of adding the unlabeled tumor and adult spleen cells shown to the assay of BALB/c Tc induced *in vitro* against MPC-11 and assayed on ^{51}Cr MPC-11. (B) The lines ●——● (MPC-11), ○——○ (MOPC-315), and △——△ (C1.18) show the results of adding the unlabeled PCT cells shown to an assay of (BALB/c × C57Bl)F$_1$ hybrid T$_C$ induced *in vitro* against MPC-11 and assayed on ^{51}Cr MPC-11. [Reproduced with permission from *J. Immunol.* 118:971 (1977).]

alloantisera were highly and specifically inhibitory of lysis at the same serum dilutions when the antigens involved were H-2 alloantigens or TNP-modified cell surface antigens on the same target cells, i.e., MPC-11 and C1.18 (Burton *et al.*, 1978).

The results of these experiments argue strongly against the hypothesis that T cells can *only* recognize modified or unmodified H-2 alloantigen determinants. They also indicate that these particular OFA and PCT TAA are not in any way related to H-2 alloantigens.

The possibility that TAA are altered H-2 antigens has been a recurrent theme in this field. An inverse relationship has been reported for the expression of H-2 antigens and tumor-associated transplantation antigens (TATA) on a series of MCA-induced sarcomas (Haywood and Mackhann, 1971), polyoma-virus-induced tumors (Ting and Herberman, 1971), and Moloney leukemia-virus-induced and spontaneous lymphomas (Cikes *et al.*, 1973). TATA solubilized from tumors induced by oncogenic viruses have been reported to have similar physical properties to soluble H-2 antigens (Drapkin *et al.*, 1974; Chang *et al.*, 1975), and, as mentioned earlier, it has been shown that alloantisera can block the lysis of certain tumor target cells by CL directed against TAA on their surface (Germain *et al.*, 1975; Schrader and Edelman, 1976). It has also been recently demonstrated that inbred rodents immunized with allogeneic cells can specifically reject certain chemically induced tumors (Parmiani and Invernizzi, 1975; Bowen and Baldwin, 1975), implying that the TATA of those tumors are foreign histocompatibility antigens. Further evidence for the depression of foreign *H-2* haplotypes in tumor cell lines has come from studies of vaccinia-virus-infected sarcoma cells (Garrido *et al.*, 1976*a*), and from experiments in which both spontaneous and chemically induced lymphomas have been treated with anti-H-2 or anti-Ia cytotoxic alloantisera (Garrido *et al.*, 1976*b*). Finally, it was shown that tumor associated and alloantigenic specificities were probably present on the same molecular moiety in the serum of A/J mice bearing a spontaneous lymphoma (Fujimoto *et al.*, 1973).

There is, however, a considerable body of evidence, in addition to the findings reported herein, which argues against the concept that TAA are always altered H-2 antigens. A report that contained evidence in support of H-2 restriction on lysis of target cells also contained data which argued against it. Thus, while spleen cells from C57B1 mice immunized with MSV could not lyse any BALB/c tumor target cells, they did lyse a DBA/2 mastocytoma (Herberman *et al.*, 1974). Furthermore, the competitive cellular inhibition assay, which was employed in those studies, demonstrated that allogeneic tumor cells, from both *in vivo* tumors and *in vitro* tissue culture lines, could block the *in vitro* lysis of a ^{51}Cr-labeled MSV tumor cell line by syngeneic spleen cells from MSV-immune mice. Analogous findings were reported in one recent paper which studied inhibition of tumor specific immunity by alloantisera. In that case lysis of a C57B1 lymphoma by BALB/c CL induced *in vitro* to TAA on a BALB/c tumor cell line was demonstrated (Schrader and Edelman, 1976). In a similar system where CL induced to TNP derivitized cells were inhibited from lysing alloantiserum-treated syngeneic target cells, CL were shown to be capable of lysing allogeneic TNP derivitized cells (Burakoff *et al.*, 1976). Furthermore, Ting and Law (1977) have demonstrated that there is no strict H-2 dependency for T-cell-mediated cytotoxicity of Friend virus induced leukemia in C57B1 or BALB/c mice. However, discordant findings were obtained when two different *in vitro* radioisotope release assays were compared. In the short-term ^{51}Cr release assay there was clear H-2 restriction, and this also applied to the other assay, a ^{125}IUdR release assay, if a short incubation time was employed. However, with long incubation times (18–24 hr) in this latter assay the H-2 restriction phenomenon was not observed.

In 1974 Davies *et al.* demonstrated that the TAA extracted from the C57B1 lymphoma EL-4 with specific rabbit antisera could be readily distinguished from H-2^b alloantigens by gel filtration and ion exchange chromatography, and the following year Kedar and Bonivida (1975) reported that two independent populations of immune lymphocytes could be isolated from BALB/c mice immunized with EL-4, one with specificity for H-2^b alloantigens and one for EL-4 TAA.

Immunofluorescence studies have also been reported in which tumor cell lines expressing TATA have had no demonstrable H-2 antigens (Birch *et al.*, 1975).

The phenomenon of the inhibition of syngeneic tumor growth in rodents immunized with allogeneic normal cells was also studied by Nakayama *et al.* (1975), who concluded that the inhibition was not due to TATA cross reactive with foreign histocompatibility antigens because lymphoid cells from immune rats could not inhibit the growth of syngeneic tumors in the Winn assay in normal rats. They speculated that the inhibition of syngeneic tumor growth might be due to nonspecific immunostimulation by alloantigens. Klein (1977) has shown that the TATA of a 3-methylcholanthrene-induced sarcoma is not a modified form of H-2 and that its structural determinants are not localized on chromosome 17, which carries the MHC, by studying a hybrid tumor cell line which had been produced by the fusion of two allogeneic tumor cells, and from which the relevant chromosome 17 had been eliminated.

It has been suggested that the studies which do not show H-2 restriction do not contradict the altered-self hypothesis, as in those instances public H-2 specificities shared between the allogeneic cells and the T_C may have been involved in the interaction or altered self antigens. There is, however, little support for this proposal from other studies. In considering the hapten modified antigen, Shearer *et al.* (1975) concluded that the major new determinants formed were restricted to private specificities, and Brondz *et al.* (1975) have shown that T_C generated against alloantigenic cells recognize *only* private H-2 specificities. A reasonable conclusion from our studies and the review of the literature reported herein is that the H-2 restriction phenomenon is *not* an absolute one. Therefore, it is proposed that although an H-2 interaction antigen (altered self) antigen may preferentially stimulate T-cell responses, non-H-2-associated surface antigens, involving for example TAA, are also capable of stimulating T cells and of acting as targets for T_C. This would be in accord with the conclusions of Germain *et al.* (1975), who suggested that antigens which arise by interaction with H-2 determinants are also likely to be strong antigens and provoke strong immune responses. A tumor cell which expressed both H-2-associated and non-H-2-associated antigens would tend to elicit an immune response which would be dominated by that of the altered H-2 antigen, and the smaller subpopulation of T_C reactive to the non-H-2-associated TAA might not be detectable under the conditions of assay. This issue will clearly only be finally resolved when biochemical studies on the nature of the TAA in different situations are resolved.

VI. COMMENTS AND CONCLUSIONS

The *in vitro* technology discussed herein has made a significant contribution to the investigation of T-cell responses to TAA. However, there is to date almost no information as to the nature of the TAA involved, and so it is important to consider other possible non-TAA when the *in vitro* responses are being analyzed. This was considered in some detail in this review in relationship to the CL which are "induced" when spleen cells are cultured without added stimulator cells. However, there are other antigens which might act as "TAA." Mycoplasma species and "irrelevant viruses" can readily contaminate tissue culture cell lines. While it is relatively easy to exclude the former, as we routinely do by testing all the cell lines by the uracil–uridine method (Schneider *et al.*, 1974), it is not possible to exclude the latter, although the results of specificity testing of T_C induced *in vitro* argue against a "universal" contaminating agent of this type. Alloantigenic differences between tumors and their strain of origin may also arise in the course of long-term tissue culture and in the breeding of inbred mice. It is possible that "unique TAA" might arise in this way; however, it is unlikely that such antigens would produce the appropriate patterns of cross reactivity of TAA seen with the viral induced tumors. Furthermore, it has not yet been possible to accomplish a primary *in vitro* induction of T_C to minor alloantigens (Gordon *et al.*, 1975).

As is often the case in cancer research, therapeutic endeavors in terminal cancer patients predated the laboratory investigations reported herein. Specific adoptive immunotherapy trials had been attempted using lymphocytes harvested from volunteers immunized with a patient's (allogeneic) tumor (Andrews *et al.*, 1967; Nadler and Moore, 1969), and also by using lymphocytes from a particular patient after they had been cocultured for a period *in vitro* with the patient's own (autochthonous) tumor (Aust *et al.*, 1970; McKhann and Jagarlamoody, 1971; Seigler *et al.*, 1972). The results were disappointing, and there was at least one death in the case of the allogeneic lymphocyte infusions which may have been due to graft-versus-host disease (Andrews *et al.*, 1967). This form of immunotherapy has been studied in experimental laboratory animals, and syngeneic mice have been partially protected against the growth of a murine tumor by the intravenous injection of syngeneic spleen cells that had been induced *in vitro* to the tumor (Treves *et al.*, 1975; Small and Trainin, 1975; Burton and Warner, 1977*b*). It has also been reported that macrophages "armed" *in vitro* by SMAF were also effective when administered in a similar fashion (Van Loveren and den Otter, 1974). These reports suggest that an animal-specific adoptive immunotherapy model is worthy of further investigation. However, since most of the intravenously injected CL appear to be sequestered in the liver and lungs (Burton and Warner, 1977*b*), necessitating the injection of very high numbers of sensitized cells, this mode of immunotherapy would not seem to have any immediate clinical application, at least until this problem is solved.

There have been a small number of *in vitro* studies of the type reported herein in fully autologous human systems. When lymphocytes from patients with Burkitt's lymphoma (Golub *et al.*, 1972), malignant melanoma (Golub and

Morton, 1974), or acute myelomonocytic leukemia (Zarling *et al.*, 1976) were cultured *in vitro* with autochthonous tumor cells, CL that were directed against the inducing tumor were detected by *in vitro* assays. Furthermore, in the case of patients with Burkitt's lymphoma and malignant melanoma, the reactivity of the CL was shown to be directed against tumors of the same type as the inducing tumor, and that normal tissue cells were not affected. One human study, however, demonstrated that *in vitro* "education" of lymphocytes on autologous human sarcoma cells generated nonspecific cytotoxicity (Martin-Chandos *et al.*, 1975).

In conclusion, the most promising directions for this type of research would seem to be:

1. To improve the technology to permit well-defined TAA rather than whole tumor cells to be used to induce T_C *in vitro*. Although soluble alloantigens are relatively ineffective in a primary *in vitro* induction, they can stimulate a secondary cytotoxic *in vitro* allograft reaction (Wagner *et al.*, 1976). In this regard we have had some success in an analogous syngeneic system with TAA, prepared from tumors by a 3MKCL extraction technique (Reisfeld *et al.*, 1971). A second technique, that of presenting soluble TAA *in vitro* on macrophages (Treves *et al.*, 1976; Hellstrom and Hellstrom, 1976), also indicates that it may be possible in the future to induce T_C *in vitro* with specificity for particular TAA.

2. Attempts to characterize the specificity of T_C induced *in vivo* or *in vitro* by C-type RNA oncogenic viral induced tumors have been successfully accomplished using whole virus or/and viral components to inhibit *in vitro* lysis of tumor target cells by these T_C (Shellam, 1974; Bruce *et al.*, 1976). It has also been shown that T lymphocytes sensitized *in vitro* to MSV-transformed cells and to purified group-specific MSV antigens are capable of protecting irradiated mice against tumor induction with MSV (Gorczynski and Knight, 1975). Studies of this type have shed some light on the specificity of T_C induced to viral-determined TAA. However, the production of highly specific antisera directed at particular oncogenic viral antigens should advance investigations in this area, as such antisera should inhibit the lysis of target cells by CL directed against the relevant antigens, when preincubated with the target cells.

3. One of the most important applications of this technology should be to the study of human TAA in fully autologous systems. The vast majority of *in vitro* research into CMI to human tumors has been conducted in allogeneic systems, where the involvement of HLA antigens cannot be rigidly excluded (Sharma and Terasaki, 1974). As mentioned above, preliminary investigations in this field have yielded promising results, and since the unequivocal demonstration of CMI to TAA demands a syngeneic or autologous system, the use of *in vitro* systems may eventually lead to a better definition of human TAA.

ACKNOWLEDGMENTS

This work was supported by The Wellcome Foundation U.K., by USPHS Research Grants CA 15600 and AM 11234, and is in part pursuant to Contract No. 1-CB-23889 from the National Cancer Institute.

Dr. Burton is a National Health and Medical Research Council postgraduate research scholar.

We are grateful to Dr. A. Harris both for his advice and also for providing a number of the tumor cell lines, and to D. Grail, G. Cousins, and J. Thompson for excellent technical assistance.

VII. REFERENCES

Andrews, G. A., Congdon, C. C., Edwards, C. L., Gengozian, N., Nelson, S., and Vodopick, H., 1967, Preliminary trials of clinical immunotherapy, *Cancer Res.* 27:2535.

Aoki, T., and Takahashi, T., 1972, Viral and cellular surface antigens of murine leukaemias and myelomas, *J. Exp. Med.* 135:443.

Aoki, T., Potter, M., and Sturm, M. M., 1973, Analysis by immunoelectron-microscopy of type-C viruses associated with primary and short-term transplanted mouse plasma cell tumors, *J. Natl. Cancer Inst.* 51:1609.

Armitage, P., 1971, *Statistical Methods in Medical Research*, Blackwell Scientific, Oxford.

Aust, J. C., Jagarlamoody, S. D., and McKhann, C. F., 1970, Immunisation of lymphocytes *in vitro* for immunotherapy of malignant disease, *Surg. Forum* 21:118.

Bach, F. H., and Voynow, K. N., 1966, One way stimulation in mixed leukocyte cultures, *Science* 153:545.

Benacerraf, B., and McDevitt, H. O., 1972, Histocompatibility linked immune response genes, *Science* 175:273.

Bernstein, I. D., Wright, P. W., and Cohen, E., 1976, Generation of cytotoxic lymphocytes *in vitro:* Response of immune rat spleen cells to a syngeneic Gross-virus induced lymphoma in mixed lymphocyte–tumor culture, *J. Immunol.* 116:1367.

Bevan, M. J., 1975, The major histocompatibility complex determines susceptibility to cytotoxic T cells directed against minor histocompatibility antigens, *J. Exp. Med.* 142:1349.

Bevan, M. J., Epstein, R., and Cohn, M., 1974, The effect of 2-mercaptoethanol on murine mixed lymphocyte cultures, *J. Exp. Med.* 139:1025.

Bevan, M. J., Langman, R. E., and Cohn, M., 1976, H-2 antigen-specific cytotoxic T cells induced by conconavalin A: Estimation of their relative frequency, *Eur. J. Immunol.* 6:150.

Birch, J. M., Moore, M., and Craig, A. W., 1975, Cell surface antigen expression on chemically induced murine leukaemias, *Brit. J. Cancer* 31:630.

Blank, K. J., Freedman, H. A., and Lilly, F., 1976, T lymphocyte response to Friend virus-induced tumour cell lines in mice of strains congenic at *H-2*, *Nature* 260:250.

Bowen, J. G., and Baldwin, R. W., 1975, Tumour-specific antigen related to rat histocompatibility antigens, *Nature* 258:75.

Brondz, B. D., Egorov, I. K., and Drizlikh, G. I., 1975, Private specificities of *H-2K* and *H-2D* loci as possible selective targets for effector lymphocytes in cell mediated immunity, *J. Exp. Med.* 141:11.

Broome, J. D., and Jeng, M. W., 1973, Promotion of replication in lymphoid cells by specific fluids and disulphides *in vitro*, *J. Exp. Med.* 138:574.

Bruce, J., Mitchison, N. A., and Shellam, G. R., 1976, Studies on a Gross-virus induced lymphoma in the rat. III. Optomisation, specificity and applications of the *in vitro* immune response, *Int. J. Cancer* 17:342.

Brunner, K. T., Manel, J., Cerottini, J. C., and Chapins, B., 1968, Quantitative assay of the lytic action of immune lymphoid cells on ^{51}Cr labelled allogeneic target cells, *Immunology* 14:181.

Brunner, K. T., Plata, F., Vasudevan, B. M., and Cerottini, J. C., 1975, in: *Proceedings of the Fifth International Symposium of the Princess Takamatsu Cancer Research Fund: Host Defence Against Cancer and Its Potentiation* (D. Mizumo, G. Chihara, F. Fukuoka, T. Yamamoto, and Y. Yakamura, eds.), p. 43, University Park Press, Baltimore.

Burakoff, S. J., Germain, R. N., and Benacerraf, B., 1976, Inhibition of cell-mediated cytolysis of trinitrophenyl-derivatized target cells by alloantisera directed to the products of the *K* and *D* loci of the *H-2* complex, *Proc. Natl. Acad. Sci. U.S.* 73:625.

Burton, R. C., and Warner, N. L., 1977a, Tumor immunity to murine plasma cell tumors. III. Detection of common tumor associated antigens on BALB/c, C3H and NZB plasmacytomas by *in vivo* and *in vitro* induction of tumor immune responses, *J. Natl. Cancer Inst.* 58:709.

Burton, R. C., and Warner, N. L., 1977b, *In vitro* induction of tumor specific immunity. IV. Specific adoptive immunotherapy with cytotoxic T cells induced *in vitro* to plasmacytoma antigens, *Cancer Immunol. Immunother.* 2:91.

Burton, R. C., and Warner, N. L., 1978a, *In vitro* induction of tumor specific immunity. V. Detection of common antigenic determinants of murine fibrosarcomas, *Brit. J. Cancer* (in press).

Burton, R. C., and Warner, N. L., 1978b, Tumor immunity to murine plasma cell tumors. IV. Influence of the responder genotype on the specificity of the immune response to plasmacytomas and T lymphomas, *Aust. J. Exp. Biol. Med. Sci.* (in press).

Burton, R. C., and Warner, N. L., 1978c, Tumor immunity to murine plasma cell tumors. V. Genetic control of the primary and secondary *in vitro* immune response to NZB plasma cell tumor antigens (submitted for publication).

Burton, R. C., Thompson, J., and Warner, N. L., 1975, *In vitro* induction of tumor specific immunity. I. Development of optimal conditions for induction and assay of cytotoxic lymphocytes, *J. Immunol. Methods* 8:133.

Burton, R. C., Chism, S. E., and Warner, N. L., 1977a, *In vitro* induction of tumor specific immunity. III. Lack of requirement for *H-2* compatibility in lysis of tumor targets by T cells activated *in vitro* to oncofetal and plasmacytoma antigens, *J. Immunol.* 118:971.

Burton, R. C., Chism, S. E., and Warner, N. L., 1977b, *In vitro* induction of tumor specific immunity. VII. Does autosensitization occur with *in vitro* culture of T lymphocytes? *J. Immunol.* 119:1329.

Burton, R. C., Scott, D., and Warner, N. L., 1978, Failure to inhibit T cell mediated lysis of plasmacytomas by anti-*H-2* sera (submitted for publication).

Cantor, H., and Boyse, E. A., 1975, Functional subclasses of T lymphocytes. 2. Cooperation between subclasses of Ly$^+$ cells in generation of killer activity, *J. Exp. Med.* 141:1390.

Cantor, H., and Boyse, E. A., 1976, Regulation of cellular and humoral immune responses by T cell subclasses, *Cold Spring Harbor Symp. Quant. Biol.* 41:23.

Canty, T. G., and Wunderlich, J. R., 1971, Quantitative assessment of cellular and humoral responses to skin and tumor allografts, *Transplantation* 11:111.

Carnaud, C., Ilfeld, D., Brook, I., and Trainin, N., 1973, Increased reactivity of mouse spleen cells sensitised *in vitro* against syngeneic tumor cells in the presence of a thymic humoral factor, *J. Exp. Med.* 138:1521.

Carnaud, C., Ilfeld, D., Levo, Y., and Trainin, N., 1974, Enhancement of 3LL tumor growth by autosensitised T lymphocytes independent of the host lymphatic system, *Int. J. Cancer* **14**:168.

Cerottini, J. C., and Brunner, K. T., 1974, Cell mediated cytotoxicity, allograft rejection and tumor immunity, *Adv. Immunol.* **18**:67.

Cerottini, J. C., Nordin, A. A., and Brunner, K. T., 1970, Specific *in vitro* cytotoxicity of thymus-derived lymphocytes sensitised to alloantigens, *Nature* **228**:1308.

Chang, K. S. S., Law, L. W., and Appella, E., 1975, Distinction between tumor-specific transplantation antigen and virion antigens in solubilised products from membranes of virus-induced leukaemic cells, *Int. J. Cancer* **15**:483.

Chism, S. E., Burton, R. C., and Warner, N. L., 1976, *In vitro* induction of tumor specific immunity. II. Activation of cytotoxic lymphocytes to murine oncofoetal antigens, *J. Natl. Cancer Inst.* **57**:377.

Chism, S. E., Burton, R. C., Graill, D. L., Bell, P. M., and Warner, N. L., 1977, *In vitro* induction of tumor specific immunity. VI. Analysis of immune response by cellular competitive inhibition. Limitations and advantages of the technique, *J. Immunol. Methods* **16**:245.

Cikes, M., Briberg, S., and Klein, G., 1973, Progressive loss of *H-2* antigens with concomitant increase of cell surface antigens determined by Moloney leukaemia virus in cultured murine lymphomas, *J. Natl. Cancer Inst.* **50**:347.

Clark, D. A., Phillips, R. A., and Miller, R. G., 1976, Characterisation of cells that suppress the cytotoxic activity of T lymphocytes. I. Quantitative measurement of inhibitor cells, *J. Immunol.* **116**:1020.

Click, R. E., Benck, L., and Alter, B. J., 1972, Enhancement of antibody synthesis *in vitro* by mercaptoethanol, *Cell. Immunol.* **3**:156.

Cohen, I. R., and Wekerle, H., 1973, Regulation of autosensitisation; the immune activation and specific inhibition of self recognising thymus derived lymphocytes, *J. Exp. Med.* **137**:224.

Cohen, I. R., Globerson, A., and Feldman, M., 1971, Autosensitisation *in vitro*, *J. Exp. Med.* **133**:834.

Davidson, W. F., Pang, T., Banden, R. V., and Doherty, P. C., 1976, "Physiological interaction" does not explain the H-2 requirement for recognition of virus-infected cells by cytotoxic T cells, *Aust. J. Exp. Biol. Med. Sci.* **54**:413.

Davies, D. A. L., Baugh, V. S. G., Buckham, S., and Maustone, A. J., 1974, Separation of the specific antigen of a mouse lymphoma from histocompatibility antigens, *Eur. J. Cancer* **10**:781.

Dennert, G., 1976, Thymus derived killer cells: Specificity of function and antigen recognition, *Transplant. Rev.* **29**:59.

Doherty, P. C., and Zinkernagel, R. M., 1975, A biological role for the major histocompatibility antigens, *Lancet* **1**:1406.

Doherty, P. C., and Zinkernagel, R. M., 1976, Specific immune lysis of paramyxovirus-infected cells by H-2 compatible thymus-derived lymphocytes, *Immunology* **31**:27.

Drapkin, M. S., Appella, E., and Law, L. W., 1974, Immunogenic properties of soluble tumor specific transplantation antigens induced by Simian virus 40, *J. Natl. Cancer Inst.* **52**:259.

Dunkley, M., Miller, R. G., and Shortman, K., 1974, A modified ^{51}Cr release assay for cytotoxic lymphocytes, *J. Immunol. Methods* **6**:39.

Evans, B., Cox, H., and Alexander, P., 1973, Immunological specific activation of macrophages armed with the specific macrophage arming factor (SMAF), *Proc. Soc. Exp. Biol. (N.Y.)* **143**:256.

Fanger, M. W., Hart, D. A., Wells, J. V., and Nisonoff, A., 1970, Enhancement by reducing agents of the transformation of human and rabbit periferal lymphocytes, *J. Immunol.* **105**:1043.

Forman, J., and Britton, S., 1973, Cytotoxic potential of mouse spleen cells on H-2 antibody treated target cells, *J. Exp. Med.* **137**:527.

Forni, G., and Green, I., 1976, Heterologous sera: A target for *in vitro* cell mediated cytotoxicity, *J. Immunol.* **116**:1561.

Friend, K., Hellstrom, I., and Hellstrom, K. E., 1976, *In vitro* sensitisation to embryonic antigens, *Int. J. Cancer* **18**:843.

Fujimoto, S., Chen, C. H., Sabbadini, E., and Sehon, A. H., 1973, Association of tumor and histocompatibility antigens in sera of lymphoma-bearing mice, *J. Immunol.* **111**:1093.

Gale, R. P., and Zighelboim, J., 1975, Polymorphonuclear leukocytes in antibody-dependent cellular cytotoxicity, *J. Immunol.* **114**:1047.

Gardner, I. D., Bowern, N. A., and Blanden, B. V., 1975, Cell mediated cytotoxicity against ectromelia virus-infected target cells. III. Role of the *H-2* gene complex, *Eur. J. Immunol.* **5**:122.

Garrido, F., Schirrmacher, V., and Festenstein, H., 1976*a*, *H-2*-like specificities of foreign haplotypes appearing on a mouse sarcoma after vaccinia virus infection, *Nature* **259**:228.

Garrido, F., Schirrmacher, V., and Festenstein, H., 1976*b*, Further evidence for derepression of *H-2* and *Ia*-like specificities of foreign haplotypes in mouse tumour cells, *Nature* **261**:705.

Germain, R. W., Dorf, M. E., and Benacerraf, B., 1975, Inhibition of T-lymphocyte mediated tumor specific lysis by alloantisera directed against the *H-2* serological specificities of the tumor, *J. Exp. Med.* **142**:1023.

Ginsberg, H., 1968, Graft versus host reaction in tissue culture. I. Lysis of monolayers of embryo mouse cells from strains differing in the H-2 histocompatibility locus by rat lymphocytes sensitised *in vitro*, *Immunology* **14**:621.

Glaser, M., Lavrin, D., and Herberman, R. B., 1976*a*, *In vivo* protection against syngeneic cross virus induced lymphoma in rats: Comparison with *in vitro* studies of cell mediated immunity, *J. Immunol.* **116**:1507.

Glaser, M., Bonnard, G. D., and Herberman, R. B., 1976*b*, *In vitro* generation of secondary cell-mediated cytotoxic response against a syngeneic cross-virus-induced lymphoma in rats, *J. Immunol.* **116**:430.

Golub, S. H., and Morton, D. L., 1974, Sensitisation of lymphocytes *in vitro* against human melanoma-associated antigens, *Nature* **251**:161.

Golub, S. H., and Zielske, J., 1975, Induction of cell-mediated cytotoxic responses against human tumor cells and fibroblasts, *Proc. Amer. Assoc. Cancer Res.* **16**:170.

Golub, S. H., Svedmyr, E. A., Hervetson, J. F., Klein, G., and Singh, S., 1972, Cellular reactions against Burkitt lymphoma cells. III. Effector cell activity of leukocytes stimulated in vitro with autoehthonous cultured lymphoma cells, *Int. J. Cancer* **10**:157.

Gomard, E., Duprez, V., Henin, Y., and Levy, J. P., 1976, H-2 region product as determinant in immune cytolysis of syngeneic tumour cells by anti-MSV T lymphocytes, *Nature* **260**:707.

Goodman, H. S., 1961, A general method for the quantitation of immune cytolysis, *Nature* **190**:269.

Gorczynski, R. M., 1976*a*, Autoreactivity developing spontaneously in cultured mouse spleen cells. I. Evidence that cytotoxicity is directed against embryo associated antigen, *Immunology* **31**:607.

Gorczynski, R. M., 1976*b*, Autoreactivity developing spontaneously in cultured mouse spleen cells. II. Comparison of cytotoxicity of cultured male and female spleen cells, *Immunology* **31**:615.

Gorczynski, R. M., and Knight, R. A., 1975, Cell mediated immunity to Moloney sarcoma virus in mice. II. Analysis of antigenic specificities involved in T lymphocyte-mediated *in vivo* rejection of murine sarcoma virus induced tumors, *Eur. J. Immunol.* **5**:148.

Gordon, R. D., Simpson, E., and Samelson, L. E., 1975, *In vitro* cell-mediated immune responses to the male specific (*H-V*) antigen in mice, *J. Exp. Med.* **142**:1108.

Green, I., 1974, Genetic control of immune responses, *Immunogenetics* **1**:4.

Harris, J. W., MacDonald, H. R., Engers, H. D., Fitch, F. W., and Cerottini, J. C., 1976, Increased cytolytic T lymphocyte activity induced by 2-mercapto-ethanol in mixed leukocyte cultures: Kinetics and possible mechanisms of action, *J. Immunol.* **116**:1071.

Hayry, P., and Defendi, V., 1970, Mixed lymphocyte cultures produce effector cells: Model *in vitro* for allograft rejection, *Science* **168**:133.

Hayry, P., Anderson, L. C., Nordberg, S., and Virolainen, M., 1972, Allograft response *in vitro*, *Transplant. Rev.* **12**:91.

Haywood, G. R., and Mackhann, C. F., 1971, Antigenic specificities of murine sarcoma cells. Reciprocal relationship between normal transplantation antigens (*H-2*) and tumor-specific immunogenicity, *J. Exp. Med.* **133**:1171.

Hellstrom, I., and Hellstrom, K. E., 1976, Specific sensitisation of lymphocytes to tumor antigens by co-cultivation with peritoneal cells exposed to such antigens, *Int. J. Cancer* **17**:748.

Herberman, R. B., Aoki, T., Nunn, M., Lavrin, D. H., Soares, N., Gazdar, A., Holden, H., and Chang, K. S. S., 1974, Specificity of ^{51}Cr release cytotoxicity of lymphocytes immune to murine sarcoma virus, *J. Natl. Cancer Inst.* **53**:1103.

Hyman, R., Ralph, P., and Sarkar, S., 1972, Cell-specific antigens and immunoglobulin synthesis of murine myeloma cells and their variants, *J. Natl. Cancer Inst.* **48**:173.

Ilfeld, D., Carnaud, C., Cohen, I. R., and Trainin, N., 1973, *In vitro* cytotoxicity and *in vivo* tumor enhancement induced by mouse spleen cells autosensitised *in vitro*, *Int. J. Cancer* **12**:213.

Ilfeld, D., Carnaud, C., and Klein, E., 1975, Cytotoxicity of autosensitised lymphocytes restricted to the H-2k end of targets, *Immunogenetics* **2**:231.

Irie, R. F., Irie, K., and Morton, D. L., 1974, Natural antibody to a neoantigen in human cultured cells grown in fetal bovine serum, *J. Natl. Cancer Inst.* **52**:1051.

Johnston, J. M., and Wilson, D. B., 1970, Origin of immunoreactive lymphocytes in rats, *Cell. Immunol.* **1**:430.

Kall, M. A., and Hellstrom, I., 1975, Specific stimulatory and cytotoxic effects of lymphocytes sensitised *in vitro* to either alloantigens or tumor antigens, *J. Immunol.* **114**:1083.

Kall, M. A., Hellstrom, I., and Hellstrom, K. E., 1976, *In vitro* generation of primary and secondary cytotoxic cell-mediated immune responses to chemically induced mouse sarcomas, *Int. J. Cancer* **18**:488.

Kasakura, S., and Lowerstein, L., 1965, The effect of irradiation *in vitro* on mixed leukocyte cultures and on leukocyte cultures with phytohaemagglutinin, in: *Histocompatibility Testing* (H. Balner, F. J. Cleton, and J. G. Eernisse, eds.), p. 211, Munksgaard, Copenhagen.

Kedar, E., and Bonivida, B., 1975, Studies on the induction and expression of T cell-mediated immunity. IV. Non-overlapping populations of allo-immune cytotoxic lymphocytes with specificity for tumor-associated antigens and transplantation antigens, *J. Immunol.* **115**:1301.

Kiessling, R., and Klein, E., 1973, Cytotoxic potential of mouse spleen cells on *H-2* antibody treated target cells, *J. Exp. Med.* **137**:527.

Kiessling, R., Klein, E., Pross, H., and Wigzell, H., 1975, "Natural" killer cells in the mouse. I. Cytotoxic cells with specificity for mouse Moloney leukaemia cells. Specificity and distribution according to genotype, *Eur. J. Immunol.* **5**:112.

Kirchner, H., Glaser, M., Holden, H. T., and Herberman, R. B., 1976, Mixed lymphocyte/

tumor-cell interaction in a murine sarcoma virus (Moloney)-induced tumor system. Comparison between lymphocyte proliferation and lymphocyte cytotoxicity, *Int. J. Cancer* 17:362.

Klein, G., 1977, Tumor-associated antigens in H-2 hemizygous isoantigenic variants of a somatic cell hybrid derived from fusion of a 3 methylcholanthrene induced sarcoma and a mammary carcinoma, *J. Natl. Cancer Inst.* 58:383.

Koszinowski, U., and Ertl, H., 1975, Lysis mediated by T cells and restricted by *H-2* antigen of target cells infected with vaccinia virus, *Nature* 255:552.

Kuperman, O., Fortner, W., and Lucas, Z. J., 1975*a*, Immune response to a syngeneic mammary adenocarcinoma. II. *In vitro* generation of cytotoxic lymphocytes, *J. Immunol.* 115:1277.

Kuperman, O., Fortner, W., and Lucas, Z. J., 1975*b*, Immune response to a syngeneic mammary adenocarcinoma. III. Development of memory and suppressor functions modulating cellular cytotoxicity, *J. Immunol.* 115:1282.

Lamon, E. W., Whitten, H. D., Skurzak, H. M., Andersson, B., and Lidin, B., 1975, IgM antibody-dependent cell-mediated cytotoxicity in the Moloney sarcoma virus system: The involvement of T and B lymphocytes as effector cells, *J. Immunol.* 115:1288.

Laux, D., and Lausch, R. N., 1974, Reversal of tumor-mediated suppression of immune reactivity by *in vitro* incubation of spleen cells, *J. Immunol.* 112:1900.

Levy, J. A., Kazan, P., Varmer, O., and Kleinmann, H., 1975, Murine xenotropic type C viruses. I. Distribution and further characterisation of the virus in NZB mice, *J. Virol.* 16:844.

Lilly, F., 1970, Fv-2: Identification and location of a second gene governing the spleen focus response to Friend leukaemia virus in mice, *J. Natl. Cancer Inst.* 45:163.

Lilly, F., 1971, The influence of *H-2* type on gross virus leukaemogenesis in mice, *Transplant. Proc.* 3:1239.

Lundak, R. L., and Raidt, O. J., 1973, Cellular immune response against tumor cells. I. *In vitro* immunisation of allogeneic and syngeneic mouse spleen cell suspensions against DBA mastocytoma cells, *Cell. Immunol.* 9:60.

Manson, L. A., and Palmer, T. C., 1975, Induction of the immune response to cell surface antigens *in vitro*, *In Vitro* 2:186.

Manson, L. A., Goldstein, L., Thorn, R., and Palmer, J., 1975, Immune response against apparently host-compatible transplantable tumors, *Transplant. Proc.* 7:161.

Martin-Chandos, M. R., Vanky, F., Carnaud, C., and Klein, E., 1975, *In vitro* "education" on autologous human sarcoma generated non-specific killer cells, *Int. J. Cancer* 15:342.

McKhann, C. F., and Jagarlamoody, S. M., 1971, *In vitro* immunization for immunotherapy, in: *Morphological and Fundamental Aspects of Immunity* (K. Lindahl-Kiessling, G. Alm, and M. G. Hanna, Jr., eds.), Plenum Press, New York.

Meltzer, M. S., 1976, Tumoricidal responses *in vitro* of peritoneal macrophages from conventionally housed and germ-free nude mice, *Cell. Immunol.* 22:176.

Miller, J. F. A. P., Brunner, K. T., Sprent, J., Russell, P. J., and Mitchell, G. F., 1971, Thymus-derived cells as killer cells in cell-mediated immunity, *Transplant. Proc.* 3:915.

Miller, R. G., and Dunkley, M., 1974, Quantitative analysis of the ^{51}Cr release cytotoxicity assay for cytotoxic lymphocytes, *Cell. Immunol.* 14:284.

Mosier, D., and Cantor, H., 1971, Functional maturation of mouse thymic lymphocytes, *Eur. J. Immunol.* 1:459.

Nadler, S. H., and Moore, G. E., 1969, Immunotherapy of malignant disease, *Arch. Surg.* 99:376.

Nakayama, M., Sendo, F., Gotohda, E., Hosokawa, M., Kodama, T., and Kobayasha, H., 1975, Studies of the mechanisms of "allogeneic cell immunity" by *in vivo* neutralisation test, *Proc. Jap. Cancer Assoc.* 34:59.

Nomoto, K., Mashiba, H., Sato, M., and Takeya, K., 1974, *In vitro* detection of tumor-specific antigens, *GANN Monogr.* **16**:211.

Nowell, P. C., 1960, Phytohaemagglutinin: An initiator of mitosis in cultures of normal human leukocytes, *Cancer Res.* **20**:462.

Ortiz de Landazuri, M., and Herberman, R. B., 1972*a*, *In vitro* activation of cellular immune response to Gross virus-induced lymphoma, *J. Exp. Med.* **136**:969.

Ortiz de Landazuri, M., and Herberman, R. B., 1972*b*, Specificity of cellular immune reactivity to virus-induced tumors, *Nature New Biol.* **238**:18.

Oth, D., Robert, F., Berebbi, M., and Meyer, G., 1976, Decreased resistance in some heterozygotes in *H-2* linked immune response to polyoma induced tumor, *Nature* **259**:316.

Parmiani, G., and Invernizzi, G., 1975, Alien histocompatibility determinants on the cell surface of sarcomas induced by methylcholanthrene. I. *In vivo* studies, *Int. J. Cancer* **16**:756.

Perlmann, P., 1972, Lymph ocyte cytotoxicity; technical aspects. Introduction, *Transplant. Proc.* **4**:295.

Plata, F., Cerottini, J. C., and Brunner, K. T., 1975, Primary and secondary *in vitro* generation of cytolytic T lymphocytes in the murine sarcoma virus system, *Eur. J. Immunol.* **5**:227.

Pollack, S., Nelson, K., and Grausz, J. D., 1975, Killer cells from murine spleen: Effectors of antibody-dependent cellular cytotoxicity, *Transplant. Proc.* **7**:477.

Reisfeld, R. A., Pellegrini, M. A., and Kahan, B. D., 1971, Salt extraction of soluble HL-A antigens, *Science* **172**:1134.

Rollinghoff, M., 1974, Secondary cytotoxic tumor immune response induced *in vitro*, *J. Immunol.* **112**:1718.

Rollinghoff, M., and Wagner, H., 1973, *In vitro* induction of tumor specific immunity: requirements for T lymphocytes and tumor growth inhibition *in vivo*, *Eur. J. Immunol.* **3**:471.

Rollinghoff, M., and Warner, N. L., 1973, Specificity of *in vivo* tumor rejection assessed by mixing immune spleen cells with target and unrelated tumor cells, *Proc. Soc. Exp. Biol. Med.* **144**:813.

Sanderson, C. J., 1976*a*, The mechanism of T cell mediated cytotoxicity. I. The release of different cell components, *Proc. Roy. Soc. Lond.* **B192**:221.

Sanderson, C. J., 1976*b*, The mechanism of T cell mediated cytotoxicity. II. Morphological studies of cell death by time-lapse micro-cinematography, *Proc. Roy. Soc. London.* **192**:241.

Sato, H., Boyse, E. A., Aoki, T., Iritani, C., and Old, L. J., 1973, Leukaemia-associated transplantation antigens related to murine leukaemia virus. The X-1 system: Immune response controlled by a locus linked to *H-2*, *J. Exp. Med.* **138**:593.

Schneider, E. L., Steinbridge, E. J., and Epstein, C. J., 1974, Incorporation of ^{3}H-uridine and ^{3}H-uracil into RNA: A simple technique for the detection of mycoplasma contamination of cultured cells, *Exp. Cell. Res.* **84**:311.

Schrader, J. W., and Edelman, G. M., 1976, Participation of the *H-2* antigens of tumor cells in their lysis by syngeneic T cells, *J. Exp. Med.* **143**:601.

Schrek, R., and Donnelly, W. J., 1961, Differences between lymphocytes of leukemic and non-leukemic patients with respect to morphologic features, mobility, and sensitivity to guinea pig serum, *Blood* **18**:561.

Seigler, H. F., Shingleton, W. W., Metzgar, R. S., Buckley, C. E., Bergoe, P. M., Miller, D. S., Fetter, B. F., and Phaup, M. B., 1972, Non-specific and specific immunotherapy in patients with melanoma, *Surgery* **72**:162.

Senik, A., Hebrero, P., and Levy, J. P., 1975, Secondary specific immune response *in vitro* to MSV tumor cells, *Int. J. Cancer* **16**:946.

Sharma, B., and Terasaki, P. I., 1974, *In vitro* immunisation to cultured human tumor cells, *Cancer Res.* 34:115.

Shearer, G., 1974, Cell mediated cytotoxicity to trinitrophenyl-modified syngeneic lymphocytes, *Eur. J. Immunol.* 4:527.

Shearer, G. M., Rehn, T. G., and Garbarino, C. A., 1975, Cell mediated lympholysis of trinitrophenyl modified autologous lymphocytes. Effector cell specificity to modified cell surface components by the H-2K and H-2D serological regions of the murine major histocompatibility complex, *J. Exp. Med.* 141:1348.

Shellam, G. R., 1974, Studies on a Gross-virus-induced lymphoma in the rat. I. The cell mediated immune response, *Int. J. Cancer* 14:65.

Shreffler, D., and David, C., 1975, *H-2* major histocompatibility complex and immune response region-genetic variation, function and organization, *Adv. Immunol.* 20:125.

Shustik, C., Cohen, I. R., Schwartz, R. C., Latham-Griffin, E., and Waksal, S. D., 1976, T cells with promiscuous cytotoxicity, *Nature* 263:701.

Small, M., and Trainin, N., 1975, Inhibition of syngeneic fibrosarcoma growth by lymphocytes sensitised on tumor cell monolayers in the presence of the thymic humoral factor, *Int. J. Cancer* 15:962.

Solliday, S., and Bach, F. H., 1970, Cytotoxicity: Specificity after *in vitro* sensitisation, *Science* 170:1406.

Stout, R. D., Waksal, S. D., and Herzenberg, L. A., 1976, Fc receptor on thymus derived lymphocytes. 3. Mixed lymphocyte reactivity and cell mediated lympholytic activity of Fc^+ and Fc^- lymphocytes, *J. Exp. Med.* 144:54.

Sulit, H. L., Golub, S. H., Reiko, F. I., Gupta, R. K., Crooms, G. A., and Morton, D. L., 1976, Human tumor cells grown in fetal calf serum and human serum; influences on the tests for lymphocyte cytotoxicity, serum blocking and serum arming effects, *Int. J. Cancer* 17:461.

Takasugi, M., and Klein, E. A., 1970, A microassay for cell-mediated immunity, *Transplantation* 9:219.

Takasugi, M., and Terasaki, P., 1973, Quantitation of the microassay for cell-mediated immunity through electronic image analysis, *Natl. Cancer Inst. Monogr.* 37:77.

Takasugi, M., Akira, D., and Kinoshita, K., 1975, Granulocytes as effectors in cell-mediated cytotoxicity of adherent target cells, *Cancer Res.* 35:2169.

Takei, F., Levy, J. G., and Kilburn, D. G., 1976, *In vitro* induction of cytotoxicity against syngeneic mastocytoma and its suppression by spleen and thymus cells from tumor-bearing mice, *J. Immunol.* 116:288.

Thorn, R. M., Palmer, J. C., and Manson, L. A., 1974, A simplified ^{51}Cr release assay for killer cells, *J. Immunol. Methods* 4:301.

Ting, C. C., and Bonnard, G. D., 1976, Cell-mediated immunity to Friend virus induced leukaemia. IV. *In vitro* generation of primary and secondary cell-mediated cytotoxic responses, *J. Immunol.* 116:1419.

Ting, C. C., and Herberman, R. B., 1971, Inverse relationship of polyoma tumour specific antigens and *H-2* histocompatibility antigens, *Nature New Biol.* 232:118.

Ting, C. C., and Law, L. W., 1977, Studies of *H-2* restriction in cell-mediated cytotoxicity and transplantation immunity to leukaemia-associated antigens, *J. Immunol.* 118:1259.

Treves, A. J., Cohen, I. R., and Feldman, M., 1975, Immunotherapy of lethal metastases by lymphocytes sensitised against tumor cells *in vitro*, *J. Natl. Cancer Inst.* 54:777.

Treves, A. J., Schechter, B., Cohen, I. R., and Feldman, M., 1976, Sensitisation of T lymphocytes *in vitro* by syngeneic macrophages fed with tumor antigens, *J. Immunol.* 116:1059.

Trinchieri, G., Aden, D. P., and Knowles, B. B., 1976, Cell mediated cytotoxicity to SV40-specific tumour associated antigens, *Nature* 261:313.

Trostmann, H., Pfizenmaier, R., Wagner, H., and Rollinghoff, M., 1976, Cell-mediated immunity to *H-2* antigens. Characteristics of the effector cells detected in the microcytotoxicity assay, *Transplantation* **21**:446.

Van Loveren, H., and den Otter, W., 1974, *In vitro* activation of armed macrophages and the therapeutic application in mice, *J. Natl. Cancer Inst.* **51**:1917.

Vasudevan, D. M., Brunner, K. T., and Cerottini, J. C., 1973, Increased cytotoxic effect of immune lymphocytes in a syngeneic tumor system following simple purification procedures, *Brit. J. Cancer* **28** (Suppl. I): 35.

Wagner, H., and Rollinghoff, M., 1973, *In vitro* induction of tumor-specific immunity. I. Parameters of activation and cytotoxic reactivity of mouse lymphoid cells immunised *in vitro* against syngeneic and allogeneic plasma cell tumors, *J. Exp. Med.* **138**:1.

Wagner, H., Harris, A., and Feldmann, M., 1972, Cell-mediated immune response *in vitro*. II. The role of thymus and thymus-derived lymphocytes, *Cell. Immunol.* **4**:39.

Wagner, H., Rollinghoff, M., and Nossal, G. J., 1973, T-cell-mediated immune responses induced *in vitro:* A probe for allograft and tumor immunity, *Transplant. Rev.* **17**:3.

Wagner, H., Hess, M., Feldmann, M., and Rollinghoff, M., 1976, Secondary cytotoxic allograft responses *in vitro*. III. The immunogenicity of allogeneic membrane fragments, *Transplantation* **21**:282.

Wainberg, M. A., Markson, Y., Weiss, D. W., and Doljanski, F., 1974, Cellular immunity against Rous sarcomas of chickens. Preferential reactivity against autochthonous target cells as determined by lymphocyte adherence and cytotoxicity tests *in vitro*, *Proc. Natl. Acad. Sci. U.S.* **71**:3365.

Warnatz, F., Scheiffarth, F., and Schmeissner, R., 1975, Studies on the cytotoxic effect of *in vivo* and *in vitro* immunised lymphocytes on liver target cells, *Clin. Exp. Immunol.* **21**:250.

Warnatz, H., and Scheiffarth, F., 1974, Cell-mediated immune response of *in vitro* sensitised lymphocytes to isogeneic methyl-cholanthrene induced tumor cell lines, *Transplantation* **18**:273.

Wigzell, H., 1965, Quantitative titrations of mouse H-2 antibodies using ^{51}Cr labelled target cells, *Transplantation* **3**:423.

Winn, H. J., 1961, Immune mechanisms in homotransplantation. II. Quantitative assay of the immunologic activity of lymphoid cells stimulated by tumor homografts, *J. Immunol.* **86**:228.

Wunderlich, J. R., and Canty, T. G., 1970, Cell mediated immunity induced *in vitro*, *Nature* **228**:63.

Zarling, J. M., Raich, P. C., Mckeogh, M., and Bach, F. H., 1976, Generation of cytotoxic lymphocytes *in vitro* against autologous human leukaemia cells, *Nature* **262**:691.

Zinkernagel, R. M., 1974, Restriction by *H-2* gene complex of transfer of cell mediated immunity to *Listeria monocytogenes*, *Nature* **251**:230.

Zinkernagel, R. M., and Doherty, P. C., 1974, Immunological surveillance against altered self components by sensitised T lymphocytes in lymphocytic choriomeningitis, *Nature* **251**:547.

Zinkernagel, R. M., and Doherty, P. C., 1975, H-2 compatibility requirement for T-cell mediated lysis of target cells infected with lymphocytic choriomeningitis virus. Different cytotoxic-T cell specificities are associated with strictures coded for on *H-2K* or *H-2D*, *J. Exp. Med.* **141**:1427.

Chapter 5

Systemic and Local Immunity in Allograft and Cancer Rejection

J. Stephen Haskill

Department of Obstetrics and Gynecology
University of North Carolina at Chapel Hill
Chapel Hill, North Carolina 27514

Pekka Häyry

Transplantation Laboratory, Department IV of Surgery
University of Helsinki
Helsinki, Finland

and

Leslie A. Radov

Department of Pharmacology
Pennwalt Corporation
Rochester, New York 14603

I. INTRODUCTION

Studies of allograft and tumor rejection have historically been closely related. Indeed, many of the studies on tumor immunity carried out in the early part of this century actually dealt with tumor allograft rejection, and the concepts derived from transplantation immunity studies have provided many useful models and concepts for tumor immunology. In this context we have reviewed the literature covering allograft rejection as well as syngeneic graft rejection, in order to provide a more complete picture of the current state of these closely

107

interrelated areas of investigation, especially as they relate to intragraft and intratumor reactions.

How the immune system mediates allograft rejection is incompletely known. Delayed hypersensitivity reactions mediated primarily by thymus-derived cytotoxic (T) lymphocytes have classically been considered the main effector pathway of allograft destruction. This concept is based on the findings obtained via classification and fractionation of immunocompetent cells, studies of the central lymphatic system, and analysis of their function *in vitro* (for a review, see Cerottini and Brunner, 1974; Bach and van Rood, 1976; Wigzell and Häyry, 1974). The immune mechanisms operating *inside* the allograft have been investigated in much less detail. Only recently has it become possible to isolate the cells infiltrating the allograft in a viable state and to analyze their functions *in vitro*. The major goal of this review is to analyze whether and to what extent the cytotoxic mechanisms operative inside the allograft resemble those detectable in the central lymphatic system of the host.

As with allograft destruction, the role of cytotoxic T cells in controlling tumor growth has been emphasized. Indeed, until recently it was generally conceded that cytotoxic T cells were advantageous to the host, whereas antibodies were thought to be disadvantageous. While several of the immune mechanisms related to systemic activation of the host's immune system toward his own tumor are already known, the events inside the tumor itself are not. This has been an area little explored. Only recently have there been reports on the isolation of various kinds of effector cells from solid tumors, which indicate great variability in host responses to solid tumors detected *in situ* and, frequently, a lack of direct relationship between measurements of systemic immunity and events inside the tumor itself (Haskill *et al.*, 1976a). We have outlined these preliminary findings, which deemphasize the role of cytotoxic T cells *in situ*, and have examined the relationships between systemic and local immunity in a number of clinical and experimental tumor systems.

II. HISTOLOGY OF ALLOGRAFT REJECTION AND HOST RESPONSE AGAINST SOLID TUMORS

A. Histology of Allograft Rejection

Several factors affect the fate of an allograft: genetic relationship between donor and recipient, species, nature of grafted tissue, anatomical position of the graft, and the status of the recipient's immune system. Likewise, the morphological features of rejection in different allografts are variable, even if one considers only the common form of allograft rejection, the acute cellular rejection.

"Mononuclear" cell infiltration is the first microscopic sign during acute rejection of most first-set allografts. For example, upon transplanting a (Lewis X BN)F$_1$ kidney to an unmodified Lewis rat (Guttmann *et al.*, 1967), mononuclear cells appear in the graft parenchyma only 2 days after transplantation. Although frequent attempts have been made, it has been exceedingly difficult to classify the different kinds of mononuclear cells directly from tissue sections. Early descriptions of allograft-infiltrating mononuclear cells examined by ordinary light microscopy (Turk *et al.*, 1966) suggested a considerable polymorphism of the cellular infiltrates. A mixture of macrophages and lymphocytes of various sizes, but very few mature plasma cells, has been found to be present in these infiltrates (Medawar, 1944; Waksman, 1963). Weiner *et al.* (1964) used electron microscopy and demonstrated both lymphocytelike and monocytelike cells in rabbit skin allografts. Monocytes with a high acid phosphatase activity have been reported to dominate the cellular infiltrates of mouse skin allografts 10 days after the transplantation (Poulter *et al.*, 1971).

Attention has also been drawn to proliferating lymphocytic cells and to the large "atypical lymphocytes" or immunoblasts sometimes present in allografts. Pedersen and Morris (1970) in sheep, and Hamburger *et al.* (1971) in man have demonstrated an increased flow of blast cells in the lymph leaving kidney allografts during rejection. We have detected proliferating blast cells in dog kidney allografts (Häyry *et al.*, 1972*b*) and in human kidney allografts (Pasternack *et al.*, 1973) by fine-needle aspiration biopsy combined with autoradiography (Fig. 1). Labeled cells and blast cells appeared in the kidney parenchyma during rejection, and the appearance of these cells often preceded clinical signs of rejection by 1–2 days (Fig. 2). Most of the labeled cells were morphologically blasts, although a fair number of them were also small lymphocytes.

In addition to mononuclear cells, neutrophils and eosinophilic polymorphs have also been found to infiltrate allografts during acute rejection. Kinkaid-Smith *et al.* (1968) described considerable infiltrations of eosinophil leukocytes in human skin allografts.

An entirely different histological picture is seen when a kidney is transplanted to a recipient with preformed allograft-directed antibodies already in the circulation. Here, the allograft destruction takes place rapidly, and the kidney ceases to function in a few minutes or hours. The histological hallmarks of hyperacute rejections are accumulations of polymorphonuclear neutrophils in glomerular and peritubular capillaries and, if the graft is left long enough *in situ*, cortical necrosis (Williams *et al.*, 1968). Concomitantly, antibodies bind to the allograft structures. In biopsies performed 10–20 minutes after transplantation, linear staining for IgG and β_1 C has been demonstrated on the luminar side of the glomerular capillary walls (Milgrom, 1977).

Transplantation of an organ is always followed by synthesis of alloantibodies. It is likely that the antibodies have a role in allograft destruction, both in acute and delayed rejections. Both renal allografts removed due to rejection and

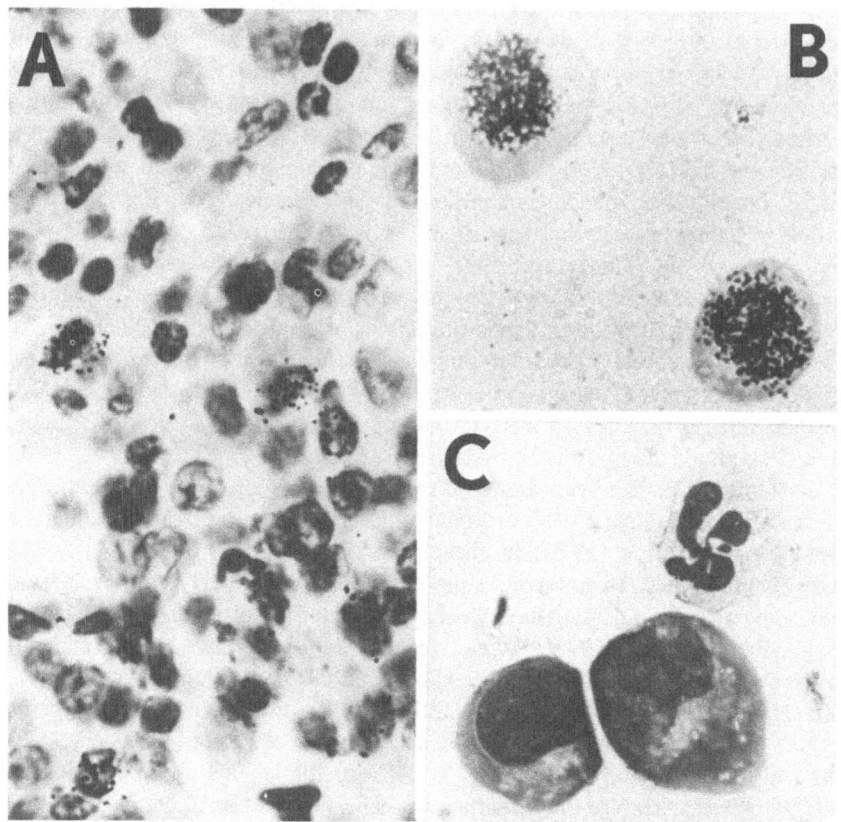

Figure 1. DNA-synthesizing (blast) ce!ls incorporating ³H-thymidine during rejection in the parenchyma of dog kidney (A), labeled (blast) cells isolated from the kidney by fine-needle aspiration biopsy (B), and two blast cells and one polymorphonuclear lymphocyte after MGG staining of the fine-needle biopsy aspirate (C).

apparently well-functioning renal allografts often display immunoglobulin deposits. Andres *et al.* (1970) and others (Rowlands *et al.*, 1970) have used fluorescein- or ferritin-labeled antiantibodies and found both IgG and IgM deposits in human renal allografts. In addition, the complement components C3, C4, and Clq have been detected (Wilson *et al.*, 1974). In some instances, the deposits may be due to recurrence of the original disease or to glomerulonephritis (Churg and Grishman, 1975), whereas in other cases some of these immunoglobulins may, in fact, be true alloantibodies directed to the organ transplant (Andres and McCluskey, 1975; McPhaul *et al.*, 1976). The functional significance of allograft-bound antibodies is discussed below.

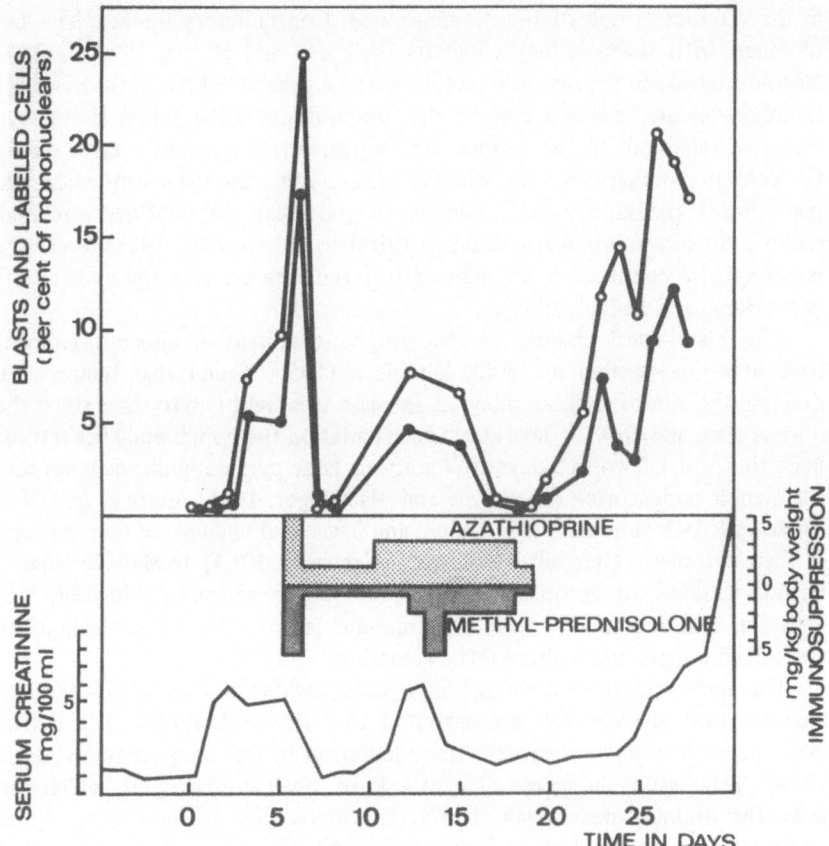

Figure 2. Appearance of blast cells (○) and ^{3}H-thymidine-incorporating cells (●) in dog kidney during three sequential rejection episodes. The rejection was monitored by the level of serum creatinine. The dog was killed on day 30.

B. Changes in the Central Lymphatic System during Allograft Rejection

A skin allograft gives rise to a proliferative reaction in the regional lymph nodes, which later extends to the spleen (Billingham *et al.*, 1954). Other types of allografts, such as kidney grafts, induce a similar reaction (Pedersen and Morris, 1970). The mechanisms of induction depend apparently on the type of graft, especially whether the graft is primarily vascularized or not. Hall (1967) transplanted skin allografts in sheep and found that there was little or no increase in the number of lymphocytes passing up the afferent lymphatic from the graft side, but a predominant increase in the flow of lymphocytes and lymphoblasts in the efferent lymph of the draining node. Contradictory findings have been obtained with sheep kidney allografts (Pedersen and Morris, 1970): a 15- to 20-fold increase in the rate of lymph flow and a substantial rise in the number of lymphocytes are observed even in the lymph draining the kidney during early stages of rejection. In the former case, sensitization apparently takes place in the central lymphatic system, whereas in the latter case the sensitization takes place inside the kidney graft. Kidney allografts can also sensitize a recipient without an intact lymphatic drainage (Strober and Gowans, 1965), even when no lymphatic connections are allowed to regenerate between the graft and the host (Hume and Egdahl, 1955).

The histological changes in the lymphatic system of allograft recipients have been investigated in detail. Mitchison (1955) found that lymph nodes draining the site of a tumor allograft increase in weight two to three times their normal size, and that 20 days after transplantation the lymph node has returned back to normal. Two to 5 days after grafting, large pyraninophilic cells appear in the lymph node cortex (Scothorne and MacGregor, 1955; Andre *et al.*, 1962). These cells lack endoplasmic reticulum and have an abundance of polyribosomes in their cytoplasm (Burwell, 1962; Andre-Schwartz, 1964). In May-Gruenwald-Giemsa staining the cytoplasm is deeply basophilic, and morphologically these cells are indistinguishable from the immunoblasts of graft-versus-host (GVH) and mixed lymphocyte culture (MLC) reactions.

The immunoblasts of draining lymph nodes divide rapidly, and ^{3}H-thymidine incorporation analysis has demonstrated that the peak proliferative activity takes place 6-8 days after skin transplantation in the rat (Tilney and Ford, 1974). This results in increased synthesis of small lymphocytes, which then leave the draining node (Hall, 1967). The blood flow in the regional lymph nodes increases fourfold, more lymphocytes pass from the blood to the lymph, and this further contributes to the increased outflow of lymphocytes from the node (Hay and Hobbs, 1977).

The proliferative response extends to the spleen (Scothorne and MacGregor, 1955). A small increase in the rate of cell division has also been claimed in nondraining lymph nodes (Micklem and Loutit, 1966). It has also been suggested that the response in the spleen takes place later than in the draining lymph nodes. Removal of the regional lymph nodes (Billingham *et al.*, 1954) or splenectomy of the recipient (Krohn and Zuckerman, 1954), however, has no effect on the tempo of skin graft rejection. This is probably due to the wide dispersal of the lymphocyte reaction in the lymphatic system of the recipient.

Although in kidney graft recipients a prominent blast response is seen inside the graft and in the central lymphatic system of the host, the blast response in the blood is usually weak and inconsistent. It is possible to detect a blast response in experimental conditions (Siciu-Foca *et al.*, 1972; Häyry *et al.*,

1972*a*), but a similar blast response has not been detected in human kidney allograft recipients, possibly owing to modification of the response by immunosuppressive therapy. Instead, for some unknown reason, myeloid precursor cells have been found to proliferate in the blood of these patients (Häyry *et al.*, 1972*a*; Dimitriu *et al.*, 1971).

C. Histology and Prognostic Significance of Host Response to Cancer

Although it is evident that the host response is necessary for the rejection of an allograft, it is far from established that the infiltration of host cells into tumor sites has a prognostic significance. Handley (1907) reported that "regressive changes due to inflammation excited by the growth may occur in melanotic sarcoma," and his contemporary, Wade (1908), studying the venerial sarcoma in dogs, concluded "that the tumors disappear by gradual cytolysis associated with the presence of, and probably caused by, lymphocytes and polyblasts." Wade also observed that the local lesion stimulated an inflammatory response "which approximates in its nature to certain of the infected granulomata such as syphilis," MacCarty (1922) reported a threefold increase in postoperative life of both breast and rectum cancer patients provided that lymphocytic infiltration, fibrosis, hyalinization, and cellular differentiation were all present in the primary tumor. Lymphocyte infiltration in the absence of the other factors also provided an extended lifetime, but he concluded that the average length of postoperative survival was greater when all the factors were present. MacCarty and Mahle (1921) suggested that patient survival was more closely related to the degree of lymphoid infiltration in the primary tumor than to the presence or absence of lymphoid metastases. They did not report the presence or absence of histiocytic infiltration in this series of patients.

These original observations went unnoticed for over 30 years, and only recently has this area been reexamined. One of the strongest arguments for an important role of lymphocytic infiltration in the control of tumor growth comes from studies on medullary carcinoma of the breast. Moore and Foote (1949), in a study of 52 medullary carcinomas, found that lymphoid infiltration was extremely common in this tumor and was not associated only with the degenerating or hemorrhagic areas. Despite the fact that these tumors display highly "malignant" cytological features and in general would be expected to have a poor long-term survival rate, the evidence suggests the opposite.

Lauder and Aherne (1972) graded lymphocyte infiltration in 23 primary neuroblastomas. Lymphocyte score correlated well with the survival time, whereas there was no obvious correlation with plasma cell infiltration. In fact, the authors observed an apparent inverse relationship between plasma cell infiltration and survival. The presence of metastases did not invalidate the correlation between lymphocyte score and survival. In a series of 165 patients with malignant melanoma, Cochran (1968) concluded that among the factors relevant to survival were dermal invasion, mitotic rate, and the presence of lymphocytes and plasma cells within the tumor. Once again (MacCarty, 1922), no single factor, including lymphocytic infiltration alone, was considered to be sufficient in controlling tumor growth.

Black's group (Black *et al.*, 1953, 1954, 1975; Black and Speer, 1958) has investigated the role of lymphoid infiltration into primary tumors and histiocytosis in the regional metastic lymph nodes. Postoperative survival in breast cancer patients appeared to be associated not only with the nuclear grade of the tumor but also with the degree of sinus histiocytosis in the draining lymph nodes. They also reported that "in approximately 40% of cases of breast cancer the axillary lymph nodes showed dilation and filling of the sinusoids by proliferation of large histiocytes" (Black *et al.*, 1953). This was associated with an almost universal survival and apparently represented a readily demonstrable expression of host resistance. Black *et al.* (1975) also drew attention to the close association between the sinus histiocytic reactions in the draining nodes and the lymphoid cell infiltrations found in the original primary tumor. According to more classical studies of delayed hypersensitivity, these two factors are interrelated, suggesting a positive role for cellular hypersensitivity in antitumor reactions in the favorably responding cancers (Brightmore *et al.*, 1970). Black's group has also examined a series of gastric carcinomas (Black *et al.*, 1954) and found that superior survival rates were obtained in those operable cases that were associated with lymphocytic infiltration of the primary tumor and/or sinus histiocytosis of the regional lymph nodes. Once again, they found that these criteria appeared to be more important to the survival than age, the microscopic growth pattern of the tumor, duration of postoperative delay, or the presence or absence of regional metastases at the time of surgery.

Conflicting results have been published concerning the role of lymphocytic infiltration in bladder carcinoma. Tanaka *et al.* (1970) reported that the prognosis was similar whether lymphocyte infiltration was present or not. Johansson and Ljungqvist (1974) observed plasma cell and lymphoid infiltration in bladder carcinomas but could not correlate such infiltration with prognosis. On the other hand, Sarma (1972) concluded that not only lymphoid cell infiltration but also epithelial proliferative reactions are important defense reactions against bladder cancer, and that, in general, bladder carcinomas with nonreactive mucosa signify a bad prognosis. Whether the disagreement on the bladder cancer studies refers to staging methods or other methodological problems is unknown.

The role of the humoral immune response in the defense against tumors has been much more controversial. It has not been possible, at least by the methods used, to build a strong case in favor of antibodies. In fact, a number of workers have concluded that the presence of antibody *in situ* is actually an indicator of a bad prognosis. As much of this information has been recently reviewed by Witz (1976), we will not consider the *in situ* antibody here.

D. Histological Studies of *in Situ* Mechanisms of Antitumor Defense

A number of laboratories have used histologic methods in attempts to understand the cellular mechanisms active in tumor growth control. Hanna and co-workers (1972, 1976) have investigated the cellular response to a transplantable guinea pig hepatoma both with and without intralesional inoculation of *Mycobacterium bovis* (BCG). Primary tumors and metastases in the draining lymph nodes could be permanently cured by injection of living BCG into the primary tumors. Histopathology of the regressing tumor and the draining lymph nodes indicated that the mechanism of BCG-induced regression is mediated by a granulomatous reaction both at the tumor site and at the site of the regional lymph node. Light and electron microscopic examination indicated that histiocytes were in frequent contact with tumor cells. The authors also observed that cellular reactions in the regional lymph nodes characteristic of delayed hypersensitivity reactions were not detrimental to tumor growth in the absence of histiocytosis. Thus the presence of a histiocyte infiltrate was favorable to the host.

In the animal model, however, the natural reactivity was insufficient to prolong survival, and BCG injections were required to induce the histiocytosis. That the histiocytes are capable of controlling tumor growth could not be concluded, however, as the authors did not isolate histiocytes from these tumors and demonstrate their activity in any functional growth inhibition or cellular cytotoxicity assay.

Russell and co-workers (1976a) studied the histology of regressor and progressor Moloney sarcomas in BALB/c mice. They observed that in regressing tumors there was a mononuclear infiltrate throughout the tumor and low numbers of mitotic figures per field. In contrast, in progressing tumors the mononuclear infiltrate was localized in the tumor periphery and had a slightly higher number of mitotic figures per field. In the central portion of the tumor, devoid of the mononuclear infiltrate, this figure was sevenfold higher. The authors concluded that there was a correlation between the presence of mononuclear cells and the inhibition of mitosis and therefore growth of the tumor. However, the calculation of mitotic index, a more direct measure of tumor growth, and that of mitotic figures per high-power field agree only if the cellular compositions of the two areas are the same. This is clearly not the case; progressors have one-fifth the proportion of macrophages per gram of tumor. Second, the morphological assessment does not at this stage distinguish among lymphocytes, macrophages, and histiocytes as being responsible for the effect. The authors have suggested the presence of both lymphocyte and macrophage effector cells in these tumors (Russell *et al.*, 1977; Gillespie *et al.*, 1978), and it would be of considerable interest to reexamine these observations with an approach which would permit identification of the different kinds of effector cells and their relationship to the mitotic tumor cells.

Kikuchi *et al.* (1976) have used a histological approach to investigate the cell-mediated immune rejection of a series of autochthonous tumors in rats. They screened 184 methylcholanthrene-induced tumors for resistance to autochthonous transplantation as compared to syngeneic normal host transplantation. They recorded 39 highly antigenic tumors (HAT) (rejected $10^4 - 10^5 : 1$ cells), 72 moderate antigenic tumors (MAT) (rejected $10^2 - 10^3 : 1$ cells), and 73 weakly antigenic tumors (LAT) (rejected $1-10:1$). HAT subcutaneous autografts were characterized by a marked mononuclear cell reaction and destruction of tumor cells, whereas progressive growth of tumor cells and decreased mononuclear cell infiltration was seen in the LAT grafts. The invading mononuclear cells first appeared around small vessels and later extended throughout the tumor. An immunofluorescence study using anti-thymus serum confirmed that the majority of mononuclear cells infiltrating and attached to the grafted tumor cells were T cells. In the LAT, the few mononuclear cells were scattered around the periphery of the tumor. In MAT, the T cells were limited to clusters in the surrounding connective tissue.

Birbeck and Carter (1972) studied infiltration in tissue sections of a metastasizing (ML) and nonmetastasizing line (NML) of hamster lymphoma. The most obvious difference in the histology of the two tumors was related to the presence of highly active macrophages in the NML and nonphagocytic macrophages in the ML. It was concluded that the ability of macrophages to infiltrate the tumor was not the deciding factor; rather, it was the lack of activation of these cells in the ML tumors. Eccles and Alexander (1974a) studied a more extensive series of rat sarcoma lines and also observed an inverse correlation between macrophage content, assessed by phagocytic properties, and metastatic ability. No attempt was made to document the presence of the nonphagocytic macrophages described by Birbeck and Carter (1972).

In addition to animal studies, histological studies have been carried out on melanoma patients following stimulation of the reticuloendothelial system by glucan. Mansell *et al.* (1975) observed that the biopsies showed evidence of tumor necrosis and infiltration by macrophages. Unlike the histiocytic cells described previously (Hanna *et al.*, 1976), these cells were highly vacuolated and "foamy" phagocytic macrophages. The macrophages localized at the interface between viable and dying tissue; polymorphonuclear leukocytes and plasma cells were also present at the tumor tissue. The authors therefore suggested an important role for direct contact between macrophages and tumor cells.

E. Changes in the Central Lymphatic System during Tumor Growth

Numerous investigators have studied the changes that occur in the lymph nodes draining human neoplasms, attempting to relate prognosis and histological appearance in the regional nodes. Although no consistent correlation has been found, sinus histocytosis has been considered by some to be a favorable prognostic sign.

Black and Speer (1958) first showed that survival of patients with breast tumors could be predicted to some degree by the amount of sinus histocytosis in the ipsilateral axillary lymph nodes. Wartman (1959) also observed a positive correlation between sinus histocytosis and survival rates in patients with carcinoma of the breast, although Dire and Lane (1963) failed to find such a relationship. Malicka (1971), like Black, observed that in patients with carcinoma of the larynx, sinus histiocytosis correlated with enhanced survival. In contrast, Bennett *et al.* (1971) did not find the same result.

There have also been attempts to correlate survival with nodal morphological features other than sinus histiocytosis. In 277 patients with breast cancer, Tsakraklides *et al.* (1974) noted that lymphocytic predominance, reflective of an active response by the cells in the thymus-dependent cortex, was common in patients with high survival rates. Lymphocyte depletion was associated with a poor prognosis. The histological appearance of the nodes of patients with intermediate survival times was characterized by either a germinal center predominance pattern (reflective of an active response of the thymus-independent germinal center of the outer cortex) or an unstimulated pattern with no discernible response of the various lymph-node regions. Fisher *et al.* (1976) in a similar study could not detect such a correlation. In studying 84 cases of squamous cell carcinoma of the head and neck, Berlinger *et al.* (1976) noted that both the lymphocyte predominance and germinal center predominance patterns were associated with a significantly greater 5-year survival rate than was the unstimulated pattern. No patient whose nodes demonstrated the depleted pattern survived for 5 years.

Active immune responses also occur during the development of neoplasia in animal models as manifested by changes in the lymphatic organs (Risdall *et al.*, 1973; Konda and Smith, 1973), a common feature being the enlargement of the spleen and draining lymph nodes (Risdall *et al.*, 1973). A marked histiocytic response in the draining lymph nodes in various animal tumors has been documented (Gorer, 1956; Amos, 1960, 1961; Weaver, 1958; Gershon *et al.*, 1967).

Russell and Cochrane (1974) studied popliteal and lumbar nodes draining an MSV-induced sarcoma. Within 14 days of inoculation, the draining nodes were significantly larger than the contralateral nodes. Proliferation of T and B cells was noted, and plasma cells appeared in the medullary cords. Following spontaneous regression of the tumor, the draining nodes diminished in size, although they remained enlarged in animals with progressively growing tumors. Alexander and Hall (1970) have observed similar changes in the draining nodes of rats bearing a syngeneic carcinoma.

In mice inoculated with Lewis lung carcinomas, the spleen increases maximally in size by 12 days after injection. Morphologically, 10–28% of the splenocytes were large lymphoid cells. In contrast to the spleen, the thymus decreased gradually in weight throughout tumor growth, and in some instances had almost disappeared at the time of death. Spleen cells obtained 4-5 days after tumor implantation inhibited tumor growth, whereas cells removed 19–23 days after implantation enhanced tumor growth. This enhancing activity was found at the same time the metastases developed. T lymphocytes apparently were responsible for this enhancing activity, which could be reduced by prior treatment with anti-theta serum and complement (Treves *et al.*, 1976).

Delorme *et al.* (1969) noted the appearance of numerous immunoblasts in the thoracic duct lymph following implantation of irradiated syngeneic sarcoma cells into rats. When viable tumor cells were implanted, the number of thoracic duct lymph immunoblasts increased initially but soon fell to normal levels (Alexander and Hall, 1970).

Lymph node cells from mice bearing large methylcholanthrene induced fibrosarcomas demonstrated elevated levels of spontaneous background nucleic acid synthesis. These lymphocytes proved incapable of further stimulation with tumor antigen *in vitro* but showed normal responses to other antigens (Burk *et al.*, 1976). The results are consistent with the hypothesis that as the tumor increases in size, a larger amount of antigen is shed into the circulation, causing lymphoid cells that were initially reactive to become refractory to further stimulation with the tumor antigen.

Although the vast majority of blastogenic assays in human neoplasia have been done using peripheral blood lymphocytes, Benninghoff and Girardet (1976) reported that thoracic duct lymphocytes from a patient with Hodgkin's disease demonstrated a normal blastogenic response to pokeweed mitogen, whereas the thoracic duct lymphocyte output was significantly diminished.

In summary, the histological observations clearly demonstrate that several types of host cells infiltrate an allograft during rejection. Histological evidence also indicates a potential role for mononuclear cells controlling tumor growth. It is not clear from these studies, however, which of the infiltrating cells function as effector cells, what subclasses of lymphocytes are present, what is the specificity of receptor structures on these cells, or what the role of antibody is in allograft and cancer destruction.

III. EFFECTOR MECHANISMS IN THE CENTRAL LYMPHATIC SYSTEM

A. Cytotoxic T Lymphocytes and Allograft Rejection

Concomitantly with the rejection of an allograft, graft-specific cytotoxic cells appear in the host (Rosenau, 1963; Brunner *et al.*, 1970). The cytotoxic cells can be removed from the sensitized population upon incubation on a target-cell monolayer (Goldstein *et al.*, 1971) or by using relevant antiidiotype sera plus complement (Binz and Wigzell, 1975). In response to a skin allograft, cytotoxic cells are detected in draining lymph nodes after 3-5 days; the peak activity takes place usually 7-8 days after grafting (Canty and Wunderlich, 1971). Cytotoxic cells are usually found in the spleen, but not substantially in the nondraining lymph nodes (Roberts, 1977). The cytotoxic cells disappear from the host 14-21 days after grafting (Canty and Wunderlich, 1971; Roberts, 1977). In secondary response the reappearance of cytotoxic cells is barely distinguishable from the primary response (Biesecker, 1973; Roberts, 1977). The cytotoxic cells disappear from the host much faster than the ability to mount a second-set transplantation rejection against a graft of the primary genetic composition (2-3 weeks as compared to 1 year).

The profile of activation of cytotoxic cells in secondary response is in some respects different from the primary response. Cytotoxic activity, which is nearly missing from the blood in the primary response, is high and biphasic in secondary response (Fig. 3). The first peak of activity takes place when the cytotoxic activity inside the graft is increasing and the second peak when it is declining. It is tempting to postulate that the first activity peak represents mobilization of "memory" cells from the periphery, and the second peak their relocalization from the graft. This postulate is not feasible, however, as very few sensitized cells of the central lymphatic system can be demonstrated during rejection inside the graft (see below).

Most investigators agree that, at least when a difference in the major histo-compatibility complex (MHC) is involved, the cytotoxic cells in the recipient's central lymphatic system, i.e., in the spleen and draining nodes, are T lympho-cytes. Anti-theta serum and complement treatment of the immune cell population eliminates the cytotoxic effect (Cerottini and Brunner, 1974), the cyto-toxic cells are not removed by procedures which eliminate highly adhesive cells or phagocytic cells, and the cytotoxic cells have the electrophoretic mobility of T lymphocytes (Andersson, 1973).

Although these experiments undoubtedly demonstrate that the central cytotoxic cells belong to the T-cell lineage, studies with velocity sedimentation have demonstrated that the cytotoxic T lymphocytes may be morphologically

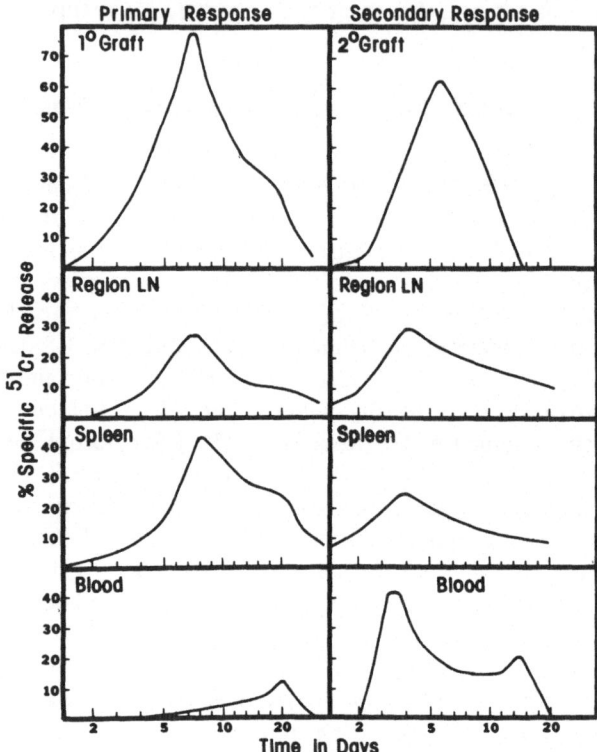

Figure 3. Appearance of killer cells inside the graft, in regional lymph nodes, in spleen, and in blood during the primary and secondary responses of a CBA mouse to DBA/2 sponge matrix allografts. Target cell, P-815; effector-to-target ratio, 25:1; exposure time, 6 hr.

large cells (blasts) or small cells (lymphocytes), depending on the timing of the response. The consistent finding (Andersson, 1973) is that during an early stage of the antiallograft response, the cytotoxic activity is primarily due to large cells (which are morphologically blasts), whereas later during the rejection the cytotoxic activity is mediated by small cells (lymphocytes). As it is known that the histocompatibility-antigen-activated T blasts later revert to small lymphocytes (Häyry, 1976), it seems reasonable to assume that the late small cytotoxic T cells are descendants of the early large cytotoxic T cells.

B. Functions of the Cytotoxic T Lymphocytes

The most simplified view, which is currently largely accepted, is that a cohort of sensitized cytotoxic cells leave the draining lymph nodes and spleen, invade the graft, and destroy it (Billingham *et al.*, 1954). There are two outstanding weaknesses in this idea. Firstly, it is evident that the allograft is infiltrated by several classes of lymphocytic and nonlymphocytic cells, and second, it has been exceedingly difficult to demonstrate relocalization of sensitized lymphocytes inside the graft.

Whether the host's cytotoxic lymphocytes contribute to the allograft-infiltrating cell population has been the subject of several studies (Najarian and Feldman, 1962; Prendergast, 1964; Lance and Cooper, 1972; Tilney and Ford, 1974; Sprent and Miller, 1976). A general agreement from these studies is that if there is any specific accumulation of lymphocytes sensitized to relevant allografts, the difference is small compared to third-party grafts or syngeneic grafts. Sprent and Miller (1976) labeled thoracic duct lymphocytes of a mouse undergoing a GVH reaction with ^{51}Cr or ^{3}H-thymidine and injected these cells into syngeneic recipients carrying either relevant or irrelevant skin grafts. They found that 0.23% of the injected lymphocytes homed into the relevant graft, as compared to 0.14% to an irrelevant graft and 0.08% into a syngeneic skin graft. Although the differences were significant, they were small, and considering that more than 98% of thoracic duct lymphocytes recovered under these conditions have responded in the GVH (and were presumably sensitized to the allograft), these experiments rather demonstrate the lack of substantial accumulation of specifically sensitized host cells to an allograft.

Lymphocytes, especially T lymphocytes, are, however, necessary for allograft rejection. Rodents devoid of the thymus and of T lymphocytes do not reject their allografts (Miller and Osoba, 1967; Wortis, 1971), but allograft rejection is triggered even in the presence of relatively small numbers of immunocompetent T lymphocytes. Extensive thoracic duct drainage (MacGregor and Gowans, 1964) or irradiation lymphopenia (Roser and Ford, 1972) does not substantially impair the rejection of allografts, and transfer of only about 1-2×10^8 lymphocytes to heavily irradiated recipients restores the competence to reject an allograft (Gowans and Knight, 1964). This suggests either that T lymphocytes are necessary only for triggering the response or that there is such a surplus of immunocompetent T lymphocytes that the rejection will take place regardless of the fact that their absolute number is only a fraction of normal.

Both *in vitro* and *in vivo* studies demonstrate that T lymphocytes can also cause an antiallograft response in an autonomous fashion, independent of the presence of other types of lymphoid cells. Cortisone-resistant lymphocytes induce splenomegaly in F_1 hybrid mice (Blomgren and Andersson, 1969), and when the MLC responder lymphocytes are separated to T and B fractions by free-flow cell electrophoresis and stimulated separately, purified T lymphocytes respond, whereas B lymphocytes do not respond (Wigzell and Häyry, 1974). Neither do T lymphocytes recruit B lymphocytes to proliferation during the MLC (Andersson *et al.*, 1973). T lymphocytes induced to proliferation by allogeneic cells produce immunologically specific T killer cells *in vivo* or *in vitro*. Sprent and Miller (1976) demonstrated that P-strain lymphocytes injected to F_1 hybrid recipients and recovered from the thoracic duct express a strong and specific cytotoxicity to the other parental strain target cells *in vitro*, and Häyry and Defendi (1970) documented that cells stimulated to proliferation in the MLC become specifically cytotoxic against target cells of the stimulator strain.

Activated T lymphocytes are probably also important as helper cells in the synthesis of alloantibodies. The IgG alloantibody response seems to be T-cell-dependent. Using congenic mouse strains differing at the *H-2* region only, Klein *et al.* (1974) demonstrated that while normal mice produced hemagglutinating and cytotoxic antibodies of both 2-mercaptoethanol-sensitive (IgM) and 2-mercaptoethanol-resistant (IgG) classes, neonatally thymectomized mice and T-deprived mice produced only 2-mercaptoethanol-sensitive (IgM) antibodies.

C. Central Effector Mechanisms in Antitumor Responses

Both humoral and cellular responses may have important cooperative as well as antagonistic interactions in host responses to growing neoplasms. A number of excellent reviews are available describing the cell types and humoral factors produced in response to neoplasms. We shall only briefly consider these various antitumor mechanisms.

It has generally been accepted that cellular immunity to neoplastic growth, especially thymus-derived lymphocytic cytotoxicity, is primarily responsible for tumor destruction both *in vivo* and *in vitro*. The evidence for this has been reviewed by numerous authors (Herberman, 1973*a,b*, 1974; Herberman *et al.*, 1976; Hellstrom, I., and Helstrom, K. E., 1974; Hellstrom, K. E., and Hellstrom, I., 1974; Henney, 1977; Cerottini and Brunner, 1974; Green and Shevach, 1974). Initial evidence for the role of T lymphocytes in controlling tumor growth came from findings that neonatally thymectomized rodents developed more primary neoplasms following infection with oncogenic viruses or treatment with chemical carcinogens (Wagner and Haughton, 1971; Ting and Law, 1976). As pointed out by Stutman (1975*a*, 1977) in two recent reviews, however, the effects of thymectomy are quite variable depending on the oncogenic agent used. In addition, there have been contradictory reports of the effects of thymectomy on systemic tumor development following treatment with chemical carcinogens (for a review, see Stutman, 1975a, 1977). Some of the contradictory effects of suppression of immunity with antilymphocyte serum treatment in animal models have been summarized by Kripke and Borsos (1974), as well as by Stutman (1975, 1977).

There is little direct evidence that cytotoxic T cells as such are directly responsible for control of existing tumors. There is, however, ample evidence of their capacity to function in transfer experiments. Allison (1972b) found that polyoma-virus-induced tumor growth could be prevented by the adoptive transfer of immune syngeneic lymphocytes, and that pretreatment of these cells with anti-theta serum and complement eliminated the protective effect. Rouse et al. (1972) noted that immune spleen cells pretreated with anti-theta serum and complement could no longer inhibit tumor development of a plasmacytoma in sublethally irradiated mice. Pretreatment of the cells with complement and serum directed against mouse Ig light chains had no effect. Similar results have been obtained by Zarling and Tevethia (1973) with lymphocytes from mice immunized with cells transformed by SV40. In the MSV system LeClerc et al. (1973) and Herberman et al. (1973) demonstrated that the cytotoxic effector cells were inactivated by prior treatment with anti-theta serum and complement. Howell et al. (1974), also using an adoptive transfer assay, found that T cells were necessary to prevent appearance of SV40 tumors.

Non-T cells have also been implicated in cytotoxic reactions against neoplastic cells. Lamon et al. (1972, 1973) reported that splenic non-T cells were responsible for the microcytotoxicity activity 1 week after transfer of MSV. O'Toole et al. (1973) reported that microcytotoxicity effector cells obtained from bladder cancer patients could be removed by passage over an anti-Ig column, suggesting that B cells were the active cell in this system.

The potential role of cells of the reticuloendothelial system in tumor growth cannot be overemphasized. Several reviews discussing the role of the "activated" and "armed" macrophages in tumor-cell destruction have been published recently (Evans, 1976; Henney, 1977; Levy and Wheelock, 1974; Hibbs, 1975; Fink, 1976). The activated macrophage has usually been found to be cytotoxic or cytostatic to a variety of neoplastic cell types. Macrophages from mice previously infected with *Toxoplasma gondii* or those given complete Freund's adjuvant have been shown to have the capacity for nonspecific destruction of a variety of tumor targets (Hibbs et al., 1971, 1972a,b). Macrophages activated *in vivo* by intraperitoneal injection of peptone, RNA, poly(IC), endotoxin, BCG, or lipid A have proved cytotoxic to tumor cells *in vitro* (Alexander and Evans, 1971; Keller, 1973, 1976; Hibbs, 1973; Meltzer et al., 1975).

Kirchner *et al.* (1975*a*,*b*) noted the presence of activated "suppressor" macrophages in the spleens of mice bearing MSV-induced tumors. Such cells inhibited lymphoma cell proliferation and incorporation of ^{3}H-thymidine. These macrophages appear to belong to the same group of cells as those capable of suppressing PHA-induced lymphocyte proliferation.

Evans and Alexander (1971, 1972), Evans (1976), Lohmann-Matthes *et al.* (1972), and Fidler (1976) have shown that macrophages could be activated ("armed") by a factor released from immune lymphocytes. The specificity of tumor cell destruction by these "armed" cells implies that they bear specific recognition sites, which may be cytophilic antibody (Granger and Weiser, 1964) or possible immune complexes. Evans *et al.* (1972) have also suggested that arming may be caused by a soluble T-cell factor, termed "specific macrophage arming factor" (SMAF).

An important aspect of macrophage–tumor interaction is the cytolytic or cytotoxic, as well as growth-inhibitory (cytostatic), effect of macrophages on tumor cell populations (Evans and Alexander, 1970; Boyle and Omerod, 1975; Keller, 1973; Krahenbuhl and Remington, 1974). Macrophage "activation" apparently is the critical process preceding the development of cytostatic ability (Keller, 1973, 1974*a*,*b*, 1975). The biochemical mechanism responsible for this process is undetermined, but the capacity of macrophages to inhibit tumor cell proliferation closely parallels the level of protein synthesis (Keller *et al.*, 1974). Keller (1974*a*) has suggested that since activated nonimmune macrophages can inhibit proliferation of most replicating malignant cells, the macrophage might serve as a homeostatic regulatory cell.

It is interesting to note that Janik (1976) has described changes in mitotic index rather than a lowering of the incorporation of ^{3}H-thymidine to be the most significant indicator of immune regulation in certain animal tumors. It is not known whether macrophages play an important role *in situ* in these model systems.

It has been shown that cell-mediated immunity against some murine tumors occurs naturally (Greenberg and Playfair, 1974; Herberman *et al.*, 1975*a*,*b*; Sendo *et al.*, 1975; Kiessling *et al.*, 1975*a*,*b*; Nunn *et al.*, 1973; Blair *et al.*, 1974). This natural killer (NK) cell appeared to be non-thymus-derived, since it was resistant to treatment with anti-theta and complement, and since athymic mice possess high levels of NK activity (Kiessling *et al.*, 1975*b*; Herberman *et al.*, 1975*b*). The NK cell is not a member of the B-cell series, since Kiessling *et al.* (1975*b*) have shown that depletion of IgG-positive cells enriched NK activity. NK cells lacked IgG or C3 receptors (Kiessling *et al.*, 1976; Herberman *et al.*, 1975*b*), had low levels of FcR (Herberman *et al.*, 1977).

Another potentially important cell-mediated mechanism for tumor cell destruction depends upon both effector cells and antibody. Antibody-dependent cell-mediated cytotoxicity (ADCC) was first described by Moller (1965) as a pathway by which murine fibrosarcoma cells could be lysed *in vitro*. Many different effector cells have been identified, depending on the system studied. A major ADCC effector cell is a non-T, nonphagocytic adherent cell bearing FcR (Allison, 1972a; Greenberg *et al.*, 1973b; Pross *et al.*, 1974; Van Boxel *et al.*, 1972; Harding *et al.*, 1971). Several other cell types have also been shown to carry out ADCC reactions. Thymus-dependent lymphocytes (Fakhri and Hobbs, 1972; Saal *et al.*, 1977; Lamon *et al.*, 1975a), macrophages and poly-morphonuclear leukocytes (Zighelboim *et al.*, 1973; Haskill and Fett, 1976; Gale and Zighelboim, 1974, 1975), B lymphocytes (Lamon *et al.*, 1975a; Zighelboim *et al.*, 1974), and normal thymocytes (Lamon *et al.*, 1975b) have all been implicated in the ADCC reaction. IgG antibody is the predominant immunoglobulin class thought to function in ADCC reactions, although IgM has also been reported to participate (Lamon *et al.*, 1975a,b,c, 1977; Blair *et al.*, 1976). The efficiency of this system may be quite high, as much less anti-body is required for cytotoxicity of this type than for complement-dependent lysis (MacLennan *et al.*, 1969). Inhibition studies using aggregated myel-oma proteins suggest that all IgG subclasses can mediate ADCC (Perlmann *et al.*, 1972; MacLennan *et al.*, 1969).

Antibody can also assist in complement-mediated lysis of tumor cells (Green *et al.*, 1959; Humphrey and Dourmashkin, 1965,1969; for a review, see Nishioka, 1971). Complement-mediated cytotoxicity is primarily significant when IgM is the class of antibody involved, and not all classes of immunoglobulins are capable of triggering complement-dependent lysis (Borsos and Rapp, 1965; Ishizada *et al.*, 1966).

Numerous manifestations of cell-mediated immunity have been attributed to the actions of soluble mediators, called lymphokines (for a review, see Yoshida and Cohen, 1974, 1977). Available evidence does suggest important biological roles for lymphokines, and certain lymphokines (lymphotoxin) can directly kill tumor cells, while others have been shown to initiate, focus, and amplify inflammatory responses.

Immunologic enhancement of tumor growth by humoral factors has been extensively studied (for a review, see Hellstrom and Hellstrom, 1977; Henney, 1977; Baldwin *et al.*, 1976; see also Hellstrom *et al.*, 1971a; Bubenik *et al.*, 1970; deVries *et al.*, 1972; Byrne *et al.*, 1973; Levy, 1973). Enhancement can act in any of the three limbs of the immune response. In the afferent limb the humoral factor prevents the host's immunization by the tumor antigen; in the efferent limb the tumor antigens are masked to prevent destruction by the host immune system; and in the central limb humoral factors suppress the host immune cells, preventing destruction of the neoplasm. Humoral blocking factors have been described in experimental animal systems and also in the sera of patients with a variety of tumors. Blocking can be due to any of the following: (1) antibodies, (2) antibody–antigen complexes, or (3) soluble antigen alone

(Hellstrom, K. E., and Hellstrom, I., 1974; Baldwin *et al.*, 1976; Thompson *et al.*, 1973; Brawn, 1971; Nepom *et al.*, 1976; Currie and Basham, 1973; Baldwin *et al.*, 1972). In addition to blocking factors, other factors, termed "unblocking," have been reported. Serum obtained from mice after regression of MSV-induced sarcomas was found to abrogate the effects of blocking sera (Hellstrom and Hellstrom, 1970; Hellstrom, K. E., and Hellstrom, I., 1974). Similarly, sera from patients following tumor removal were found to possess unblocking activity (Hellstrom *et al.*, 1971 *b*). The evidence suggests that such material can be either antigen or antibody directed against the respective tumor antigen.

The strong T-cell dependency of both allograft rejection and host resistance to transplantable tumors is well established. Although it is often possible to arm primarily noncommitted blood mononuclear cells to carry out ADCC against allogeneic target cells, the predominant allograft-directed killer cell in the central lymphatic system seems to be a T lymphocyte. Both cytotoxic T lymphocytes and non-T lymphocytic or moncytic cells, including the so-called "natural killer cells" with specificity to cultured tumor cells, have been demonstrated in the circulation or in the central lymphatic system of tumor-bearing hosts. These studies, however, do not demonstrate whether and to what extent these cellular elements participate in actual rejection of the allograft or control of tumor growth. To answer this question it is necessary to analyze the types of cells and antibodies present in allografts and tumors *in situ* and to elucidate their functions.

IV. ISOLATION OF INFILTRATING CELLS AND ANTIBODIES FROM ALLOGRAFTS AND TUMORS

It has been rather difficult to isolate allograft-infiltrating cells in a functionally viable state. The greatest success has been in isolating the cells from conventional allografts, such as skin grafts. Jakobisiak and co-workers (1971) exchanged subpannicular skin grafts 10 mm in diameter between histoincompatible mouse strains. They dissected the graft separate from the graft bed, scraped away loose tissue from the graft dermis, and finally treated the material with trypsin and collagenase. A total of 1–2.5×10^6 cells were recovered from a 10-day allograft with excellent viability. The use of proteolytic enzymes in the recovery of the cells may, of course, destroy their surface receptors and can make it difficult (or impossible) to use such cells in functional assays and for classification of the lymphocyte subclass.

Tilney *et al.* (1975, 1976) isolated infiltrating cells from rat cardiac allografts, and Strom *et al.* (1975) from human kidney allografts. An excellent yield of infiltrating cells (160×10^6 cells per gram of myocardium on day 7 after transplantation) was found when proteolytic enzymes were applied to the cardiac allografts. Much smaller recoveries, only $0.1-1 \times 10^6$ viable cells per gram of tissue, were obtained by mechanical dissection and DNase, and the procedure also required a one-step density centrifugation over Ficoll–Isopaque. Eight to 12 cardiac allografts transplanted on two consecutive days had, therefore, to be pooled to obtain adequate numbers of cells for a single determination. This method, however, gave ample numbers of infiltrating cells from human kidney allografts.

It is also possible to recover a sample of allograft-infiltrating cells by fine-needle aspiration biopsy. The method is especially applicable to repeated assays in human patients. A thin needle, 0.8 mm in external diameter, is inserted directly into the organ parenchyma, and a sample of 10–20-μl volume is pulled from the parenchyma by suction. In over 1000 biopsies performed from human kidney allografts at the University of Helsinki Hospital, not a single serious complication has taken place.

Tumor allografts may also be used in the analysis of the allograft-infiltrating cells. The large size of some tumor cells (e.g., 1699 mouse carcinoma) makes it possible to separate them from the infiltrating cells by unit gravity velocity sedimentation (Haskill *et al.*, 1975*a,b*).

In order to produce large numbers of infiltrating cells for experimentation we have developed the so-called "sponge matrix" allograft method (Roberts and Häyry, 1976*b*). A spongy matrix tissue (in our case a viscous cellulose sponge $3 \times 3 \times 3$ mm) is infiltrated by strain-X fibroblasts, and the sponge is placed subcutaneously into the neck of strain-Y mice. The sponge behaves as an allograft and generates an alloimmune response. Cytotoxic cells appear in the draining lymph node and in the spleen of the recipient, and the sponge is quickly infiltrated by the host cells. Compression of the sponge then liberates practically all infiltrating cells. Centrifugation over a one-step 35% BSA "gradient" removes dead cells and all tissue debris from the sample but leaves behind more than 90% of the original viable graft-infiltrating cells. This method allows us to produce approximately 3×10^6 infiltrating cells from a single mouse with a minimal experimental effort.

Analysis of cells infiltrating solid tumors has been facilitated by the use of combinations of enzymes to disperse the various cell types. Recovery of cells can be quite high, and the majority of cell markers and receptors can be left at detectable levels. Russell *et al.* (1976*b*) have carried out an exhaustive study of this problem and have concluded that enzymatic digestion with collagenase and trypsin provides the most convenient and efficient way to break down relatively firm tumors such as the Moloney sarcoma. Cell yields using trypsin collagenase and DNase were as high as 50% (measured as DNA recovered in cell suspensions). This general approach has been utilized by most workers as the most efficient way to obtain single-cell suspensions of tumor-infiltrating cells.

V. IDENTIFICATION OF INFILTRATING CELLS IN ALLOGRAFTS AND TUMORS

A. Composition of Cellular Infiltrates in Allografts

Jakobisiak (1971) has performed differential counts on the various white cell types infiltrating a mouse skin graft during rejection. On day 10 after transplantation, the largest cell population was macrophage (41%) and the second largest was lymphocyte (24%). Neutrophils were also present in considerable numbers (13%), as were mononuclear cells with "deeply basophilic and pyraninophilic cytoplasm" (15%). The last cell population was considered to be similar to the "graft rejection cells" defined by electron microscopy in rabbit skin grafts by Weiner *et al.* (1964). Very few mature plasma cells, classical blast cells, or mast cells were seen in the infiltrates. The lymphocytes, basophilic cells, and macrophages appeared in the allografts between days 4 and 6; the neutrophils appeared slightly later.

Identification of subclasses of mononuclear cells, especially subclasses of lymphocytes, is extremely difficult to perform from tissue sections. Balch *et al.* (1973) used fluoresceinated antisera to rat thymocytes and demonstrated abundant numbers of T lymphocytes in early Lewis renal allografts in BN rats, and similar findings were reported by Billingham *et al.* (1976); however, no numerical quantitation was possible from these preparations.

A detailed classification of mononuclear cell subtypes in rat heart allografts was performed by Tilney *et al.* (1975). Four to 5 days after transplantation, 41% of the cells infiltrating a heart allograft carried detectable amounts of surface Ig, and 45% of them had the Fc receptor on their surface. Macrophages were present in significant numbers both in early (3-4 day) and late (5-6 day) allografts (27% and 17%, respectively). Notable was the nearly complete absence of complement receptor-carrying lymphocytes in the allograft infiltrates.

A similar study was performed using cellular infiltrates of human kidney allografts removed due to rejection (Strom *et al.*, 1975, 1978). In this case, 75-90% of the cells recovered at the Ficoll–Isopaque interphase were lymphocytes, with only 1-10% neutrophils. Lymphocytes expressing surface Ig (B lymphocytes) ranged from 18 to 73% in 10 individual infiltrates. E-rosette-forming cells (T lymphocytes were present in most cases in significant numbers (36-72%). In three separate determinations, EA-rosette-forming (Fc receptor-carrying) cells were found in 7-47%. This corresponds well to the percent of cells binding aggregated Ig on their surface (8-53%).

We have performed a detailed analysis of cells infiltrating a 3 X 3 X 3 mm sponge matrix allograft during peak of rejection (day 8) and compared the infiltrates with those from a syngeneic graft and from a sponge alone (Roberts and Häyry, 1977). As seen in Table I, the recovery of infiltrating cells from an allograft was approximately tenfold that of a syngeneic graft. The largest single-cell population infiltrating the allograft was lymphocytes. Monocytes and granulocytes were also present in significantly elevated numbers, as were blast cells, which were completely lacking from the controls.

In accordance with morphological evidence suggesting the presence of monocytes, macrophages, and (some) granulocytes among the sponge matrix allograft-infiltrating cells, ample numbers of phagocytic cells have been documented in these infiltrates. Of the host cells infiltrating DA sponge grafts in Lewis rats, 45% ingested latex particles (Binz et al., 1976), and approximately 30% of the cells infiltrating DBA/2 sponge grafts in CBA mice ingested heat-killed particles of baker's yeast (unpublished). Several of the infiltrating cells also expressed the FcR on their surface. In conditions where 15% of CBA spleen cells formed rosettes with sheep erythrocytes coated lightly with anti-SRBC IgG, nearly 38% of allograft-infiltrating cells were rosette-forming (Roberts and Häyry, 1977). When the graft-infiltrating lymphocytic cells (after removal of phagocytic cells with yeast phagocytosis and centrifugation over 35% BSA) were treated with anti-brain T-cell serum and complement, only one-third of the graft-infiltrating cells were lysed, as compared with 70% in the draining lymph node and 50% in the spleen.

Table I. Cellular Infiltrates from Allogeneic and Syngeneic Sponge Matrix Grafts and from Control Sponges 7 Days after Subcutaneous Transplantation to the Neck

| Type of graft | Cells per graft X 10^{6} [a] | | | | |
	Blasts	Lymphocytes	Granulocytes	Monocytes/ macrophages	Total
Allogeneic	0.94 ± 0.41	3.12 ± 1.08	1.59 ± 0.36	1.40 ± 0.55	7.04 ± 1.24
Syngeneic	0.0	0.056 ± 0.019	0.461 ± 0.248	0.283 ± 0.020	0.80 ± 0.23
Sponge alone	0.0	0.068 ± 0.028	0.151 ± 0.040	0.031 ± 0.016	0.25 ± 0.08

[a]Mean ± S.D. for triplicate determinations. The infiltrating cells were released by compression, differential cell counts of viable cells were performed from MGG-stained cytocentrifuged cell smears, and the actual number of different types of cells per 3 X 3 X 3 mm graft were calculated on the basis of viable cell counts. [From P. J. Roberts and P. Häyry, Cell. Immunol. 26:160–167 (1976), by courtesy of the publisher.]

B. Receptor Specificity of Allograft-Infiltrating Cells

Development of anti-idiotypic antisera presumably directed to the antigen-recognizing part of alloantibody or T-lymphocyte receptor(s) (Binz *et al.*, 1974; Binz and Wigzell, 1975) has enabled direct visualization of the cell receptor idiotype in the rat system. Such visualization is achieved by the use of the specific antiidiotypic antibodies selectively reacting with B and T lymphocytes carrying idiotypic receptors, signifying reactivity against a certain alloantigen.

In order to quantitate the number of cells infiltrating an allograft and carrying the relevant idiotypic receptors against the graft antigens, we transplanted DA, Lewis, or BN sponge matrix allografts to Lewis or DA rats (Binz *et al.*, 1976). The recipients were killed 7 or 8 days later, and their grafts and draining and nondraining lymph nodes and spleen were removed. The percentages of cells displaying idiotypic receptors fo Lewis anti-DA specificity in the various cell populations were analyzed using FITC-conjugated anti-(anti-DA)-IgG antibodies. Some of the results are shown in Table II. A low "background noise" staining was observed in the control DA rats (highest percentage "positive" cells being 1.3% in the most macrophage-rich population). In normal Lewis rats, 4.5% of the lymph node cells and 5.2% of the spleen cells carried receptors to DA alloantigens. In Lewis rats which had received DA allografts, the number of DA-directed cells was elevated both in draining lymph nodes and in the spleen (25.1% and 9.1%, respectively). Still higher percentages (56%) of DA-directed cells were observed inside the allograft. Normal levels of DA-directed cells were

Table II. Expression of Anti-DA Idiotypic Receptors on Graft-Infiltrating Cells, Cells from Draining and Nondraining Lymph Nodes, and Spleen Cells 7 Days after Grafting of a Syngeneic or Allogeneic Sponge Matrix Graft

Animal	Source of cells[a]			
	Graft	Draining lymph nodes	Nondraining lymph nodes	Spleen
Lewis-carrying DA graft	56.0	25.1	4.51	9.1
DA-carrying Lewis graft	1.3	0.7	0.0	0.1
Lewis-carrying Lewis graft	2.0	5.8	5.0	4.9
Lewis-carrying BN graft	3.9	7.5	5.4	5.7
Normal Lewis rat	ND	ND	4.5	5.2
Normal DA rat	ND	ND	0.1	0.2

[a]Figures refer to the percentages of cells stained by direct immunofluorescence with FITC-conjugated anti-(anti-DA)-antiserum. ND, not done.

found within a BN allograft transplanted into a Lewis rat, and in the central lymphatic system of BN graft recipients.

As demonstrated above, T lymphocytes make up at most only 30% of the cells infiltrating a sponge matrix allograft 7–8 days after transplantation. The fact that more than 55% of the infiltrating cells carry relevant idiotypic receptors to the graft antigens suggests that some of these cells are non-T (B) lymphocytes and monocytes. Macrophages equipped with anti-DA receptors were also directly demonstrated by simultaneous visualization of the receptor structure and *in vitro* ingested Latex particles inside the cell (Binz *et al.*, 1976).

C. Immunological Analysis of Tumor-Infiltrating Cells from Histological Sections of Solid Tumors

In the previous section we described histological evidence suggesting a relationship between host inflammatory cells and the control of tumor growth. The purpose of this section is to subdivide these inflammatory cells into categories with the aid of immunological tests.

It has been possible to use rosette techniques employing IgG-coated erythrocytes or IgM- and complement-coated erythrocytes to detect FcR and C′3 receptor-carrying cell populations within frozen sections of tumors. Melgrom *et al.* (1968) observed antibody-mediated opsonic absorption of erythrocytes to tumor sections, and concluded that the binding was mediated by cytophilic antibodies with an affinity for tumor cells. The authors could not distinguish whether absorption was due to the malignant cells, inflammatory cells, or both. Tønder *et al.* (1974) continued this approach and concluded that there were receptors for sensitized erythrocytes on tumor cells, similar to the Fc receptors present on lymphocytes and monocytes. Roubin *et al.* (1975) have attempted to characterize the mononuclear cell infiltrates in human malignant melanoma. Nonphagocytic mononuclear cells represented a major component of the infiltrate. When these cells were in contact with a malignant melanocyte, the tumor cell underwent ultrastructural changes. Using rosette techniques and frozen sections, the authors demonstrated that in 3 of the 10 cases EA-IgG rosette-forming cells were identified inside the tumor. These cells showed morphologic similarities to a subpopulation of cells in the blood that were capable of acting in the ADCC effector assay *in vitro*.

Edelson *et al.* (1975) devised methods for differentiating between B cells, T cells, and histiocytes in frozen sections of melanotic lesions, primary and metastatic melanoma, and halo and giant pigmented nevi. A spectrum of cellular subtypes was detected. Although the techniques involved did not permit the identification of T lymphocytes *in situ*, disruption of the tumors and rosetting with uncoated sheep erythrocytes provided evidence that at least two of the six primary melanomas contained viable infiltrating T lymphocytes. The authors also observed that most of the cells infiltrating the metastatic sites were histiocytes, as detected by ultrastructural appearance and the presence of the Fc receptor on their surface. Of more interest was that in six primary melanomas, as well as in six halo nevi, the majority of infiltrating cells lacked the complement receptors characteristic of histiocytes. Some of these cells were presumably T lymphocytes. Focal aggregates of B lymphocytes and plasma cells were identified in sections of a giant pigmented nevus. The authors concluded that the type of infiltrating cell is probably related to the type of lesion. Husby *et al.* (1976) used immunofluorescence to study the T and B lymphocytes infiltrating primary and metastatic tumors. The majority of these tumors were carcinomas of epithelial origin arising in a variety of anatomic sites. The authors observed lymphocytic infiltration in 24 of 29 primary tumors and 5 of 8 metastatic lesions. T lymphocytes predominated in the infiltrate of primary tumors, the average value being 80%. In contrast, B cells identified using anti-Fab$_2$ reagent were identified at the margins of 2 of 5 tumor metastases. Mononuclear cells bearing Fc receptors were not readily identified in either primary tumors or metastases.

Interest and controversy have recently centered around the origin and characterization of Fc receptor (FcR)-bearing cells in solid tumors. Cohen *et al.* (1971) reported that disaggregated transmissible dog venereal tumor cells bound antibody-coated erythrocytes, and concluded that the reacting cells were probably tumor cells and not phagocytic cells. Although up to 30% of the cells in the suspension had adherence characteristics, these authors considered it improbable that such a high percentage of nontumor cells could be present. Such a finding is by no means uncommon. Studies by Evans (1972, 1976) indicate that many tumors contain high percentages of macrophages. Kerbel *et al.* (1975) and Kerbel and Pross (1977) have described FcR-positive cells in a wide variety of experimental tumors as being of host origin. Most of the FcR-positive cells were capable of ingesting the antibody-coated erythrocytes used in the Fc receptor assay. Based on data derived from transplantation studies using F$_1$ hybrid recipients and alloantisera, the authors concluded that the FcR assay was a reliable marker for quantitating the host lymphoreticular infiltration of solid tumors. Moore and Moore (1977) have also provided evidence that most infiltrating cells are of host rather than tumor origin. Szymaniec and James (1976) demonstrated the presence of high levels of FcR-bearing cells of both phagocytic and nonphagocytic varieties in a murine fibrosarcoma.

There is evidence that not only inflammatory cells but also some tumor cells may express Fc receptors. Although Tønder *et al.* (1974, 1976) and Husby *et al.* (1976) have described the presence of FcR on tumor cells, these authors have not proved that the FcR-positive cells were of malignant origin. Until this is done, the available evidence supports the FcR assay as a valid measure of host lymphoreticular infiltration.

Table III. Cellular Composition of the "Host Fraction"[a]

Spontaneous tumor number	% Theta-positive	% Forming EA rosettes	% Bearing surface Ig	% Phagocytic for latex
22	16	15	<1	10
26	4.5	46	<1	ND
33	30	24	<1	15
38	45	8.5	<1	13

[a]Host fraction cells were isolated by collagenase dispersion and sedimentation velocity fractionation as described previously (Haskill *et al.*, 1975). C3H spontaneous mammary tumors were used between the third and sixth passages.

Attempts have been made to identify B cells in dispersed tumor-cell suspensions. Richters and Kaspersky (1975) investigated the presence of surface immunoglobulin positive lymphocytes in 10 primary human breast cancer patients. Five of the cancers contained no positive cells, and in the other five both IgG- and IgM-positive lymphocytes were found in variable proportions.

Thymus-derived lymphocytes have also been identified in certain melanotic lesions following dispersion of the cells (Edelson *et al.*, 1975), and Jondal *et al.* (1975) have identified T cells in biopsies of Burkitt's lymphoma. In the MSV tumor system, Plata *et al.* (1975) have observed both T and B lymphocytes infiltrating the tumors. The results, however, show a far higher percentage of B lymphocytes than that reported by Holden *et al.* (1976) in a similar tumor system. As the method of isolation of the cells (mechanical vs. enzymatic) was different, it is possible that the result simply reflects an increased survival of B-cell populations. Pross and Kerbel (1976) observed a wide variation in the percentages of phagocytic cells and T cells in original and early passages of methylcholanthrene-induced tumors. Haskill *et al.* (1975*b*) performed a similar study for T cells and FcR-positive cells in a series of spontaneous mammary adenocarcinomas in C3H mice, and also observed significant variations in the relative proportions of T lymphocytes and FcR-positive cells (Table III).

VI. EFFECTOR MECHANISMS INSIDE ALLOGRAFTS AND TUMORS

A. Functional Analysis of the Allograft-Infiltrating Cells

Histological and cytological studies represent, at their best, only a static point in the series of dynamic changes taking place inside the allograft during rejection. The allograft-infiltrating cells have recently been isolated and functionally characterized *in vitro*. During the past five years a substantial armamentarium of methods has been developed for these purposes [for details the reader is referred to review articles by, e.g., Cerottini and Brunner (1974), Wigzell and Häyry (1974).]

Treatment with anti-Ig plus complement did not remove the cytotoxic activity of cells infiltrating rat cardiac allografts (Tilney *et al.*, 1975). The cytotoxic activity was also resistant to 10 mg/ml trypsin. Treatment of the effector cells with anti-brain T serum plus complement almost completely destroyed direct target cell lysis (Strom *et al.*, 1978). Cells nonadherent to nylon wool were also more effective than adherent cells in producing the target lysis. On this basis it was concluded that the predominant killer cell inside rat cardiac allografts is a T lymphocyte. In addition to T lymphocytes, the cardiac allograft also contains cells capable of mounting an ADCC type of cytotoxicity against alloantibody-coated cells. ADCC could not be demonstrated with fresh cells, but was found following overnight recovery of the effector cells. Although FcR-carrying T lymphocytes can also perform ADCC (Kimura *et al.*, 1977), it is conceivable to conclude that at least two types of effector cells reside inside rat cardiac allografts.

When cells infiltrating human renal allografts were similarly studied, different results were obtained (Strom *et al.*, 1975). In three out of four cases, E-rosette depletion did not substantially reduce the lytic activity. In the fourth case E-rosette depletion abolished the lytic activity. Adherence of effector cells to glass beads did not reduce lytic activity, demonstrating that most of the killer cells infiltrating human kidney allograft were nonadherent. Although (nonadherent) monocytes also bear the FcR (Wigzell and Häyry, 1974), this suggested to the authors that most of the killer cells inside a human kidney allograft are B lymphocytes.

We have fractionated the sponge matrix allograft-infiltrating cells by density centrifugation, unit-gravity velocity sedimentation, and preparative free-flow cell electrophoresis, and have treated the infiltrating cells with anti-T-cell serum plus complement (Roberts and Häyry, 1977). In both velocity sedimentation and density centrifugation the lytic activity distributed over a wide range, suggesting that several cell classes are active. When monocytic cells were then separated from the nonmonocytic cells via yeast particle phagocytosis or via the high-affinity Fc receptor combined with unit-gravity velocity sedimentation, both the monocytic and the nonmonocytic cells were lytic to relevant target cells (Roberts and Häyry, 1977). When the nonphagocytic cell fractions (consisting of more than 95% lymphocytes) were fractionated in free-flow cell electrophoresis, the predominant lytic activity of the graft-infiltrating lymphocytic cells was confined to the B area of the electrophoretic profile (Fig. 4). Only one-third of the activity resided in the T area, although most, if not all, of the lymph-node lymphocytes of the same recipient mice displayed lytic activity in the T-cell peak only. This finding was confirmed by treatment of the lympho-

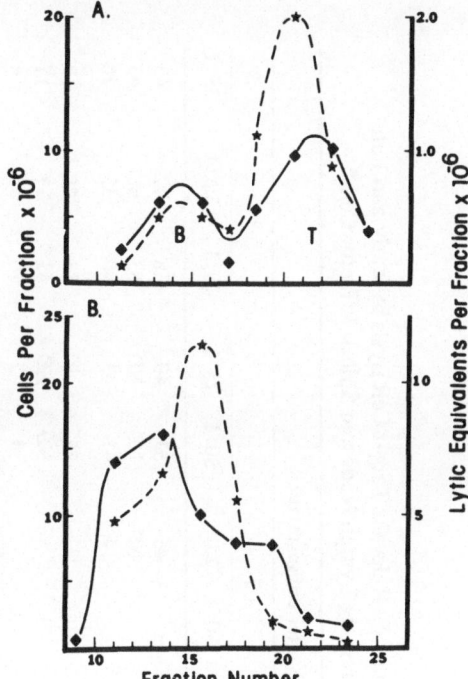

Figure 4. Electrophoretic fractionation of immune lymph node cells (A) and graft-infiltrating cells (B) 8 days after transplantation of a DBA/2 sponge matrix allograft to a CBA mouse. Solid lines: distribution of cells (in lymph nodes the B and T areas of the electrophoretic profile are indicated). Dashed lines: distribution of cytotoxic activity. Target cell, P-815; exposure time, 6 hr; effector-to-target ratio, 25:1.1

cytic effector cells with anti-brain T serum plus complement. The treatment with anti-T plus complement completely abolished the lytic activity of the allograft-infiltrating cells. We therefore concluded that in sponge matrix allografts both lymphocytic and nonlymphocytic (i.e., monocytic) cells can perform target lysis, and that B lymphocytes are more active than T lymphocytes in this respect.

Although it has been almost universally accepted that the main effector cell in the central lymphatic system of alloimmune mice or rats is the T lymphocyte (or blast), it seems that several types of effector cells are active inside an allograft during rejection. The comparisons between rat heart, human kidney, and mouse sponge matrix allografts also suggest that different effector mechanisms are operative in the different types of grafts. It is also possible that different effector mechanisms are operative inside a given type of graft, depending on the timing of the antiallograft response. We investigated this possibility by treating the sponge matrix allograft-infiltrating cells with anti-brain T-cell serum plus complement at different times after transplantation. The results of these preliminary studies are shown in Table IV. Shortly after transplantation most of the lytic effect was removed by the antiserum treatment, whereas when the rejection

Table IV. Effect of Anti-T Serum Plus Complement on Relevant Target-Cell Lysis by Early and Late Allograft-Infiltrating Effector Cells and by Draining Lymph Node and Spleen Effector Cells[a]

Source of effector cells	Treatment	Days after transplantation[b]									
		4		6	7		8		8		9
		25:1	12.5:1	50:1	50:1	25:1	50:1	25:1	25:1	12.5:1	25:1
Graft	None	18	5	38		45	51	49	58	42	43
	NS + C	17	7	ND		ND	ND	ND	83	68	43
	Anti-T + C'	-1	-1	3		14	41	43	40	32	40
Draining lymph node	None	36	11	55	25		26	9	43	28	19
	NS + C'	38	ND	ND	21		ND	ND	63	37	17
	Anti-T + C'	1	3	0	0		4	2	10	5	4
Spleen	None	15	8	17	18	5	56	34	28	17	28
	NS + C'	ND	ND	ND	18	7	ND	ND	54	24	29
	Anti-T + C'	1	1	0	7	5	3	2	-1	-2	-2
Syngeneic graft	None	-2	ND	0	ND		ND		-5	-2	-2
Syngeneic spleen	None	-2	ND	0	ND		ND		3	-2	-2

[a] Transplantation, DBA/2 SMG to CBA. Controls, CBA SMG to CBA.
[b] Specific ^{51}Cr release from DBA/2 P-815 target cells, exposure time 6–10 hr. ND, not done.

process proceeded, the allograft-infiltrating effector cells became notably more resistant. The effector cells in the spleen and in the draining node were sensitive to anti-T cell serum plus complement throughout the response.

There is currently no evidence suggesting that non-T (or "B") lymphocytes or monocytes/macrophages are able to function as specific killer cells via their own receptor, synthetized by these cells themselves. There are, however, several pathways, documented mainly by *in vitro* experiments, by which antigen-specific T or B cells can "instruct" or "arm" primarily noncommitted non-T lymphocytes, monocytes, and macrophages to become specifically cytotoxic killer cells. Evans *et al.* (1972) have shown that peritoneal macrophages from nonimmune mice become specifically cytotoxic to allogeneic cells after incubation with either immune T cells or supernatants from cultures containing sensitized T lymphocytes plus specific target cells. The factor appearing in the supernatants has been called "specific macrophage arming factor." Perlmann *et al.* (1972) and MacLennan (1972) have described *in vitro* arming of noncommitted lymphocytic and monocytic ("K") cells to specific killer cells via antibody attached to the target cells. The arming antibody seems to belong to the IgG class, and the different K effector cells, whether monocytes or lymphocytes, have somewhat different affinities to different subclasses of IgG (Wigzell and Häyry, 1974). As the antibody-dependent arming of noncommitted cells has also been amply demonstrated to take place in histocompatibility systems *in vitro*, we consider it possible that the graft-infiltrating non-T lymphocytic and monocytic cells demonstrating proper idiotypic specificity have been armed by mechanisms such as these. As the "K"-cell activity is not readily demonstrable in the central lymphatic system, it is possible that the "arming" takes place inside the allograft via *in situ* alloantibody.

B. Role of Antibody in Allograft Destruction

The evident role of preformed alloantibody in the hyperacute rejection of an allograft is well established (Milgrom, 1977) and will not be discussed here. Instead, we will attempt to analyze the role of the often-encountered immunoglobulin and complement deposits (Andres *et al.*, 1970; Rowlands *et al.*, 1970) in acute rejection, delayed rejection, or possibly in the protection of the organ transplant from rejection.

Both IgG and IgM deposits (Andres *et al.*, 1970), and C3-4 and C'lq have been demonstrated in renal allografts, but the mere presence of the antibody and complement components does not correlate with the outcome of the transplant. It is, therefore, plausible to assume that allograft-infiltrating antibodies are not always harmful to the graft, and sometimes may in fact be protective.

Two approaches have been used to elucidate the role of antibodies in allograft rejection: the antibodies have been eluted from the graft, or the allograft recipient has been perfused with antibody in order to induce graft rejection. Finally, the presence or absence of antibody in the circulation has been correlated with graft prognosis. In all these studies it is naturally important to resolve both the class and receptor specificity of the antibody involved.

The frequent formation of rheumatoid factor by most human renal allograft recipients has been described (Kano and Milgrom, 1969). Some of the immunoglobin deposits in, e.g., kidney allografts are probably immune complexes, especially as circulating immune complexes have been demonstrated in kidney allograft recipients (Milgrom, 1977). In cases where the glomerular lesions resemble immune complex nephritis, the recurrence of the original disease may be involved.

On other occasions, however, the immunoglobulin deposits may represent true alloantibodies directed to the histocompatibility antigens of the allograft. Alloantibodies appear in the circulation promptly after rejection or surgical removal of the graft (Williams *et al.*, 1968). Alloantibodies have also been eluted from several allografts after surgical removal, as well as from grafts with excellent function (Kano and Milgrom, 1969).

Little is known of the functions of the various classes of alloantibodies in allograft rejection or protection. Voisin *et al.* (1969) analyzed anti-H2 alloantibodies in hyperimmune mouse sera. No biological effects could be demonstrated to IgM alloantibodies; IgG_1 and IgG_2 caused direct hemagglutination reactions; IgG_2 alloantibodies were active in complement-dependent cytotoxicity; and enhancing ability was mainly confined to IgG_1. Harris and Harris (1973) also found IgG_2 alloantibodies to be active in complement-dependent cytotoxicity, whereas Takasugi and Klein (1971) found both IgG_1 and IgG_2 alloantibodies to enhance the growth of CBA tumors in A.SW mice.

It is not known either how or to what extent complement-dependent cytotoxic effects are responsible for allograft destruction (Fearon *et al.*, 1977). Renal graft recipients with clinically recognized rejection episodes have unstable serum levels of C4 and C3 (Carpenter *et al.*, 1969), and uncontrollable rejection may lead to persistent depression of C2 and C3 (Austen *et al.*, 1966; Carpenter *et al.*, 1967). Consumption rather than depression of complement production is anticipated, as deposits of C3 and C1q appear concomitantly in the renal allograft (Andres *et al.*, 1970).

Antibody may also trigger cell-mediated cytotoxicity via ADCC activation of primarily noncommitted cells to specific killer cells (Perlmann *et al.*, 1972). That an alloantibody can perform a similar activation event *in vivo* has been elegantly demonstrated by Johnson *et al.* (1977), who isolated IgG_1 alloantibody from hyperimmune B6 serum immunized with 6 C3HED lymphoma. The IgG_1 was suppressive to the tumor growth both in allogeneic (B6) and syngeneic

(C3H) recipients, and the suppressive activity was thermostable. The effect was not demonstrable in lethally irradiated mice, but was restored by simultaneous infusion of platelets or macrophages (but not lymphocytes). On the average, $5-13 \times 10^4$ alloantibody molecules were necessary per tumor cell for 50% suppression of syngeneic tumor growth.

It is also possible that all alloantibodies directed to the MHC antigens are not equally detrimental to allograft survival. Ettenger *et al.* (1977) have identified B-lymphocyte-directed cytotoxic antibodies during rejection in human renal allograft recipients. However, there was no hyperacute rejection if the graft recipient possessed preformed antibodies to B lymphocytes but not to T lymphocytes. The anti-B-cell antibodies were not enhancing to allograft survival either. The presence of these antibodies—defined as "anti-Ia" antibodies—in patients who experienced rejection was confirmed by Suthanthiran *et al.* (1978), whereas the antibodies were absent in patients with no rejection episodes. The anti-Ia antibodies were also eluted from rejected human kidney allografts (Garovoy *et al.*, 1978). Eight of nine eluates presenting a predominantly "humoral" pattern of rejection possessed the anti-Ia antibody, suggesting a pathogenetic role of these antibodies. Ia antigens are also demonstrable in addition to B lymphocytes on vascular endothelium, suggesting that they may be linked to the IgG deposits in cases of predominantly "humoral" rejection. As the same type of antibodies are protective to the transplant in rat kidney allografting experiments (Solillou *et al.*, 1976) and in mouse skin-grafting experiments (Davies and Staines, 1976), different roles for this type of antibody in predominantly "cellular" and predominantly "humoral" rejections may be anticipated. The enhancement phenomenon has recently been reviewed (e.g., see Davies and Staines, 1976) and will not be considered here.

C. Functional Analysis of Effector Cell Populations in Tumor Infiltrates

1. Lymphocyte Reactivity

Several cell types play important roles in cellular resistance to infection, and as we have seen in allograft rejection, a variety of effector cells can be isolated from different allografted tissues or organs. It is to be expected, therefore, that different classes of lymphocytes, monocytes, and macrophages with functional activity against tumor cells should be isolated from both regressing and progressing tumors.

Naim *et al.* (1971a) appear to have been the first to attempt to define lymphocyte activity *in situ*. Using time-lapse cinematography, they were unable to demonstrate tumor cell destruction by lymphocytes isolated along with tumor cells from a single human skin carcinoma, in spite of the observation that autologous peripheral lymphocytes were specifically cytotoxic. These studies have been extended to a large series of both colonic (Nairn *et al.*, 1971*b*) and malignant melanoma patients (Nind *et al.*, 1973). Their results scarcely provide an enthusiastic support for the role of cytotoxic lymphocytes *in situ*. All of 10 patients with colonic carcinoma and 5 with malignant melanoma failed to show *in vitro* cytotoxicity against autologous target cells, in spite of the fact that more than half had peripheral blood activity. Lymph node anergy in this test was also observed. The authors concluded that lymphocyte inhibition rather than selective changes in the infiltrating cells had occurred.

The first attempts to isolate lymphocyte populations from solid tumors is attributed to Zettergren *et al.* (1973), who separated lymphocytes from disaggregated mouse malignant neoplasms using sequential adherence, velocity, and isopycnic sedimentation. They reported purities of 76.3 to 96.8%. Although no functional tests were applied to these lymphocytes, their results stimulated others to test the functions of lymphocytes from a variety of solid tumors.

T cells isolated from a Burkitt's lymphoma (Jondal *et al.*, 1975) were capable of killing not only the autologous tumor cells but also three other tumor cell lines carrying EBV antigens. These studies were expanded to include nasopharyngeal carcinomas (Klein *et al.*, 1976). Specific cytotoxic effector cells were isolated from some of these tumors.

Plata and co-workers (Plata *et al.*, 1975; Plata and Sordat, 1977) isolated cytotoxic T lymphocytes from MSV-induced tumors. The specific activity of the effector cells varied with the age of the tumor. Highest activity was detected at the peak of tumor regression, but unlike the activity in the spleen, as the tumor disappeared the effector cells also disappeared. Holden *et al.* (1976) also found cytotoxic T cells in MSV-induced tumors and demonstrated that these effector cells were significantly smaller than the effector cells in the spleen.

Finally, Gillespie *et al.* (1978) identified cytotoxic T cells in regressing MSC tumors and observed that similar levels of lytic activity per 10^6 effector cells were obtained in regressing and progressing tumors at time of peak tumor size. As regression occurred, the specific activity of T cells isolated from regressing tumors increased dramatically, whereas the cells isolated from progressor tumors showed a marked decrease in activity. Whether this important observation is due to blocking of cytotoxic T cells, suppression of the immune response, or dilution of cytotoxic effector cells by other lymphocyte populations is not known.

If there should be parallels between the immune response to infectious agents characterized by granulomata formation and immune responses to growing neoplasms, delayed hypersensitivity responses should be demonstrable *in situ*. We have recently demonstrated that delayed hypersensitivity effector lymphocytes can be isolated from the T1699 mammary adenocarcinoma (Haskill *et al.*, 1976*b*). Two populations of effector cells were identified, one of which consisted of T lymphocytes. Similar results have also been obtained in a number of early transplant lines of spontaneous mammary adenocarcinomas in C3H mice (Radov and Haskill, unpublished observation).

2. Natural Killer Cells

Klein *et al.* (1976) and Becker and Klein (1976) have isolated natural killer (NK) cells from regressing MSV tumors. The highly NK-reactive CBA strain had the highest level of active NK cells *in situ*, whereas the low-reactive A/Sn strain had considerably lower levels of active cells. Cytotoxic T cells were not identified, although the tumors regressed. Recent experiments (Fig. 5) (Haskill and Becker, 1978) have indicated that the A/Sn strain tumors contain two distinct effector cells, a slow-sedimenting cell active against target cells isolated from the same tumor as the effector cells and another faster-sedimenting cell active in the NK assay. The slower-sedimenting cell is apparently not a T cell. These data raise the important question of the *in vivo* role of both the NK and cytotoxic T cell in spontaneous regression of MSV-induced tumors in ASn mice. If these cells fail to influence the survival of autologous target cells, what role do they perform *in situ*?

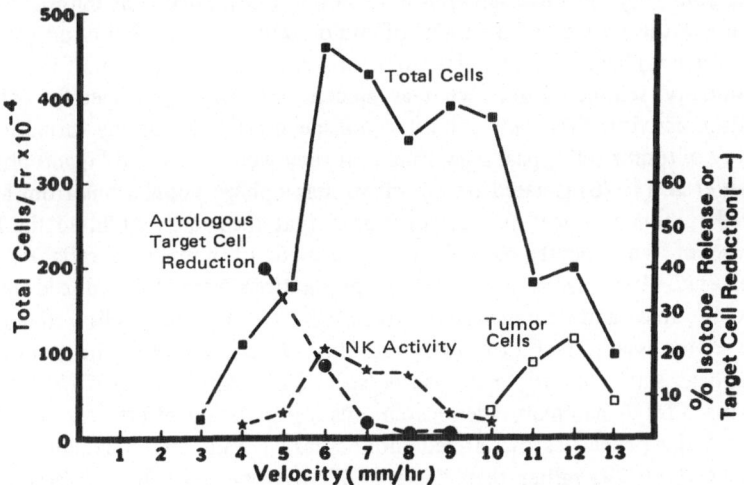

Figure 5. Velocity sedimentation separation of two distinct effector cell populations from MSV-induced tumors in A/Sn mice. Six tumors yielded approximately 90×10^6 "host fraction" cells after collagenase digestion. Sedimentation velocity was carried out at unit gravity as described previously (Haskill *et al.*, 1975*b*). To test for killing of autologous target cells, target cells were isolated from the high-velocity (10–13 mm/hr) fractions and cultured overnight prior to addition of effector cells at a 500:1 ratio. Natural killer cell activity was assayed using YAC target cells and a 30:1 ratio of effector to target cells (for details, see Becker and Klein, 1976).

3. Macrophages

A major stimulus to the identification of effector mechanisms inside solid tumors originates from the pioneering work of Evans and Alexander on the role of macrophages in the host defense against growing neoplasms. This extensive work has recently been reviewed by Evans (1976). The percentage of tumor-infiltrating cells identifiable as macrophages varied greatly from tumor to tumor. It should be noted, however, that some tumors with at least 50% macrophages still fail to regress spontaneously. Thus it is possible that the presence of several additional types of mononuclear cells, lymphocytes, monocytes, and histiocytes, as well as antibody or other soluble factors, may be obligatory for the induction of regression. Macrophages are not limited to animal tumors but have also been identified in human tumors (Gauci and Alexander, 1975). These macrophages are quite heterogeneous in size, probably representing both blood monocyte and macrophage populations. For example, we have been able to demonstrate physically separable FcR-positive macrophage populations in a number of specimens of human ovarian tissue (Fig. 6) (Haskill and Korn, unpublished observations).

A variety of functions have been identified for tumor-infiltrating macrophages. Evans (1973) isolated macrophages from enzymatically dispersed rat fibrosarcomas by selective adherence to Petri dishes. Such cells inhibited nonspecifically the growth of a variety of tumor cells. Also, Haskill *et al.* (1975*a*) isolated macrophages from similar tumors by enzymatic dispersion of the tumor and velocity sedimentation. Whereas spleen cells displayed specific colony-inhibition activity, these cells inhibited nonspecifically the colony formation of a variety of tumor cell types, suggesting that they were "activated" macrophages. Holden *et al.* (1976) isolated FcR-positive macrophage populations from MSV-induced tumors in mice, and demonstrated that these cells inhibited the PHA response of lymphocytes as well as the growth of lymphoma cells *in vitro*. Russell *et al.* (1977) isolated macrophage populations from MSC-induced tumors in BALB/c mice and demonstrated cytotoxicity to the tumor cells with a chromium release assay. The lytic growth-inhibiting effect induced by the monocyte-macrophage series of cells may also be specific. Haskill *et al.* (1975*b*) isolated from the T1699 mammary adenocarcinoma a population of effector cells with many of the properties of "armed monocytes" (Evans and Alexander, 1971; Evans *et al.*, 1972) rather than "activated" macrophages. These effector cells have high levels of Fc receptors, are adherent, accumulate in the tumor of thymectomized irradiated marrow-reconstituted animals, and are capable of demonstrating specific growth inhibition of the T1699 adenocarcinoma cell *in vitro*. An additional blood-borne bone-marrow-derived monocyte was also present in the T1699 tumor and was active either in an *in vitro* ADCC assay or against *in vivo* isolated tumor cells (Haskill and Fett, 1976; Haskill, 1977).

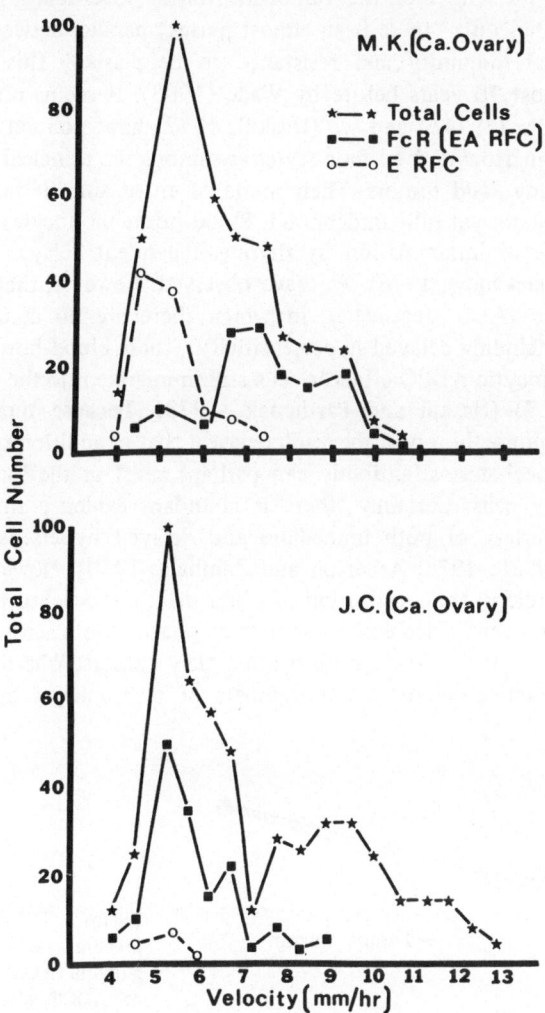

Figure 6. Sedimentation velocity profiles of total, monocyte–macrophage (EARFC), and T-lymphocyte populations. Human ovarian tumors were dispersed in collagenase and separated as the mouse tumors in Fig. 5. (The level of antibody coating on the sheep erythrocytes used for EARFC has been shown to detect cells belonging mainly to the monocyte–macrophage series.)

What is the origin of the tumor-infiltrating macrophages? As Mackaness (1976) pointed out, "there is an almost perfect parallel between cell-mediated anti-microbial immunity and resistance to neoplasia." This conclusion was reached almost 70 years before by Wade (1908). It seems possible, as Eccles and Alexander (1974b) and we (Haskill, 1977) have pointed out, that blood-borne bone-marrow-derived monocytes are among the principal effector cells infiltrating many solid tumors. Their mode of entry and the factors controlling the influx are not yet fully understood. Blood-borne monocytes may be directed into the site of inflammation by thymus-dependent delayed hypersensitivity reactions (Mackaness, 1976). We have observed, however, that in immunosuppressed mice (ALG treatment), in which there are no demonstrable T-cell responses (including delayed hypersensitivity), these blood-borne bone-marrow-derived monocytic ADCC effector cells still immigrate into the tumor in normal levels (Fig. 7) (Haskill and Parthenais, 1978). Because there is a residual antibody response, however, the results suggest that in addition to delayed hypersensitivity mechanisms, antibody can perhaps assist in the localization of the inflammatory cells. Certainly, there is abundant evidence that antibody can mediate a variety of both immediate and delayed hypersensitivity reactions (Askenase *et al.*, 1976; Asherson and Zembala, 1970). However, the thymus may play a role in the localization of other macrophages. Stutman (1975b) has reported significantly decreased numbers of phagocytic macrophages per tumor in *nu/nu* compared to *nu/+* mice bearing MSV tumors. Whether this reflects a decrease in activation or in net numbers of macrophages infiltrating is not known.

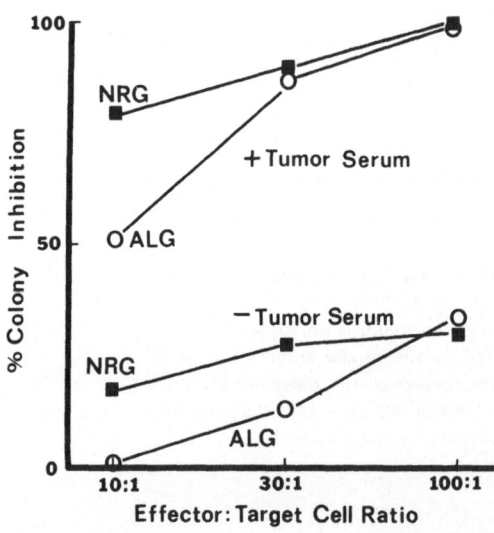

Figure 7. Effect of immunosuppression with antilymphocyte globulin (ALG) on the localization of ADCC effector cells in the T1699 mammary adenocarcinoma. Infiltrating cells were isolated from collagenase-dispersed tumors, and ADCC assays were carried out as described previously (Haskill and Fett, 1976). Tumor bearers received 0.3 ml of either ALG or normal rat globulin on days 0, 3, and 5 after tumor inoculation, and tumors were harvested at day 12.

Another possible way for macrophages to accumulate in tumors is by pro-liferation of tissue-derived macrophages or histiocytes, as is the case for some granulomas (Spector and Mariano, 1975). There is little information as to whether this is also true in solid tumors. Eccles and Alexander (1974b) have claimed that most, if not all, macrophages are derived not by *in situ* self-replication but by blood-borne infiltration. Haskill *et al.* (1975a) observed the presence of colony-forming macrophages in some of these rat fibrosarcomas, but the tissue or bone marrow origin of these cells was not identified. It was possible, however, to demonstrate the presence of two different kinds of colonies: one with a colony morphology typical of cells derived from bone marrow colony-forming units, and the other with a more histocytic morphology. *In vitro* proliferation of these cells was blocked by the simultaneous presence of tumor cells. It is therefore possible that in certain tumors, not only blood-borne monocytes but also tissue-derived macrophages and perhaps bone-marrow-stem-cell-derived macrophages play an important role. Parthenais *et al.* (unpublished observations) have observed that 12–18% of the large macrophages in the T1699 tumor incorporate a 1-hr pulse of ^{3}H-TdR, suggesting that macro-phage proliferation *in situ* may be an important source of inflammatory cells in this tumor.

The one area which surprisingly has not been investigated, and which from the classical histological studies seems to be promising, is the role of the histio-cyte in controlling tumor growth. Histologic studies clearly implicate a positive role for large nonphagocytic histiocytes in tumor responses. In the immunother-apy studies reported by Hanna *et al.* (1976), regressing tumors were heavily in-filtrated with histiocytes, and yet there has been no evidence that such cells after isolation from tumors are capable of causing *in vitro* effects either by cyto-toxicity or by tumor growth inhibition. It is clearly an area which should be investigated.

D. Role of Antibody in Solid Tumors

Antibodies have been reported to have a variety of roles, both beneficial and detrimental, in the host's response to growing tumors. Here we shall discuss only the evidence for antibodies localizing in syngeneic tumors and the possible roles these antibodies can play *in situ*. Most of this area has been well discussed in a recent review by Witz (1976). There is ample evidence for immunoglobulin localization in tumors, and sometimes these immunoglobulins clearly have anti-tumor specificity.

Studies by Cochran (1968) on malignant melanoma indicated that whereas *in situ* lymphocyte levels were correlated with good prognosis, the presence of plasma cells was inversely related, suggesting that *in situ* antibodies may have a potentially detrimental role in survival. Ran and Witz (1972) eluted tumor-associated immunoglobulins with low-pH buffers and found them to have tumor-enhancing activities. When such eluates were mixed with limiting dilutions of tumor cells, they enhanced tumor growth in syngeneic mice. Sjogren *et al.* (1972) eluted blocking factors from a number of human tumors. They concluded that a variety of human tumors contained blocking factors which inhibited cyto-toxic effects of lymphocytes in an *in vitro* assay. Bansal *et al.* (1972) demon-strated that low-pH eluates of polyoma tumor tissue, when injected into rats grafted with polyoma, enhanced tumor growth. Similar material could also be isolated from sera of tumor-bearing rats. In contrast, Johansson and Ljungqvist (1974) found that in 3 of 12 urinary bladder tumors IgM and cellular infiltra-tion were missing; these tumors showed marked invasive tendencies, whereas the remaining 9 tumors were devoid of cellular infiltration and yet did not display invasion. Their conclusion was that infiltration of IgM-positive cells appeared to be independent of the invasive characteristics of the tumor. Vanky *et al.* (1973, 1975) observed a good inverse correlation between tumor-bound immunoglobulins (detected by a radioiodinated antiimmunoglobulin reagent) and *in vitro* tumor cell stimulation of autologous lymphocytes. Izsak *et al.* (1974) have also attempted to correlate prognosis, pathological features, and the pres-ence or absence of cell surface immunoglobulin. They observed an apparent association of high malignant potential with the presence of membrane-associated immunoglobulin. Fourteen of 25 specimens had immunoglobulin-coated tumor cells, and of the 12 highly malignant tumors, 9 had Ig coating.

All antibodies need not be detrimental to the host. Ran *et al.* (1976) demon-strated that the SEYF-a polyoma-induced tumor stimulates a strong antibody response. The ascites tumor cells are coated with antibodies and the addition of complement results in lysis of tumor cells. We have studied antibody localization in the T1699 mammary adenocarcinoma. Mechanically dispersed tumor cells were sensitive to macrophage destruction *in vitro*, whereas tumor cells from im-munologically depressed animals with low antibody responses (ALG or ATX BM) were not destroyed by macrophages (Haskill and Fett, 1976; Haskill *et al.*, 1977). Immunofluorescence with indirect techniques demonstrated that low amounts of antibodies were present *in situ*, although only the IgG_{2a} and IgG_{2b} subclasses were readily detected. The level of fluorescence was only 10% of that of the same cells after exposure to autologous serum. Material with specificity for T1699 in the ADCC assay was eluted from the tumor cells by low-pH buffers, and ef-fector cells active in this ADCC assay could also be isolated from the same tumor.

In contrast, Lewis *et al.* (1976) studied a group of tumors obtained from 37 patients with malignant melanoma. They concluded that very little antibody was associated with the tumor cells, and that most of it was found on the infiltrating inflammatory cells.

Functional *in vivo* analyses of allograft and cancer infiltrates clearly indicate a multitude of cellular effector mechanisms in addition to classical T-cell-mediated cytotoxicity. It is possible that different types of allografts and different tumors are rejected by different effector pathways. It is equally possible, however, that different effector mechanisms dominate in a given type of graft at different stages of the immune response, as is clearly seen in sponge matrix allografts. Consequently, the importance of this phenomenon should be investigated in the other models.

VII. CORRELATIONS BETWEEN LOCAL AND SYSTEMIC IMMUNITY

A. In Antiallograft Responses

As we have discussed above, the predominant allograft-directed cytotoxic cell present during rejection in the central lymphatic system is the cytotoxic T lymphocyte. Although a multitude of cellular effector mechanisms may apparently be operative inside the allograft, it is important from a practical point of view to understand to what extent local immune activation inside the allograft is reflected in the activation of killer cells in the central immune system of the graft recipient, and vice versa. This would facilitate "immunological monitoring" of the allograft recipient, and possibly permit early detection of rejection episodes in clinical kidney transplantation.

Many attempts have been made to detect the activation of blood lymphocytes against antigens. A blast response can be detected in the recipient's blood in certain experimental conditions where no immunosuppressive therapy is used (Häyry et al., 1972b). In humans, however, possibly because of immunosuppressive therapy, it has been exceedingly difficult to demonstrate any substantial blast response in the blood of allograft recipients (Häyry et al., 1972a; Dimitriu et al., 1971). Although proliferating cells have been reported to be present in the blood of renal allograft recipients (Hersh et al., 1970), later analyses (Dimitriu et al., 1971; Häyry et al., 1972a) have demonstrated that the majority of these cells are myeloid precursor cells, and that the proliferating activity in the blood is not indicative of rejection episodes or the condition of the graft. Instead, a blast-cell activation to the antiallograft response is readily detected inside the graft (Pasternack et al., 1973) or in the lymph draining the allograft (Hamburger et al., 1971).

When a relevant second "sponge matrix" graft is provided to the primary host, a rapid flux of cytotoxic cells appears in the circulation of the graft recipient (Roberts, 1977). As most rejection episodes taking place beyond the immediate posttransplant period in human renal transplantation may be considered "secondary," it should thus be possible to detect graft-directed cytotoxic cells in the recipient's circulation shortly before and during the rejection. In fact, this has been demonstrated in kidney transplantation in man. Grunnet and Kristensen (1975) have shown that killer cells with specificity for the graft antigens appear in the circulation of kidney graft recipients during rejection, and that this event may be successfully used for the monitoring of rejection episodes in transplant recipients.

Also, the appearance of antibody may in certain cases correlate to rejection. As mentioned above, Ettenger *et al.* (1977) have demonstrated anti-B-cell lymphotoxins in the systemic circulation in cases of human renal allograft rejection. This finding has been confirmed by Suthanthiran *et al.* (1977). The "anti-Ia" antibodies directed to B lymphocytes were detected in 41 of 43 assays performed during acute or sustained rejection, whereas a positive finding was obtained in only 6 of 36 assays performed in the absence of rejection episodes.

Altogether, it seems to be possible to define correlations between central and systemic immunity reflecting activation of allograft rejection. To what extent this will lead to practical applications and improve immunological detection of rejection episodes remains to be seen.

B. In Antitumor Responses

1. Cellular Mechanisms

It is also important to determine to what extent *in vivo* assays of immunity using peripheral blood cells or serum factors can be expected to reflect local immunity inside a cancer. At this stage it is not evident that any set of assessments of systemic immunity show a good correlation with prognosis. The reasons for this are evident. Phenomena taking place in the spleen, nodes, and blood are not only physiologically distinct from the tumor environment but may also be related only indirectly to the actual defense mechanisms prevalent *in situ*. For example, we have already emphasized the potential role of lymphocytes, and macrophages or histiocytes, in the control of tumor growth *in situ*; however, neither macrophages nor histiocytes are likely to be found in peripheral blood. Therefore, indirect measures of *in situ* immunity must also be considered. Since some of the tumor-infiltrating cells may be T cells, and since the infiltrating macrophages may be activated by T cells, then presumably *in vitro* assays for T-cell activation can be utilized as a possible measure of *in situ* macrophage activity. A relationship between serum lysozyme levels and macrophage content of tumors has recently been described (Currie and Eccles, 1976; Bordin and Young, 1976), and this might also serve as an estimate of macrophage infiltration into tumors.

At present, however, our experience is still insufficient to determine to what extent the mere presence of effector cells in the circulation indicates their localization *in situ* (see Summary, Table V). Klein *et al.* (1976) investigated the ability of lymphocytes isolated from a human osteosarcoma to undergo blast trans-formation *in vitro* with autologous tumor cells. Whereas peripheral blood cells responded, the *in situ* lymphocytes did not, although they were reactive to PHA. As the antigen extract induced skin reactivity, it appears that the specific antigen-reactive lymphocytes, while present systemically, were absent *in situ*. Three lung tumor patients gave different results. Neither peripheral blood nor tumor lym-phocytes responded to autologous tumor cell antigens. Human ovarian tumor-associated lymphocytes failed to respond in mitogen stimulation assays. In each of the four cases, peripheral blood responses were normal (Haskill and Korn, un-published observations).

Radov *et al.* (1978) have made use of a passive transfer assay to study the distribution of delayed hypersensitivity effector T cells in a series of C3H spon-taneous mammary adenocarcinomas (Fig. 8). In this study the effector cells were found either in the tumor or in the draining nodes or in both, depending on the particular tumor. Such a wide variation in results casts considerable doubt on the premise that measures of systemic T-cell immunity necessarily reflect *in situ* immunity.

Nairn *et al.* (1971*a*) appear to have been the first to attempt to define lym-phocyte activity *in situ*. Using time-lapse cinematography, they were unable to demonstrate tumor cell destruction by lymphocytes isolated along with tumor cells from a single human skin carcinoma, in spite of the observation that autol-ogous peripheral lymphocytes were specifically cytotoxic. These studies have been extended to a large series of both colonic (Nairn *et al.*, 1971*b*) and malig-nant melanoma patients (Nind *et al.*, 1973). Their results scarcely provide an enthusiastic support for the role of cytotoxic lymphocytes *in situ*. All of 10 patients with colonic carcinoma and 5 with malignant melanoma failed to show *in vitro* cytotoxicity against autologous target cells in spite of the fact that more than half had peripheral blood activity. Lymph node anergy in this test was also observed. The authors concluded that lymphocyte inhibition rather than selec-tive changes in the infiltrating cells had occurred.

Studies by Jondal *et al.* (1975) and Klein *et al.* (1976) suggest that in some instances, cytotoxic T cells may be active *in situ*. However, as both Burkitt's lymphoma and nasopharyngeal carcinomas may contain normal lymphoid tissue, it is possible that the origin of the cytotoxic cells is the normal tissue and not the tumor infiltrate. A number of other investigations have failed to isolate cytotoxic T cells from solid tumors. In methylcholanthrene-induced tumors, cytotoxic T cells can be detected in the peripheral lymph nodes; however, neither Evans (personal communication) nor Cornain and Klein (personal communication) have been able to detect the presence of cytotoxic T cells *in situ*. Similarily, Haskill *et al.* (1975*a*) found activated macrophages but not cytotoxic effector cells in two different rat fibrosarcomas. On the other hand, *in situ* delayed hypersensitivity T cells have been detected in the T1699

Table V. Summary: Reported Relationships between Systemic and *in Situ* Antitumor Effector Cells[a]

Tumor type (Reference)[b]	T lymphocytes								Macrophages/monocytes						"Natural killer" cells	
	Cytotoxic		DHR		Mitogen				Activated (nonspecific)		"Armed" (specific)		ADCC			
					PHA		ATC									
	S	T	S	T	S	T	S	T	S	T	S	T	S	T	S	T
Mouse																
T1699 (a)																
Syngeneic	−	−	+	+					−	−	−	+	+	+		
Allogeneic	+	+									−	−				
MSV																
C57BL/6 (b)	+	+							+	+					+	+
BALB/c (c)	+	+							+							
A/Sn, CBA (d)	−	−													+	+
C57BL/6 (e)	+	+														
Spontaneous mammary,																
C3H (f)			+,−	+,−												
MCA-induced (g)	+	−														

Rat								
MC-1, HSH fibrosarcomas (h)	+	−					−	+
Various fibrosarcomas (i)	+	−					−	+
Human								
Osteosarcoma (j)			2+	2+	2+	2−		
Lung carcinoma (j)			3+	3+	3−	3−		
Ovarian carcinoma (k)			4+	4−				
Squamous cell carcinoma (l)	1+	1−						
Burkitt's lymphoma (l)	2−	2+,1−						
Nasopharyngeal carcinoma (l)	18−	2+,8−						
Colonic carcinoma (m)	6+,4−	10−						
Malignant melanoma (m)	5+	5−						
Breast carcinoma (n)							4+	4−
Lung, nasopharyngeal carcinomas (o)							17+, 15	1+,13−

[a] Abbreviations: S, systemic lymphoid cells (spleen cells in animals, peripheral blood lymphocytes in humans); T, tumor-infiltrating cells; PHA, nonspecific mitogen response; ATC, autologous tumor cell response; DHR, delayed hypersensitivity response.

[b] References: a, Haskill *et al.* (1975b); b, Holden *et al.* (1976); c, Russell *et al.* (1977); d, Becker and Klein (1976); e, Plata *et al.* (1975); f, Radov (unpublished); g, Cornain and Evans (personal communication); h, Haskill *et al.* (1975a); i, Evans (1976); j, Klein *et al.* (1976); k, Haskill and Korn (unpublished); l, Jondal *et al.* (1975); m, Nind *et al.* (1973); n, Blomgren *et al.* (1973); o, Vose *et al.* (1977).

murine mammary adenocarcinoma (Haskill *et al.*, 1976*b*), and it is expected that such T cells may well be involved in the localization of various inflammatory cells found in both infectious and malignant granulomata. That delayed hypersensitivity T cells can be detected *in situ* whereas cytotoxic T cells cannot argues against the fact that the cytotoxic T cells are actually present in the tumors but are blocked by antigen. It should be noted that in the T1699 model, syngeneic hosts fail to produce either systemic or *in situ* cytotoxic T cells, although both are found in allogeneic recipients of the same tumor (Haskill *et al.*, 1975*b*).

Natural killer cells have also been detected in the peripheral lymphoid organs, and there are reports that these effector cells can be detected *in situ* (Klein *et al.*, 1976; Becker and Klein, 1976). Whether there is a direct relationship between systemic and *in situ* natural killer cell "immunity" has not been determined, nor has the actual effector role of these cells in the regulation of tumor growth been determined.

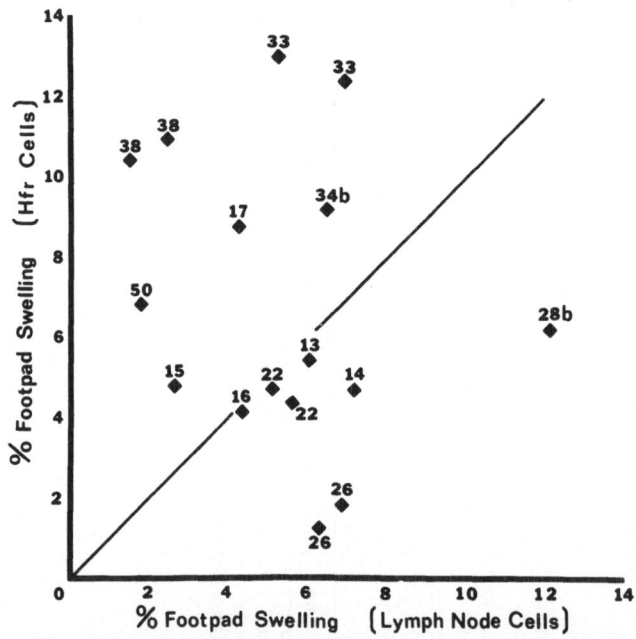

Figure 8. Relationship between DHR effector cells in draining lymph nodes and tumor-infiltrating cells from C3H mice bearing spontaneous mammary tumors after the first and second passages. Control cells or 3 M KCl extracts of the autologous tumor (2×10^6 cells) were transferred into the footpads of normal syngeneic mice, and swelling was measured after 18 hr (see Haskill *et al.*, 1976*b*, for further details).

2. Antibody-Dependent Mechanisms

In both allograft and tumor graft destruction, the role of antibody *in situ* has been subject to much less investigation in terms of effector mechanism than perhaps is warranted. Many investigators have eluted blocking factors from a variety of solid tumors. The fact that they can inhibit cytotoxic lymphocyte activity *in vitro* is interesting, but in fact if such cytotoxic T cells cannot be identified in tumors, what is the value of such blocking complexes? Saksela *et al.* (1975) and Greenberg *et al.* (1973*a*) have shown that immune complexes can arm K cells; it would therefore appear possible that rather than being a detriment to the host, such immune complexes could, in some cases at least, act in favor of the host. Until such mechanisms are looked at and excluded, it is difficult to conclude otherwise. *In situ* antibody-coated tumor cells can clearly be demonstrated in a number of tumor systems. If the antibodies are of the correct class or subclass to activate an ADCC-type reaction, and if appropriate effector cells can also localize *in situ*, there seems to be no reason why an ADCC mechanism cannot be considered to be important *in situ*. In addition, antibody-coated tumor cells can be susceptible to complement destruction, provided that necessary complement components can find their way *in situ* and are all active *in situ*.

The relationship between serum and *in situ* antibody has been an area of considerable interest. Two particular points are worth consideration. Witz (1976) has recently reviewed the evidence for the preferential localization of the IgG_2 subclass antibody *in situ* in a variety of animal tumors. This implies that the type of immune response detected in the circulation need not reflect events taking place inside the tumor. Not only may the antibodies be unequally localized *in situ*, but some of these antibodies may be selectively degraded as a result of proteolytic enzymes released by either inflammatory cells or by the tumor cells (Witz, 1976; Sobczak and deVaux Saint Cyr, 1971). Such processes carried out *in situ* would clearly alter the systemic and *in situ* antibody levels independently. In addition, the relatively high concentration of tumor antigen released *in situ* probably causes imbalances in the relative levels of free and complexed antibody *in situ* and in the circulation.

VIII. CONCLUDING REMARKS

Altogether, recent results on both allograft and tumor immunity suggest that largely different effector mechanisms may operate in the host's central lymphatic system and *in situ*. These observations are probably important, and they contribute to the understanding of the immunological mechanisms operating in both allograft and tumor immunity.

Cytotoxic T lymphocytes are also the predominant, if not exclusive, allograft-directed killer cells in the central lymphatic system of the host. In contrast, the killer cells actually infiltrating the allograft may be predominantly T lymphocytes (as is the case with rat heart allografts), non-T ("B") lymphocytes (human kidney allografts), or a mixture of "B" lymphocytes, monocytes, and T lymphocytes (sponge matrix allografts). At any rate, these findings show considerable heterogeneity in the allograft-infiltrating killer population, and it appears that the concept of allograft destruction solely via activated (T) lymphocytes must be revised. Sequential studies using sponge matrix allografts also suggest that the killer cells initially present inside the graft are T lymphocytes, but that non-T lymphocytes and even monocytes subsequently infiltrate the site and participate in graft destruction.

In the case of tumor rejection, Wade observed in 1907 that regression of canine infective sarcomas was accompanied by infiltration of lymphocytes and lymphoblasts. He noted that the tumor lesions resembled inflammatory changes produced during the formation of syphilitic granulomata. Almost 70 years later, Mackaness (1976), in reviewing the role of macrophages in neoplasia, reached a similar conclusion. During the intervening years there has been very little progress in our assessment of the role of the immune system *in situ*, in spite of the vast literature on immunological mechanisms accounting for *in vitro* destruction or prophylactic inhibition of tumor growth. One of the most striking observations from histologic studies is the apparent importance of histiocytic infiltration, expecially in regressing tumors; however, experimental studies have so far failed to provide any evidence for a role of histiocytes in tumor cell destruction. Thus, although pathologists have inferred a role for such effector mechanisms in tumor regression, experimental immunologists have failed to follow up in this area.

There is little doubt that tumor defense mechanisms may well depend upon T cells, but how the T cells are involved is still very much in question. The central role of cytotoxic T cells in tumor immunity, as in the main pathway of allograft destruction, is already in question, and with the exception of MSV tumors and some examples of Burkitt's lymphoma and nasopharyngeal carcinomas (also of possible viral etiology and possibly containing normal lymphoid tissue), there is little real evidence that cytotoxic T cells play an important role in tumor cell destruction *in situ*.

The presence of monocytes and macrophages is common in several tumors, and it may well be that our experimental approaches have been biased in favor of cytotoxic lymphocytes, with the result that we have heretofore strayed away from examining other potentially important effector mechanisms.

Probably none of these mechanisms function independently. It must be considered that a simple test using peripheral blood cells or serum to describe host immune response to either allografts or cancers can only be disappointing, as the *in situ* mechanisms involved in control of tumor growth or allograft rejection depend upon a multitude of factors. It is also clear that before our eventual goal —i.e., the development of practical methods to enhance or suppress host immunity toward cancers or allografts—can be attained, we must further explore the various mechanisms involved in systemic and *in situ* resistance, their relationships, and their overall significance in the process of rejection.

ACKNOWLEDGMENTS

The experimental work was financed by National Cancer Institute Contract NO1-CB-64032 (to P.H.), USPHS grant CA-17694, and ACS grant IM-84 (to J.S.H.). Part of the investigations were done during the tenure of Dr. Haskill at the Transplantation Laboratory, University of Helsinki, funded by a UICC International Cancer Research Technology Transfer Award. We thank Charles L. Smith for editorial assistance.

IX. REFERENCES

Alexander, P., and Evans, R., 1971, Endotoxin and double stranded RNA render macrophages cytotoxic, *Nature New Biol.* 232:76–78.

Alexander, P., and Hall, J. G., 1970, The role of immunoblasts in host resistance to immunotherapy of primary sarcomata, *Adv. Cancer Res.* 13:1–37.

Allison, A. C., 1972a, Interactions of antibodies and effector cells in immunity against tumours, *Ann. Inst. Pasteur* 22:619–631.

Allison, A. C., 1972b, Immunity and immunopathology in virus infections, *Ann. Inst. Pasteur* 23:585–608.

Amos, D. B., 1960, Possible relationships between the cytotoxic effects of isoantibody and host cell function, *Ann. N.Y. Acad. Sci.* 87:273–292.

Amos, D. B., 1961, Host response to ascites tumors, in: *Mechanism of Cell and Tissue Damage Produced by Immune Reactions* (2nd International Symposium on Immunopathology), (N. Grabar and P. Miesher, eds.), pp. 210–222, Benno Schwabe & Co., Basel.

Andersson, L. C., 1973, Size distribution of killer cells during allograft response, *Scand. J. Immunol.* 2:75–88.

Andersson, L. C., Nordling, S., and Hayry, P., 1973, Proliferation of T and B cells in mixed lymphocyte cultures, *J. Exp. Med.* 138:324–329.

Andre, J. A., Schwartz, R. S., Mitus, W. J., and Dameshek, W., 1962, The morphologic response of the lymphoid system to homografts. I. First and second-set responses in normal rabbits, *Blood* 19:313.

Andre-Schwartz, J., 1964, The morphological responses of the lymphoid system to homografts. III. Electron microscopy study, *Blood* 24:113.

Andres, G. A., and McCluskey, R. T., 1975, Tubular and interstitial renal disease due to immunologic mechanisms, *Kidney Int.* 7:271–289.

Andres, G. A., Accinni, L., Hsu, K. C., Penn, I., Porter, K. A., Rendall, J. M., Seegal, B. C., and Starzl, T. E., 1970, Human renal transplants. III. Immunopathologic studies, *Lab. Invest.* 22:588–604.

Asherson, G. L., and Zembala, M., 1970, Contact sensitivity in the mouse. IV. The role of lymphocytes and macrophages in passive transfer and the mechanism of their interaction, *J. Exp. Med.* **132**:1–15.

Askenase, P. W., Haynes, J. D., and Hayden, B. J., 1976, Antibody-mediated basophil accumulations in cutaneous hypersensitivity reactions of guinea pigs, *J. Immunol.* **117**:216–224.

Austen, K. G., *et al.*, 1966, Detection of renal allograft rejection in man by demonstration of a reduction in the serum concentration of the second component of complement, *Ann. N.Y. Acad. Sci.* **129**:657.

Bach, F. H., and van Rood, J. J., 1976, The major histocompatibility complex, *New Engl. J. Med.* **295**:806, 872, 927.

Balch, C. M., Wilson, C. B., Lee, S., and Feldman, J. D., 1973, Thymus-dependent lymphocytes in tissue sections of rejecting rat renal allograft, *J. Exp. Med.* **138**:1584–1590.

Baldwin, R. W., Price, M. R., and Robins, R. A., 1972, Blocking of lymphocyte-mediated cytotoxicity for rat hepatoma cells by tumor-specific antigen-antibody complexes, *Nature New Biol.* **238**:185–186.

Baldwin, R. W., Path, F. R., and Price, M. R., 1976, Tumor antigens and tumor–host relationship, *Ann. Rev. Med.* **27**:151–163.

Bansal, S. C., Hargreaves, R., and Sjogren, H. O., 1972, Facilitation of polyoma tumor growth in rats by blocking sera and tumor eluate, *Int. J. Cancer* **9**:97–108.

Becker, S., and Klein, E., 1976, Decreased "natural killer" effect in tumor-bearing mice and its relation to the immunity against oncorna virus-determined cell surface antigens, *Eur. J. Immunol.* **6**:892–898.

Bennett, S. H., Futrell, J. W., Roth, J. A., Hoye, R. C., and Ketcham, A. S., 1971, Prognostic significance of histologic host response in cancer of the larynx or hypopharynx, *Cancer* **28**:1255–1265.

Benninghoff, D. L., and Girardet, R., 1976, Lymphocyte function in Hodgkin's disease, *Lymphology* **9**:39–42.

Berlinger, N. T., Tsakraklides, V., Pollak, K., Adams, G. L., Yang, M., and Good, R. A., 1976, Immunological assessment of regional lymph node histology in relation to survival in head and neck carcinoma, *Cancer* **37**:697–705.

Biesecker, J. L., 1973, Cellular and humoral immunity after allogeneic transplantation in the rat. I. Cellular and humoral imminity as measured by ^{51}Cr cytotoxicity assay after allogeneic tumor and renal transplantation, *Transplantation* **15**:298–307.

Billingham, M., Warnke, R., and Weissman, I. L., 1976, The cellular infiltrate in cardiac allograft rejection in mice, *Transplantation* **23**:171–176.

Billingham, R. E., Brent, L., and Medawar, P. B., 1954, Quantitative studies on tissue transplantation immunity. II. The origin, strength and duration of actively and adoptively acquired immunity, *Proc. Roy. Soc. London* **B143**:58–80.

Binz, H., and Wigzell, H., 1975, Shared idiotypic determinants on B and T lymphocytes reactive against the same antigenic determinants. IV. Isolation of two groups of naturally occurring, idiotypic molecules with specific antigen-binding activity in the serum and urine of normal rats, *Scand. J. Immunol.* **4**:591–598.

Binz, H., Lindenmann, J., and Wigzell, H., 1974, Cell-bound receptors for alloantigens on normal lymphocytes. I. Characterization of receptor-carrying cells by the use of antibodies to alloantibodies, *J. Exp. Med.* **139**:877–887.

Binz, H., Wigzell, H., and Hayry, P., 1976, Correlation between specific cytolysis and expression of idiotypic receptors of allograft-infiltrating cells, *Nature* **259**:401–403.

Birbeck, M. S. C., and Carter, R. L., 1972, Observations on the ultrastructure of two hamster lymphomas with particular reference to infiltrating macrophages, *Int. J. Cancer* **9**:249–257.

Black, M. M., and Speer, F. D., 1958, Sinus histocytosis of lymph nodes in cancer, *Surg. Gynecol. Obstet.* **106**:163–175.

Black, M. M., Kerpe, S., and Speer, F. D., 1953, Lymph node structure in patients with cancer of the breast, *Amer. J. Pathol.* **29**:505–521.

Black, M. M., Opler, S. R., and Speer, F. D., 1954, Microscopic structure of gastric carcinomas and their regional lymph nodes in relation to survival, *Surg. Gynecol. Obstet.* **98**:725–734.

Black, M. M., Barclay, T. H. C., and Hankey, B. F., 1975, Prognosis in breast cancer utilizing histologic characteristics of the primary tumor, *Cancer* **36**:2048–2055.

Blair, P. B., Lane, M. A., and Yagi, M. J., 1974, *In vitro* detection of immune responses to MTV-induced mammary tumors: Activity of spleen cell preparations from both MTV-free and MTV-infected mice, *J. Immunol.* **112**:693–705.

Blair, P. B., Lane, M. A., and Mar, P., 1976, Antibody in the sera of tumor-bearing mice that mediates spleen cell cytotoxicity toward the autologus tumor, *J. Immunol.* **116**:606–609.

Blomgren, H., and Andersson, B., 1969, Evidence for a small pool of immunocompetent cells in the mouse thymus, *Exp. Cell. Res.* **57**:185–192.

Blomgren, H., Glas, U., Franzen, S., and Granberg, P. O., 1973, Lymphoid cells in carcinoma of the breast, *Acta Radiol.* **12**:434–442.

Bordin, S., and Young, E. T., 1976, Tumor-associated macrophages as the primary source of lysozyme in the urine of mice bearing GPC-II, a transplantable reticulum cell sarcoma, *J. Natl. Cancer Inst.* **57**:827–833.

Borsos, T., and Rapp, H. J., 1965, Complement fixation on cell surfaces by 19S and 7S antibodies, *Science* **150**:505–506.

Boyle, M. D. P., and Omerod, M. G., 1975, The destruction of allogeneic tumour cells by peritoneal macrophages from immune mice: Purification of lytic effector cells, *Cell. Immunol.* **17**:247–258.

Brawn, R. J., 1971, Evidence for association of embryonal antigen(s) with several 3-methylcholanthrene-induced murine sarcomas, in: *Proceedings of the 1st Conference and Workshop on Embryonic and Fetal Antigens in Cancer* (N. G. Anderson and J. H. Coggins, eds.), pp. 143–149, Oak Ridge National Laboratory, Oak Ridge, Tenn.

Brightmore, T. G. J., Greening, W. P., and Hamlin, I., 1970, An analysis of clinical and histopathological features in 101 cases of carcinoma of breast in women under 35 years of age, *Brit. J. Cancer* **24**:644–669.

Brunner, K. T., Mauel, J., Rudolf, H., and Chapuis, B., 1970, Studies of allograft immunity in mice. I. Introduction, development and *in vitro* assay of cellular immunity, *Immunology* **18**:501–515.

Bubenik, J., Perlmann, P., Helmstein, K., and Moberger, G., 1970, Cellular and humoral immune responses to human urinary bladder carcinomas, *Int. J. Cancer* **5**:310–319.

Burk, M. W., Yu, S., and McKhann, C. F., 1976, Tumor-specific immune responsiveness of the tumor-bearing host, in: *Immunological Parameters of Host-Tumor Relationships*, Vol. 4 (D. W. Weiss, ed.), pp. 80–88, Academic Press, New York.

Burwell, R. G., 1962, Studies of the primary and the secondary immune responses of lymph nodes draining homografts of fresh cancellous bone (with particular reference to mechanisms of lymph node reactivity), *Ann. N.Y. Acad. Sci.* **99**:821–860.

Byrne, M., Heppner, G., Stolbach, L., Cummings, F., McDonough, E., and Calabresi, P., 1973, Tumor immunity in melanoma patients as assessed by colony inhibition and microcytotoxicity methods: A preliminary report, *Natl. Cancer Inst. Monogr.* **37**:3–8.

Canty, T. G., and Wunderlich, J. R., 1971, Quantitative assessment of cellular and humoral responses to skin and tumor allografts, *Transplantation* 11:111–116.

Carpenter, C. B., Gill, T. J., III, Merrill, J. P., and Dammin, G. J., 1967, Alterations in human serum B_{1c}-globulin (C'3) in renal transplantation, *Amer. J. Med.* 43:854–867.

Carpenter, C. B., Ruddy, S., Shehadeh, I. H., Merrill, J. P., Austen, K. F., and Muller-Eberhard, H. J., 1969, Metabolism of radiolabelled C'3 and C'4 in human renal allograft recipients, *Transplant. Proc.* 1:279–282.

Cerottini, J. C., and Brunner, T., 1974, Cell mediated cytotoxicity, allograft rejection and tumor immunity, *Adv. Immunol.* 18:67–132.

Churg, J., and Grishman, E., 1975, Ultrastructure of glomerular disease: A review, *Kidney Int.* 7:254–270.

Cochran, A. J., 1968, Histology and prognosis in malignant melanoma, *J. Pathol.* 97:459–468.

Cohen, D., Gurner, B. W., and Coombs, R. R. A., 1971, A phenomenon resembling opsonic adherence shown by disaggregated cells of the transmissible venereal tumour of the dog, *Brit. J. Exp. Pathol.* 52:447–451.

Currie, G. A., and Basham, C., 1973, Serum mediated inhibition of the immunological reactions of the patient to his own tumour: A possible role for circulating antigen, *Brit. J. Cancer* 26:427–438.

Currie, G. A., and Eccles, S. A., 1976, Serum lysozyme as a marker of host resistance. I. Production by macrophages resident in rat sarcomata, *Brit. J. Cancer* 33:51–59.

Davies, D. A. L., and Staines, U. A., 1976, A cardinal role for I-region antigens (Ia) in immunological enhancement and the clinical implications, *Transplant. Rev.* 30:18–39.

Delorme, E. J., Hodgett, J., Hall, J. G., and Alexander, P., 1969, The cellular immune response to primary sarcomata in rats. I. The significance of large basophilic cells in the thoracic duct lymph following antigenic challenge, *Proc. Roy. Soc. London* B174:229–236.

deVries, J. E., Rumke, P., and Bernheim, J. L., 1972, Cytotoxic lymphocytes in melanoma patients, *Int. J. Cancer* 9:567–576.

Dimitriu, A., Debray-Sachs, M., Descamps, B., Sultan, C., and Hamburger, J., 1971, Triated thymidine incorporation in blood leukocytes of renal allograft recipients, *Transplant. Proc.* 3:1577–1583.

Dire, J. J., and Lane, N., 1963, The relation of sinus histiocytosis in axillary lymph nodes to surgical curability of carcinoma of the breast, *Amer. J. Clin. Pathol.* 40:508–515.

Eccles, S. A., and Alexander, P., 1974a, Macrophage content of tumors in relation to metastatic spread and host immune reaction, *Nature* 250:667–669.

Eccles, S. A., and Alexander, P., 1974b, Sequestration of macrophages in growing tumors and its effect on the immunological capacity of the host, *Brit. J. Cancer* 30:42–49.

Edelson, R. L., Hearing, V. J., Dellon, A. L., Frank, M., Edelson, E. K., and Green, I., 1975, Differentiation between B cells, T cells, and histiocytes in melanocytic lesions: Primary and metastatic melanoma and halo and giant pigmented nevi, *Clin. Immunol. Immunopathol.* 4:557–568.

Ettenger, R. B., Terasaki, A. T., Malekzadeh, M. H., Pennisi, A. J., Uittenbogaart, C. H., and Fine, R. N., 1977, Role of antibodies to B lymphocytes in renal transplantation, *Transplant. Proc.* 9:751–753.

Evans, R., 1972, Macrophages in syngeneic animal tumours, *Transplantation* 14:468–473.

Evans, R., 1973, Preparation of pure cultures of tumor macrophages, *J. Natl. Cancer Inst.* 50:271–273.

Evans, R., 1976, Tumor macrophages in host immunity to malignancies, in: *The Macrophage in Neoplasia* (M. Fink, ed.), pp. 27–42, Academic Press, New York.

Evans, R., and Alexander, P., 1970, Cooperation of immune lymphoid cells with macrophages in tumour immunity, *Nature* 228:620–622.

Evans, R., and Alexander, P., 1971, Rendering macrophages specifically cytotoxic by a factor released from immune lymphoid cells, *Transplantation* 12:227–229.

Evans, R., and Alexander, P., 1972, Mechanism of immunologically specific killing of tumour cells by macrophages, *Nature* 236:168–170.

Evans, R., Grant, C. K., Cox, H., Steele, K., and Alexander, P., 1972, Thymus-derived lymphocytes produce and immunologically specific macrophage-arming factor, *J. Exp. Med.* 136:1318–1322.

Fakhri, O., and Hobbs, J. R., 1972, Target cell death without added complement after cooperation of 7S antibodies with non-immune lymphocytes, *Nature New Biol.* 235:177–178.

Fearon, D. T., Daha, M. R., Strom, T. B., Weiler, J. M., Carpenter, C. B., and Austen, K. F., 1977, Pathways of complement activation in membranoproliferative glomerulonephritis and allograft rejection, *Transplant. Proc.* 9:729–739.

Fidler, I. J., 1976, Macrophage deficiency in tumor bearing animals: Control of experimental metastasis with macrophages activated *in vitro*, in: *The Macrophage in Neoplasia* (M. Fink, ed.), pp. 245–257, Academic Press, New York.

Fink, M. A., 1976, *The Macrophage in Neoplasia*, Academic Press, New York.

Fisher, E. R., Gregorio, R., Redmond, C., Dekker, A., and Fisher, B., 1976, Pathologic findings from the national surgical adjuvant breast project (protocol no. 4). II. The significance of regional node histology other than sinus histiocytosis in invasive mammary cancer, *Amer. J. Clin. Pathol.* 65:21–30.

Gale, R. P., and Zighelboim, J., 1974, Modulation of polymorphonuclear leukocyte-mediated antibody-dependent cellular cytotoxicity, *J. Immunol.* 113:1793–1800.

Gale, R. P., and Zighelboim, J., 1975, Polymorphonuclear leukocytes in antibody-dependent cellular cytotoxicity, *J. Immunol.* 114:1047–1051.

Garovoy, M. R., Suthanthiran, M., Gailiunas, P., Carpenter, C. B., Graves, M., Busch, G., and Tilney, N. L., 1978, Anti-"*Ia*" antibody eluted from rejected human renal allografts, *Transplant. Proc.* (in press).

Gauci, C. L., and Alexander, P., 1975, The macrophage content of some human tumors, *Cancer Lett.* 1:29–32.

Gershon, R. K., Carter, R. L., and Lane, N. J., 1967, Studies on homotransplantable lymphomas in hamsters. IV. Observations on macrophages in the expression of tumor immunity, *Amer. J. Pathol.* 51:1111–1133.

Gillespie, G. Y., Hansen, C. B., Hoskins, R. G., and Russell, S. W., 1978, Inflammatory cells in solid murine neoplasms. IV. Cytolytic T lymphocytes isolated from regressing or progressing Moloney sarcomas, *J. Immunol.* 119: 564–570.

Goldstein, P., Svedmyr, E. A. J., and Wigzell, H., 1971, Cells mediating specific *in vitro* cytotoxicity. I. Detection of receptor-bearing lymphocytes, *J. Exp. Med.* 134:1385–1402.

Gorer, P. A., 1956, Some recent work on tumor immunity, *Adv. Cancer Res.* 4:149–186.

Gowans, J. L., and Knight, E. J., 1964, The route of re-circulation of lymphocytes in the rat, *Proc. Roy. Soc. London* 159:257–282.

Granger, G. A., and Weiser, R. S., 1964, Homograft target cells: Specific destruction *in vitro* by contact interaction with immune macrophages, *Science* 145:1427–1429.

Green, H., Barrow, P., and Goldberg, B., 1959, Effect of antibody and complement on permeability control in ascites tumor cells and erythrocytes, *J. Exp. Med.* 110:699–713.

Green, I., and Shevach, E. M., 1974, Cellular aspects of tumor immunity, in: *Mechanisms of Cell-Mediated Immunity* (R. T. McCluskey and S. Cohen, eds.), pp. 221–225, John Wiley and Sons, Inc., New York.

Greenberg, A. H., and Playfair, J. H. L., 1974, Spontaneously arising cytotoxicity to the P-815-Y mastocytoma in NZB mice, *Clin. Exp. Immunol.* **16**:99–110.

Greenberg, A. H., and Shen, L., 1973, A class of specific cytotoxic cells demonstrated *in vitro* by arming with antigen–antibody complexes, *Nature New Biol.* **245**:283–285.

Greenberg, A. H., Hudson, L., Shen, L., and Roitt, I. M., 1973*a*, Antibody-dependent cell-mediated cytotoxicity due to a "null" lymphoid cell, *Nature New Biol.* **242**:111–113.

Greenberg, A. H., Shen, L., and Roitt, I. M., 1973*b*, Characterization of the antibody-dependent cytotoxic cell: A non-phagocytic monocyte?, *Clin. Exp. Immunol.* **15**: 251–259.

Grunnet, N., and Kristensen, T., 1975, Direct cell mediated lympholysis by peripheral blood lymphocytes from renal allograft recipients, *Scand. J. Urol. Nephrol. Suppl.* **29**:41–44.

Guttmann, R. D., Lindquist, R. R., Parker, R. M., Carpenter, C. B., and Merrill, J. P., 1967, Renal transplantation in the inbred rat. I. Morphologic, immunologic, and functional alterations during acute rejection, *Transplantation* **5**:668–681.

Hall, J. G., 1967, Studies of the cells in the afferent and efferent lymph of lymph nodes draining the site of skin homografts, *J. Exp. Med.* **125**:737–754.

Hamburger, J., Dimitriu, A., Bankir, I., Debray-Sacho, M., and Auvert, J., 1971, Collection of lymph from kidneys homotransplanted in man: Cell transplantation *in vivo*, *Nature* **232**:633–634.

Handley, W. S., 1907, The pathology of melanotic growths in relation to their operative treatment, *Lancet* **1**:927–933.

Hanna, M. G., Jr., Snodgrass, J. M., Zbar, B., and Rapp, H. J., 1972, Histopathology of mycobacterium bovis (BCG)-mediated tumor regression, *Natl. Cancer Inst. Monogr.* **35**:345–357.

Hanna, M. G., Jr., Bucana, C., Hobbs, B., and Fidler, I. J., 1976, Morphologic aspects of tumor cell cytotoxicity by effector cells of the macrophage-histiocyte compartment: *In vitro* and *in vivo* studies in BCG-mediated tumor regression, in: *The Macrophage in Neoplasia* (M. A. Fink, ed.), pp. 113–134, Academic Press, New York.

Harding, B., Pudifin, D. J., Gotch, F., and MacLennan, I. C. M., 1971, Cytotoxic lymphocytes from rats depleted of thymus processed cells, *Nature New Biol.* **232**:80–81.

Harris, T. N., and Harris, S., 1973, Fate of skin allografts in normal mice injected with anti-graft strain globulin in relation to the IgG1 and IgG2 class of the antibodies, *Immunology* **25**:409–421.

Haskill, J. S., 1977, ADCC effector cells in a murine adenocarcinoma. I. Evidence for blood-borne bone-marrow-derived monocytes, *Int. J. Cancer* **20**:432–440.

Haskill, J. S., and Becker, S., 1978, *Proceedings of Erwin Riesch Symposium on Cytotoxic Cell-Interaction and Immunostimulation* (in press).

Haskill, J. S., and Fett, J. W., 1976, Possible evidence for antibody-dependent macrophage-mediated cytotoxicity directed against murine adenocarcinoma cells *in vivo*, *J. Immunol.* **117**:1992–1998.

Haskill, J. S., and Parthenais, E., 1978, Immunological factors influencing the intra-tumor localization of ADCC effector cells, *J. Immunol.* (in press).

Haskill, J. S., Proctor, J. W., and Yamamura, Y., 1975*a*, Host responses within solid tumors. I. Monocytic effector cells within rat sarcomas, *J. Natl. Cancer Inst.* **54**:387–393.

Haskill, J. S., Yamamura, Y., and Radov, L., 1975*b*, Host responses within solid tumors: Non-thymus-derived specific cytotoxic cells within a murine mammary adenocarcinoma, *Int. J. Cancer* **16**:798–809.

Haskill, J. S., Yamamura, Y., Radov, L., and Parthenais, E., 1976*a*, Discussion paper: Are peripheral and *in situ* tumor immunity related?, *Ann. N.Y. Acad. Sci.* **276**:373–380.

Haskill, J. S., Radov, L. A., Yamamura, Y., Parthenais, E., Korn, J. H., and Ritter, F. L.,

1976*b*, Experimental solid tumors: The role of macrophages and lymphocytes as effector cells, *J. Reticuloendothel. Soc.* 20:233–241.

Haskill, J. S., Radov, L. A., Fett, J. W., and Parthenais, E., 1977, The antibody response to the T1699 murine adenocarcinoma. Antibody class and subclass heterogeneity detected in serum and in situ, *J. Immunol.* 119:1000–1005.

Hay, J. B., and Hobbs, B. B., 1977, The flow of blood to lymph nodes and its relation to lymphocyte traffic and the immune response, *J. Exp. Med.* 145:31–44.

Häyry, P., 1976, Anamnestic responses in mixed lymphocyte culture-induced cytolysis (MLC-CML) reaction, *Immunogenetics* 3:417–453.

Häyry, P., and Defendi, V., 1970, Mixed lymphocyte cultures produce effector cells. An *in vitro* model for allograft rejection, *Science* 68:133–135.

Häyry, P., Lalla, M., Pasternack, A., and Virolainen, M., 1972*a*, Proliferation of white blood cells in the blood of human renal allograft recipients. Lack of correlation with acute rejection episodes, *Ann. Clin. Res.* 4:100–109.

Häyry, P., Lindstrom, B. L., Virolainen, M., Pasternack, A., and Lindfors, O., 1972*b*, Immunobiological diagnosis of rejection in dogs with renal allografts, *Surgery* 71:494–506.

Hellstrom, I., and Hellstrom, K. E., 1970, Colony inhibition studies on blocking and non-blocking serum effects on cellular immunity to Moloney sarcomas, *Int. J. Cancer* 5:195–201.

Hellstrom, I., and Hellstrom, K. E., 1974, Cell-mediated immune reactions to tumor antigens with particular emphasis on immunity to human neoplasms, *Cancer* 34:1461–1468.

Hellstrom, I., Sjogren, H. O., Warner, G., and Hellstrom, K. E., 1971*a*, Blocking of cell-mediated tumor immunity by serum from patients with growing neoplasms, *Int. J. Cancer* 7:226–237.

Hellstrom, I., Hellstrom, K. E., Sjogren, H. O., and Warner, G. A., 1971*b*, Serum factors in tumor-free patients cancelling the blocking of cell-mediated tumor immunity, *Int. J. Cancer* 8:185–191.

Hellstrom, K. E., and Hellstrom, I., 1974, Lymphocyte-mediated cytotoxicity and blocking serum activity to tumor antigens, *Adv. Immunol.* 18:209–277.

Hellstrom, K. E., and Hellstrom, I., 1977, Immunologic enhancement of tumor growth, in: *Mechanisms of Tumor Immunity* (I. Green, S. Cohen, and R. T. McCluskey, eds.), pp. 147–174, John Wiley and Sons, New York.

Henney, C. S., 1977, Mechanisms of tumor cell destruction, in: *Mechanisms of Tumor Immunity* (I. Green, S. Cohen, and R. T. McCluskey, eds.), pp. 55–86, John Wiley and Sons, New York.

Herberman, R. B., 1973*a*, Cellular immunity to human tumor-associated antigens: A review, *Isr. J. Med. Sci.* 9:300–307.

Herberman, R. B., 1973*b*, Immunologic reactions of experimental animals to tumor-associated cell-surface antigens, *Pathobiol. Ann.* 3:291–307.

Herberman, R. B., 1974, Cell-mediated immunity to tumor cells, *Adv. Cancer Res.* 19:207–263.

Herberman, R. B., Nunn, M. E., Lavin, D. H., and Asofsky, R., 1973, Effect of antibody to O-antigen on cell-mediated immunity induced in syngeneic mice by murine sarcoma virus, *J. Natl. Cancer Inst.* 51:1509–1512.

Herberman, R. B., Nunn, M. E., and Avrin, D. H., 1975*a*, Natural cytotoxic reactivity of mouse lymphoid cells against syngeneic and allogenic tumors. I. Distribution of reactivity and specificity, *Int. J. Cancer* 16:216–229.

Herberman, R. B., Nunn, M. E., Holden, H. T., and Avrin, D. H., 1975*b*, Natural cytotoxic reactivity of mouse lymphoid cells against syngeneic and allogenic tumors. II. Characterization of effector cells, *Int. J. Cancer* 16:230–239.

Herberman, R. B., Kirchner, H., Holden, H. T., Glaser, M., Haskill, S., and Bonnard, G. D., 1976, Cell-mediated immunity in murine virus tumor systems, in: *Tumor Virus Infections and Immunity* (R. L. Crowell, H. Friedman, and J. E. Prier, eds.), pp. 147–164, University Park Press, Baltimore.

Herberman, R. B., Bartram, S., Haskill, J. S., Nunn, M., Holden, H. T., and West, W. H., 1977, Fc receptors on mouse effector cells mediating natural cytotoxicity against tumor cells, *J. Immunol.* 119:322–326.

Hersh, E. M., Butler, W. T., Rossen, R. D., and Morgan, R. O., 1970, Lymphocyte activation: A rapid test to predict allograft rejection, *Nature* 226:757–758.

Hibbs, J. B., Jr., 1973, Macrophage nonimmunologic recognition: Target cell factors related to contact inhibition, *Science* 180:868–870.

Hibbs, J. B., Jr., 1975, Role of macrophages in host defense against cancer, in: *Immunological Aspects of Neoplasia*, Vol. 26, pp. 305–327, Williams & Wilkins, Baltimore.

Hibbs, J. B., Jr., Lambert, L. H., Jr., and Remington, J. S., 1971, Resistance to murine tumors conferred by chronic infection of intracellular protozoa, *Toxoplasma gondii* and *Besnoitia jellisoni*, *J. Infect. Dis.* 124:587–592.

Hibbs, J. B., Jr., Lambert, L. H., Jr., and Remington, J. S., 1972a, Adjuvant induced resistance to tumor development in mice, *Proc. Soc. Exp. Biol. Med.* 139:1053–1056.

Hibbs, J. B., Jr., Lambert, L. H., Jr., and Remington, J. S., 1972b, Control of carcinogenesis: A possible role for the activated macrophage, *Science* 177:998–1000.

Holden, H. T., Haskill, J. S., Kirchner, H., and Herberman, R. B., 1976, Two functionally distinct anti-tumor effector cells isolated from primary murine sarcoma virus-induced tumors, *J. Immunol.* 117:440–446.

Holtermann, O. A., Casale, G. P., and Klein, E., 1972, Tumor cell destruction by macrophages, *J. Med. (Basel)* 3:305–309.

Howell, S. B., Dean, J. H., Esber, E. C., and Law, L. W., 1974, Cell interactions in adoptive immune rejection of a syngeneic tumor, *Int. J. Cancer* 14:662–674.

Hume, D. M., and Egdahl, R. H., 1955, Progressive destruction of renal homografts isolated from the regional lymphatics of the host, *Surgery* 38:194–214.

Humphrey, J. H., and Dourmashkin, R. R., 1965, Electron microscope studies of immune cell analysis, in: *Ciba Foundation Symposium on Complement* (G. E. W. Wolstenholme and J. Knight, eds.), pp. 175–186, Churchill, London.

Humphrey, J. H., and Dourmashkin, R. R., 1969, The lesions in cell membranes caused by complement, *Adv. Immunol.* 11:75–115.

Husby, G., Hoagland, P. M., Strickland, R. G., and Williams, R. C., Jr., 1976, Tissue T and B cell infiltration of primary and metastatic cancer, *J. Clin. Invest.* 57:1471–1482.

Ishizaka, T., Ishizaka, K., Borsos, T., and Rapp, H. J., 1966, C'1 fixation by human isoagglutinins: Fixation of C'1 by gamma-G and gamma-M but not by gamma-A antibody, *J. Immunol.* 97:716–726.

Izsak, F. C., Brenner, H. J., Landes, E., Ran, M., and Witz, I. P., 1974, Correlation between clinicopathological features of malignant tumors and cell surface immunoglobulins, *Isr. J. Med. Sci.* 10:642–646.

Jakobisiak, M., 1971, Quantitative data concerning the development of the cellular infiltration of skin allograft in mice, *Transplantation* 12:364–367.

Jakobisiak, M., Kossowaka, B., Moskalewski, S., and Rymaszewska-Kossokowska, T., 1971, Isolation of cells infiltrating the skin allograft in mice, *Transplantation* 11:354–356.

Janik, P., 1976, Are the tumor cells of G_2 period of the cell cycle sensitive to the immune pressure?, *Neoplasma* 23:31–36.

Johansson, B., and Ljungqvist, A., 1974, Localization of immunoglobulins in urinary bladder tumours, *Acta. Pathol. Microbiol. Scand.* A82:559–563.

Johnson, R. J., Pasternack, G. R., and Shin, H. S., 1977, Antibody-mediated suppression of tumor growth: I. *J. Immunol.* 118:489-504.

Jondal, M., Svedmyr, E., Klein, E., and Singh, S., 1975, Killer T cells in a Burkitt's lymphoma biopsy, *Nature* 255:405-407.

Kano, K., and Milgrom, F., 1969, Relation of anti-γ-globulin antibodies to transplantation antibodies in human renal allograft recipients, *Transplantation* 7:281-289.

Keller, R., 1973, Cytostatic elimination of syngeneic rat tumor cells *in vitro* by nonspecifically activated macrophages, *J. Exp. Med.* 138:625-644.

Keller, R., 1974a, Modulation of cell proliferation by macrophages: A possible function apart from cytotoxic tumour rejection, *Brit. J. Cancer* 30:401-415.

Keller, R., 1974b, Mechanisms by which activated normal macrophages destroy syngeneic rat tumour cells *in vitro*. Cytokinetics, non-involvement of T lymphocytes, and effect of metabolic inhibitors, *Immunology* 27:285-298.

Keller, R., 1975, Major changes in lymphocyte proliferation evoked by activated macrophages, *Cell. Immunol.* 17:542-551.

Keller, R., 1976, Cytostatic and cytocidal effects of activated macrophages, in: *Immunobiology of the Macrophage* (D. S. Nelson, ed.), pp. 487-508, Academic Press, New York.

Kerbel, R. S., and Pross, H. F., 1977, Fc receptor-bearing cells as a reliable marker for quantitation of host lumphoreticular infiltration of progressively growing solid tumors, *Int. J. Cancer* 18:432-438.

Kerbel, R. S., Pross, H. F., and Elliott, E. V., 1975, Origin and partial characterization of Fc receptor-bearing cells found within experimental carcinoms and sarcomas, *Int. J. Cancer* 15:918-932.

Kiessling, R., Klein, E., and Wigzell, H., 1975a, "Natural" killer cells in the mouse. I. Cytotoxic cells with specificity for mouse Moloney leukemia cells. Specificity and distribution according to genotype, *Eur. J. Immunol.* 5:112-117.

Kiessling, R., Klein, E., Pross, H., and Wigzell, H., 1975b, "Natural" killer cells in the mouse. II. Cytotoxic cells with specificity for mouse Moloney leukemia cells. Characteristics of the killer cell, *Eur. J. Immunol.* 5:117-121.

Kiessling, R., Petranyi, G., Karre, K., Jondal, M., Tracey, D., and Wigzell, H., 1976, Killer cells: A functional comparison between natural, immune T-cell and antibody-dependent *in vitro* systems, *J. Exp. Med.* 143:722-780.

Kikuchi, K., Ishii, Y., Ueno, H., and Koshiba, H., 1976, Cell-mediated immunity involved in autochthonous tumor rejection in rats, *Ann. N.Y. Acad. Sci.* 276:188-206.

Kimura, A. K., Rubin, B., and Andersson, L. C., 1977, Evidence for "K" cell killing by Fc receptor bearing alloactivated cytotoxic T lymphocytes, *Scand. J. Immunol.* 6:787-796.

Kincaid-Smith, P., Morris, P. J., Saker, B. M., Ting, A., and Marshall, V. C., 1968, Immediate renal-graft biopsy and subsequent rejection, *Lancet* 2:748-750.

Kirchner, H., Holden, H. T., and Herberman, R. B., 1975a, Inhibition of *in vitro* growth of lymphoma cells by macrophages from tumor-bearing mice, *J. Natl. Cancer Inst.* 55:971-975.

Kirchner, H., Muchmore, A. V., Chused, T. M., Holden, H. T., and Herberman, R. B., 1975b, Inhibition of proliferation of lymphoma cells and T lymphocytes by suppressor cells from spleens of tumor-bearing mice, *J. Immunol.* 114:206-210.

Klein, E., Becker, S., Svedmyr, E., Jondal, M., and Vanky, F., 1976, Tumor infiltrating lymphocytes, *Ann. N.Y. Acad. Sci.* 276:207-216.

Klein, J., Livnat, S., Hauptfeld, V., Jerabek, L., and Weissman, I., 1974, Production of anti-H-2 antibodies in thymectomized mice, *Eur. J. Immunol.* 4:41-44.

Konda, S., and Smith, R. T., 1973, The effects of tumor bearing upon changes in cell distribution and membrane antigen characteristics in murine, spleen and thymus cell subpopulations, *Cancer Res.* 33:1878-1884.

Krahenbuhl, J. L., and Remington, J. S., 1974, The role of activated macrophages in specific and nonspecific cytostasis of tumor cells, *J. Immunol.* 113:507–516.

Kripke, M. L., and Borsos, T., 1974, Immunosuppression and carcinogenesis: A review, *Isr. J. Med. Sci.* 10:888–903.

Krohn, P. L., and Zuckerman, A., 1954, The effect of splenectomy on the survival of skin homografts in rabbits and on the response to cortisone, *Brit. J. Exp. Pathol.* 35:223–226.

Krzymanski, M., Quadracci, L., Ringden, O., and Lundgren, G., 1975, Lymphocyte subpopulations in uremics and in transplanted patients, *Scand. J. Urol. Nephrol. Suppl.* 29:37–40.

Lamon, E. W., Skurzak, H. M., Klein, E., and Wigzell, H., 1972, *In vitro* cytotoxicity by a nonthymus-processed lymphocyte population with specificity for a virally determined tumor cell surface antigen, *J. Exp. Med.* 136:1072–1079.

Lamon, E. W., Wigzell, H., Klein, E., Andersson, B., and Skurzak, H. M., 1973, The lymphocyte response to primary Moleney sarcoma virus tumors in BALB/c mice, *J. Exp. Med.* 137:1472–1493.

Lamon, E. W., Whitten, H. D., Lidin, B., and Fudenberg, H. H., 1975a, IgM-induced tumor cell cytotoxicity mediated by normal thymocytes, *J. Exp. Med.* 142:542–547.

Lamon, E. W., Whitten, H. D., Skurzak, H. M., Andersson, B., and Lidin, B., 1975b, IgM antibody-dependent cell-mediated cytotoxicity in the Moloney sarcoma virus system: the involvement of T and B lymphocytes as effector cells, *Immunology* 115:1288–1294.

Lamon, E. W., Skurzak, H. M., Andersson, B., Whitten, H. D., and Klein, E., 1975c, Antibody-dependent lymphocyte cytotoxicity in the murine sarcoma virus system: Activity of IgM and IgG with specificity for MLV determined antigen(s), *J. Immunol.* 114:1171–1176.

Lamon, E. W., Shaw, M. W., Goodson, S., Lidin, B., Walia, A. S., and Fuson, E. W., 1977, Antibody-dependent cell-mediated cytotoxicity in the Moloney sarcoma virus system: Differential activity of IgG and IgM with different subpopulations of lymphocytes, *J. Exp. Med.* 145:302–313.

Lance, E. M., and Cooper, S., 1972, Homing of specifically sensitized lymphocytes to allografts of skin, *Cell. Immunol.* 5:66–73.

Lauder, I., and Aherne, W., 1972. The significance of lymphocytic infiltration in neuroblastoma, *Brit. J. Cancer* 26:321–330.

LeClerc, J. C., Gomard, E., Plata, F., and Levy, J. P., 1973, Cell-mediated immune reaction against tumors induced by oncornaviruses. II. Nature of the effector cells in tumor-cell cytolysis, *Int. J. Cancer* 11:426–432.

Levy, M. H., and Wheelock, E. F., 1974, The role of macrophages in defense against neoplastic disease, *Adv. Cancer Res.* 20:131–163.

Levy, N. L., 1973, Use of an *in vitro* microcytotoxicity test to assess human tumor-specific cell-mediated immunity and its serum-mediated abrogation, *Natl. Cancer Inst. Monogr.* 37:85–92.

Lewis, M. G., Proctor, J. W., Thomson, D. M., Rowden, G., and Phillips, T. M., 1976, Cellular localization of immunoglobulin within human malignant melanomata, *Brit. J. Cancer* 33(3):260–266.

Lohmann-Matthes, M. L., Schipper, H., and Fisctier, H., 1972, Macrophage-mediated cytotoxicity against allogeneic target cells *in vitro*, *Eur. J. Immunol.* 2:45–49.

MacCarty, W. C., 1922, Factors which influence longevity in cancer, *Ann. Surg.* 76:9–12.

MacCarty, W. C., and Mahle, A. E., 1921, Relation of differentiation and lymphocytic infiltration to postoperative longevity in gastric carcinoma, *J. Lab. Clin. Med.* 6:473–480.

MacGregor, D. D., and Gowans, J. L., 1964, Survival of homografts of skin in rats depleted of lymphocytes by chronic drainage from the thoracic duct, *Lancet* 1:629–632.

Mackaness, G. B., 1976, Role of macrophages in host defense mechanisms, in: *The Macrophage in Neoplasia* (M. A. Fink, ed.), pp. 3–13, Academic Press, New York.

MacLennan, I. C. M., 1972, Antibody in the induction and inhibition of lymphocyte cytotoxicity, *Transplant. Rev.* 13:67–90.

MacLennan, I. C. M., Loewi, G., and Howard, A., 1969, A human serum immunoglobulin with specificity for certain homologous target cells, which induces target cell damage by normal human lymphocytes, *Immunology* 17:897–910.

Macphail, S., 1976, The class of antibody involved in the antibody-dependent cell-mediated lysis of chicken erythrocytes, *Immunology* 31:697–705.

Malicka, K., 1971, Attempt at evaluation of defensive activity of lymph nodes on the basis of microscopic and clinical studies in cases of laryngeal cancer, *Pol. Med.* 10:154–164.

Mansell, P. W. A., Ichinose, H., Reed, R. J., Krementz, E. T., McNamee, R., and DiLuzio, N. R., 1975, Macrophage-mediated destruction of human malignant cells *in vivo, J. Natl. Cancer Inst.* 54:571–580.

McPhaul, J. J., Lordon, R. E., Thompson, A. L., and Mullins, J. D., 1976, Nephritogenic immunopathologic mechanisms and human renal transplants: The problem of recurrent glomerulonephritis, *Kidney Int.* 10:135–138 (editorial).

Medawar, P. B., 1944, Behavior and fate of skin autografts and skin homografts in rabbits, *J. Anat.* 78:176–199.

Melgrom, F., Humphrey, L. J., Tonder, O., Yasuda, J., and Witebsky, E., 1968, Antibody-mediated hemadsorption by tumor tissues, *Int. Arch. Allergy Appl. Immunol.* 33:478–492.

Meltzer, M. S., Tucker, R. W., Sanford, K. K., and Leonard, E. J., 1975, Interaction of BCG-activated macrophages with neoplastic and nonneoplastic cell lines *in vitro:* Quantitation of the cytotoxic reaction by release of triated thymidine from prelabelled target cells, *J. Natl. Cancer Inst.* 54:1177–1184.

Micklem, H. S., and Loutit, J. F., 1966, Tissue transplantation in normal animals, in: *Tissue Grafting and Radiation*, pp. 1–31, Academic Press, New York.

Milgrom, F., 1977, Role of humoral antibodies in transplantation, *Transplant. Proc.* 9:721–727.

Miller, J. F. A. P., and Osoba, D., 1967, Current concepts of immunological functions of the thymus, *Physiol. Rev.* 477:437–520.

Mitchison, N. A., 1955, Studies on the immunological response to foreign tumor transplants in the mouse. I. The role of lymph node cell in conferring immunity by adoptive transfer, *J. Exp. Med.* 102:157–177.

Moller, E., 1965, Contact-induced cytotoxicity by lymphoid cells containing foreign isoantigens, *Science* 147:873–874; 879.

Moore, K., and Moore, M., 1977, Intra-tumor host cells of transplanted rat neoplasms of different immunogenicity, *Int. J. Cancer* 19:803–813.

Moore, O. S., Jr., and Foote, F. W., Jr., 1949, The relatively favorable prognosis of medullary carcinoma of the breast, *Cancer* 2:635–642.

Nairn, R. C., Nind, A. P. P., Guli, E. P. G., Muller, H. K., Rolland, J. M., and Minty, C. C. J., 1971a, Specific immune response in human skin carcinoma, *Brit. Med. J.* 4:701–705.

Nairn, R. C., Nind, A. P. P., Guli, E. P. G., Davies, D. J., Rolland, J. M., McGiven, A. R., and Hughes, E. S. R., 1971b, Immunological reactivity in patients with carcinoma of colon, *Brit. Med. J.* 4:706–709.

Najarian, J. S., and Feldman, J. D., 1962, Passive transfer of transplantation immunity. I.

Triated lymphoid cells. II. Lymphoid cells in millipore chambers, *J. Exp. Med.* 115:1083–1093.

Nepom, J. T., Hellstrom, I., and Hellstrom, K. E., 1976, Purification and partial characterization of a tumor-specific blocking factor from sera of mice with growing chemically induced sarcomas, *J. Immunol.* 117:1846–1852.

Nind, A. P. P., Nairn, R. C., Rolland, J. M., Guli, E. P. G., and Hughes, E. S. R., 1973, Lymphocyte anergy in patients with carcinoma, *Br. J. Cancer* 28:108–117.

Nishioka, K., 1971, Complement and tumor immunology, *Adv. Cancer Res.* 14: 231–292.

Nunn, M., Djeu, J., Lavrin, D., and Herberman, R., 1973, Natural cytotoxic reactivity of rat lymphocytes against syngeneic Gross leukemia, *Proc. Amer. Assoc. Cancer Res.* 14:87.

O'Toole, C., Perlmann, P., Wigzell, H., Unsgaard, B., and Zetterlund, C. G., 1973, Lymphocyte cytotoxicity in bladder cancer. No requirement for thymus-derived effector cells?, *Lancet* 1:1085–1088.

Pasternack, A., Virolainen, M., and Häyry, P., 1973, Fine-needle aspiration biopsy in the diagnosis of human renal allograft rejection, *J. Urol.* 109:167–172.

Pedersen, N. C., and Morris, B., 1970, The role of the lymphatic system in the rejection of homografts: A study of lymph from renal transplants, *J. Exp. Med.* 131:936–969.

Perlmann, P., Perlmann, H., and Wigzell, H., 1972, Lymphocyte mediated cytotoxicity *in vitro*. Induction and inhibition by humoral antibody and nature of effector cells, *Transplant. Rev.* 13:91–114.

Plata, F., and Sordat, B., 1977, Murine sarcoma (MSV)-induced tumors in mice. I. Distribution of MSV-immune CTL *in vivo*, *Int. J. Cancer* 19:205–211.

Plata, F., MacDonald, H. R., and Sordat, B., 1975, Studies on the distribution and origin of cytolytic T lymphocytes present in mice bearing Moloney murine sarcoma virus (MSV)-induced tumors, *Bibliotheca Haematol.* 43:274–277.

Poulter, L. W., Bradley, N. J., and Turk, J. L., 1971, The role of macrophages in skin allograft rejection. I. Histochemical studies during first-set rejection, *Transplantation* 12:40– 44.

Prendergast, R. A., 1964, Cellular specificity in the homograft reaction, *J. Exp. Med.* 119:377–388.

Pross, H. F., and Kerbel, R. S., 1976, An assessment of intratumor phagocytic and surface marker-bearing cells in a series of autochthonous and early passaged chemically induced murine sarcomas, *J. Natl. Cancer Inst.* 57:1157–1167.

Pross, H. F., Tracey, D. E., Wigzell, H., and Scherrmacher, V., 1974, Antibody-dependent cell-mediated cytotoxicity in the mouse. I. Surface characteristics of an effector cell, *Scand. J. Immunol.* 3:769–780.

Radov, L. A., Haskill, J. S., Korn, J. H., and Fett, J. W., 1978, Correlation between tumor-specific systemic and *in situ* immunity as manifested by the delayed hypersensitivity response, *J. Natl. Cancer Inst.* (in press).

Ran, M., and Witz, I. P., 1972, Tumor-associated immunoglobulins. Enhancement of syngeneic tumors by IgG2-containing tumor eluates, *Int. J. Cancer* 9:242–247.

Ran, M., Klein, G., and Witz, I. P., 1976, Tumor-bound immunoglobulins. Evidence for the *in vivo* coating of tumor cells by potentially cytotoxic anti-tumor antibodies, *Int. J. Cancer* 17:90–97.

Richters, A., and Kaspersky, C. L., 1975, Surface immunoglobulin positive lymphocytes in human breast cancer tissue and homolateral axillary lymph nodes, *Cancer* 35:129–133.

Risdall, R. J., Aust, J. C., and McKhann, C. F., 1973, Immune capacity and response to antigenic tumors, *Cancer Res.* 33:2078–2085.

Roberts, P. J., 1977, Effector mechanisms in allograft rejection. III. Kinetics of killer cell activity inside the graft and in the immune system during primary and secondary allograft immune responses, *Scand. J. Immunol.* 6:635–640.

Roberts, P. J., and Häyry, P., 1976a, Sponge matrix allografts. A model for analysis of killer cells infiltrating mouse allografts, *Transplantation* 21:437–445.

Roberts, P. J., and Häyry, P., 1976b, Effector mechanisms in allograft rejection. I. Assembly of "sponge matrix" allografts, *Cell. Immunol.* 26:160–167.

Roberts, P. J., and Häyry, P., 1977, Effector mechanisms in allograft rejection. II. Density-, electrophoresis- and size fractionation of allograft-infiltrating cells demonstrating several classes of killer cells, *Cell. Immunol.* 30:236–253.

Rosenau, W., 1963, Interaction of lymphoid cells with target cells in tissue culture, in: *Cell Bound Antibodies* (B. Amos and H. Koprowski, eds.), pp. 75–88, Wistar Institute Press, Philadelphia.

Roser, B. J., and Ford, W. L., 1972, Prolonged lymphocytopenia in the rat. The immunological consequences of lymphocyte depletion following injection of ^{185}W tungsten trioxide into the spleen or lymph node, *Aust. J. Exp. Biol. Med. Sci.* 50:185–198.

Roubin, R., Cesarini, J. P., Fridman, W. H., Pavie-Fisher, J., and Peter, H. H., 1975, Characterization of the mononuclear cell infiltrate in human malignant melanoma, *Int. J. Cancer* 16:61–73.

Rouse, B. T., Rollinghoff, M., and Warner, N. L., 1972, Anti-theta serum-induced suppression of the cellular transfer of tumour-specific immunity to a syngeneic plasma cell tumour, *Nature New Biol.* 238:116–117.

Rowlands, D. T., Burkholder, P. M., Bossen, E. H., and Lin, H. H., 1970, Renal allografts in HLA matched recipients, *Amer. J. Pathol.* 61:177–229.

Russell, S. W., and Cochrane, C. G., 1974, The cellular events associated with regression and progression of murine (Moloney) sarcomas, *Int. J. Cancer* 13:54–63.

Russell, S. W., Doe, W. F., and Cochrane, C. G., 1976a, Number of macrophages and distribution of mitotic activity in regressing and progressing moloney sarcomas, *J. Immunol.* 116:164–166.

Russell, S. W., Doe, W. F., Hoskins, R. G., and Cochrane, C. G., 1976b, Inflammatory cells in solid murine neoplasms. I. Tumor disaggregation and identification of constituent inflammatory cells, *Int. J. Cancer* 18:322–330.

Russell, S. W., Gillespie, G. Y., and McIntosh, A. T., 1977, Inflammatory cells in solid murine neoplasms. III. Cytotoxicity mediated *in vitro* by macrophages recovered from disaggregated regressing moloney sarcomas, *J. Immunol.* 118:1574–1579.

Saal, J. G., Rieber, E. P., Hadam, M., and Riethmuller, G., 1977, Lymphocytes with T-cell markers cooperate with IgG antibodies in the lysis of human tumour cells, *Nature* 265:158–160.

Saksela, E., Imir, T., and Makela, O., 1975, Specifically cytotoxic human and mouse lymphoid cells induced with antibody or antigen–antibody complexes, *J. Immunol.* 115:1488–1492.

Sarma, K. P., 1972, Proliferative and lymphoid reactions in bladder cancer, *Invest. Urol.* 10:199–207.

Scothorne, R. J., and MacGregor, I. A., 1955, Cellular changes in lymph nodes and spleen following skin homografts in the rabbit, *J. Anat.* 89:283–292.

Sendo, F., Aoki, T., Boyse, E. A., and Buafo, C. K., 1975, Natural occurrence of lymphocytes showing cytotoxic activity to BALB/c radiation leukemia RLo1 cells, *J. Natl. Cancer Inst.* 55:603–609.

Siciu-Foca, N., Buda, J. A., and Thiem, T., 1972, Serial determination of blast cell count during allograft rejection in rats, *Transplantation* 14:711–715.

Sjogren, H. O., Hellstrom, I., Bansal, S. C., Warner, G. A., and Hellstrom, K. E., 1972,

Elution of "blocking factors" from human tumors, capable of abrograting tumor-cell destruction by specifically immune lymphocytes, *Int. J. Cancer* 9:274–283.

Sobczak, E., and deVaux Saint Cyr, C., 1971, Study of the *in vivo* fixation of antibodies on tumors provoked in hamsters by injection of SV40-transformed cells (TSV$_5$Cl$_2$), *Int. J. Cancer* 8:47–52.

Solillou, J. P., Carpenter, C. B., d'Apice, A. J. F., and Strom, T. B., 1976, The role of non-classical, Fc receptor-associated, Ag-B antigens (*Ia*) in rat allograft enhancement, *J. Exp. Med.* 143:405.

Spector, W. G., and Mariano, M., 1975, Macrophage behavior in experimental granulomas, in: *Mononuclear Phagocytes in Immunity, Infection and Pathology* (R. van Furth, ed.), pp. 927–942, Blackwell Scientific, Oxford.

Sprent, J., and Miller, J. F. A. P., 1972, Interaction of thymus lymphocytes with histo-incompatible cells. III. Immunological characteristics of recirculating lymphocytes derived from activated thymus cells, *Cell. Immunol.* 3:213.

Sprent, J., and Miller, J. F. A. P., 1976, Fate of H2-activated T lymphocytes in syngeneic hosts. II. Residence in recirculating lymphocyte pool and capacity to migrate to allografts, *Cell. Immunol.* 21:303–313.

Strober, S., and Gowans, J. L., 1965, The role of lymphocytes in the sensitization of rats to renal homografts, *J. Exp. Med.* 122:347–360.

Strom, T. B., Nicholas, L. T., Carpenter, C. B., and Busch, G. J., 1975, Identity and cytotoxic capacity of cells infiltrating renal allografts, *New Engl. J. Med.* 292:1257–1263.

Strom, T. B., Tilney, N. L., Paradysz, J. M., Bancewisz, J., and Carpenter, C. B., 1978, The cellular components of allograft rejection. The identity, specificity and cytotoxic function of cells accumulating within acutely rejecting allografts (in press).

Stutman, O., 1975*a*, Immunodepression and malignancy, *Adv. Cancer Res.* 22:261–422.

Stutman, O., 1975*b*, Delayed tumour appearance and absence of regression in nude mice infected with murine sarcoma virus, *Nature* 253:142–144.

Stutman, O., 1977, Immunodeficiency and cancer, in: *Mechanisms of Tumor Immunity* (I. Green, S. Cohen, and R. T. McCluskey, eds.), John Wiley and Sons, Inc., pp. 27–53, New York.

Suthanthiran, M., Gailiunas, P., Fagan, G., Strom, T. B., Carpenter, C. B., and Garovoy, M. R., 1978, Detection of anti-donor "Ia" antibodies: A strong correlation of rejection, *Transplant. Proc.* (in press).

Szymaniec, S., and James, K., 1976, Studies on the Fc-receptor bearing cells in a transplanted methylcholanthrene-induced mouse fibrosarcoma, *Brit. J. Cancer* 33:36–50.

Takasugi, M., and Klein, E., 1971, The role of blocking antibodies in immunological enhancement, *Immunology* 21:675–684.

Tanaka, T., Cooper, E. H., and Anderson, C. K., 1970, Lymphocyte infiltration in bladder carcinoma, *Rev. Eur. Études Clin. Biol.* 15:1081–1089.

Thompson, D. M. P., Steele, K., and Alexander, P., 1973, The presence of tumour-specific membrane antigen in the serum of rats with chemically induced sarcomata, *Brit. J. Cancer* 27:27–34.

Tilney, N. L., and Ford, W. L., 1974, The migration of rat lymphoid cells into skin grafts. Some sensitized cells localize preferentially in specific allografts, *Transplantation* 17:12–21.

Tilney, N. L., Strom, T. B., MacPherson, S. G., and Carpenter, C. B., 1975, Surface properties and functional characteristics of infiltrating cells harvested from acutely rejecting cardiac allografts in inbred rats, *Transplantation* 20:323–330.

Tilney, N. L., Strom, T. B., MacPherson, S. G., and Carpenter, C. B., 1976, Studies on infiltrating host cells harvested from acutely rejecting rat cardiac allografts, *Surgery* 79:209–217.

Ting, R. C., and Law, L. W., 1976, Thymic function and carcinogenesis, *Prog. Exp. Tumor Res.* 9:165–191.

Tønder, O., Morse, P. A., Jr., and Humphrey, L. J., 1974, Similarities of Fc receptors in human malignant tissue and normal lymphoid tissue, *J. Immunol.* 113:1162–1168.

Tønder, O., Krishnan, E. C., Jewell, W. R., Morse, P. A., Jr., and Humphrey, L. J., 1976, Tumor Fc receptors and tumor-associated immunoglobulins, *Acta. Pathol. Microbiol. Scand.* C84:105–111.

Treves, A. J., Cohen, I. R. and Feldman, 1976, A syngeneic metastatic tumor model in mice: The natural immune response of the host and its manipulation, in: *Immunological Parameters of Host-Tumor Relationships*, Vol. 4 (D. W. Weiss, ed.), pp. 89–103, Academic Press, New York.

Tsakraklides, V., Olson, P., Kersey, J. H., and Good, R. A., 1974, Prognostic significance of the regional lymph node histology in cancer of the breast, *Cancer* 34:1259–1267.

Turk, J. L., Heather, C. J., and Diengdoh, J. V., 1966, A histochemical analysis of mononuclear cell infiltrates of the skin with particular reference to delayed hypersensitivity in the guinea pig, *Int. Arch. Allergy Appl. Immunol.* 29:278–289.

Van Boxel, J. A., Stobo, J. D., Paul, W. E., and Green, I., 1972, Antibody-dependent lymphoid cell-mediated cytotoxicity: No requirement for thymus-derived lymphocytes, *Science* 175:194–195.

Vanky, F., Stjernsward, J., Klein, G., Steiner, L., and Lindberg, L., 1973, Tumor-associated specificity of serum-mediated inhibition of lymphocyte stimulation by authochthonous human tumors, *J. Natl. Cancer Inst.* 51:25–32.

Vanky, F., Trempe, G., Klein, E., and Stjernsward, J., 1975, Human tumor-lymphocyte interaction *in vitro*: Blastogenesis correlated to detectable immunoglobulin in the biopsy, *Int. J. Cancer* 16:113–124.

Voisin, G. A., Kinsky, R., Jansen, F., and Bernard, C., 1969, Biological properties of antibody classes in transplantation immune sera, *Transplantation* 8:618–632.

Vose, B. M., Vanky, F., Argov, F., and Klein, E., 1977, Natural cytotoxicity in man: Activity of lymph node and tumour infiltrating lymphocytes, *Eur. J. Immunol.* 7:753–757.

Wade, H., 1908, An experimental investigation of infective sarcoma of the dog, with a consideration of its relationship to cancer, *J. Pathol. Bacteriol.* 12:385–425.

Wagner, J. L., and Haughton, G., 1971, Immunosuppression by anti-lymphocyte serum and its effect on tumors induced by 3-methylcholanthrene in mice, *J. Natl. Cancer Inst.* 46:1–10.

Waksman, B. H., 1963, The pattern of rejection in rat skin homografts and its relation to the vascular network, *Lab. Invest.* 12:46–57.

Wartman, W. B., 1959, Sinus cell hyperplasia of lymph nodes regional to adenocarcinoma of the breast and colon, *Brit. J. Cancer* 13:389–397.

Weaver, J. M., 1958, Destruction of mouse ascites tumor cells *in vivo* and *in vitro* by homologous macrophages, lymphocytes and cell-free antibodies, *Proc. Amer. Cancer Res.* 2:354.

Weiner, J., Spiro, D., and Russell, P. S., 1964, An electron microscopic study of the homograft reaction, *Amer. J. Pathol.* 44:319–347.

Wigzell, H., and Häyry, P., 1974, Specific fractionation of immunocompetent cells. Application to the analysis of effector cells involved in cell-mediated lysis, *Current Top. Microbiol. Immunol.* 67:1–42.

Williams, G. U., Hume, D. M., and Hudson, R. P., 1698, "Hyperacute" renal-homograft rejection in man, *New Engl. J. Med.* 279:611–618.

Witz, I. P., 1976, Tumor bound immunoglobulins in situ expressions of humoral immunity, *Adv. Cancer Res.* 25:95–141.

Wortis, H. H., 1971, Immunological responses of "nude" mice, *Clin. Exp. Immunol.* 8:305–317.

Yoshida, T., and Cohen, S., 1974, *In vivo* manifestations of lymphokine and lymphokine-like activity, in: *Mechanisms of Cell-Mediated Immunity* (R. T. McCluskey and S. Cohen, eds.), pp. 43–60, John Wiley and Sons, New York.

Yoshida, T., and Cohen, S., 1977, Lymphokines in tumor immunity, in: *Mechanisms of Tumor Immunity* (I. Green, S. Cohen, and R. T. McCluskey, eds.), pp. 87–108, John Wiley and Sons, New York.

Zarling, J. M., and Tevethia, S. S., 1973, Transplantation immunity to simian virus 40-transformed cells in tumor-bearing mice. II. Evidence for macrophage participation at the effector level of tumor cell rejection, *J. Natl. Cancer Inst.* 50:149–157.

Zettergren, J. G., Luberoff, D. E., and Pretlow, T. G., 1973, Separation of lymphocytes from disaggregated mouse malignant neoplasms by sedimentation in gradients of Ficoll in tissue culture medium, *J. Immunol.* 111:836–840.

Zighelboim, J., Bonavida, B., and Fahey, J. L., 1973, Evidence for several cell populations active in antibody-dependent cellular cytotoxicity, *J. Immunol.* 111:1737–1742.

Zighelboim, J., Gale, R., Chiu, A., Bonavida, B., Ossoris, R. C., and Fahey, J. L., 1974, Antibody-dependent cellular cytotoxicity: cytotoxicity mediated by non T-lymphocytes, *Clin. Immunol. Immunopathol.* 3:193–200.

Chapter 6

Natural Killer Cells in the Mouse: An Alternative Immune Surveillance Mechanism?

Rolf Kiessling

Department of Tumor Biology
Karolinska Institute
S-104 01 Stockholm 60, Sweden

and

Otto Haller

Department of Immunology
Uppsala University, Box 582
S-751 23 Uppsala, Sweden

I. INTRODUCTION

During the last 10 years the number of effector cell types active in growth inhibition or cytolysis of tumor cells has steadily increased. Although the importance of immune T cells in tumor rejection, measured by cytolytic or cytostatic activity *in vitro*, is firmly established, there is an increasing amount of evidence showing that tumor resistance also could be mediated by non-T-cell-dependent mechanisms. Some of these alternatives to T-cell cytotoxicity involve tumor killing by activated macrophages (Keller, 1976) or by antibody-dependent cellular cytotoxicity (ADCC) (Perlmann *et al.*, 1972) carried out by a variety of nonimmune effector cells. The phenomenon of natural cell-mediated immunity to be discussed in this article will add further to the complexity of this field. The purpose of this chapter is, however, to convince the reader that this phenomenon, although still poorly understood, is a factor which must be seriously considered when discussing immune surveillance mechanisms against tumors.

171

Cytostatic and cytotoxic effects mediated by leukocytes from nonimmune donors have been observed for quite some time. Initially, however, these effects were disregarded as representing nonspecific background noise, and no efforts were made to assess their possible biological significance. In fact, nonimmune leukocytes were often used as the "baseline" when assessing cytotoxicity of immune cells. Thus much of earlier reports of specific antitumor-related activities could probably rather be attributed to the use of control leukocytes with low background levels of natural cell-mediated effects than actual presence of "true" immune effector cells.

The notion of natural cell-mediated immunity as a nonspecific background effect without any biological significance is, however, no longer valid. Several reports from human as well as rodent systems recently have described strong cytolytic effects with leukocytes from normal nonimmunized donors (for a review, see Herberman and Holden, 1978). Moreover, in some of these systems there is now evidence that these effects are directed against specific target structures on the tumor cells. It has been shown mainly in human systems that natural cell-mediated cytotoxicity and conventional specific immune activities can coexist in leukocyte populations from the same patient (Svedmyr and Jondal, 1975). Much effort has been directed to find methods of discrimination between these two groups of activities. In the mouse, however, it has been found relatively easy to define natural cell-mediated immunity as a component of the lymphoid system separate from conventional immune reactivities.

In the present article we will discuss natural cell-mediated immunity in the mouse. We will summarize work which has been carried out in our group in this field. Some pertinent data from other groups of investigators will also be mentioned. However, for a more complete overlook of this expanding research area, the reader is referred to a recent review article by Herberman and Holden (1978).

Our studies in this field started with the observation that certain mouse lymphomas were highly sensitive to lysis in a ^{51}Cr release assay using nonimmune spleen cells from some mouse strains as effector cells (Kiessling *et al.*, 1975*a*). Although the cell donors had experienced no previous immunization, their spleen cells were found to be highly active in short-term cytolytic assays. It was soon realized that this activity revealed a number of unusual characteristics, which distinguished this kind of killing from other known cell-mediated activities. We have chosen to call the responsible cell type natural killer cell (NK cell), as an analogy to the phenomenon of natural antibodies which has been studied extensively in mice (Aoki *et al.*, 1966; Ihle *et al.*, 1973; Nowinski and Kaehler, 1974; Aaronson and Stephenson, 1974; Martin and Martin, 1975).

It soon became clear that this NK cell could be influenced by a number of genetic as well as nongenetic factors. Our efforts to analyze some of these factors will be described with particular emphasis focused on the genetic analysis. We will discuss further the important question of whether the NK activity should be regarded as an immunological phenomenon. Thus we will touch upon questions about the nature of NK specificity and the possibility of specifically enhancing or suppressing NK activity. Experiments leading to the conclusion that NK cells might represent a "new" type of lymphocyte-generated autonomously from bone marrow precursor cells will be described. The implications of recent findings of receptors for the hemagglutinin *Helix pomatia* (HP) on the surface of NK cells will be discussed.

Finally, we will document and discuss the positive relationship between levels of *in vitro* measured cytolytic activity of NK cells and the subsequent *in vivo* tumor resistance of the cell donors. We will also draw the readers' attention to the possibility that NK cells, besides being active against malignant cells, could also play an important role in rejection of nonmalignant hemopoietic grafts.

II. GENERAL CHARACTERISTICS OF THE NK SYSTEM

The initial reason why we became interested in NK cells, to a large extent, was dependent upon our early choice of YAC-1 as a most frequently used target cell. This is a Moloney-leukemia-virus (MLV)-induced mouse T lymphoma of strain A/Sn origin and it is adapted to tissue culture (Cikes *et al.*, 1973). Initially, we intended to use this cell as a target for studying immune T cells. It proved, however, to be a comparatively poor target for immune killer cells, but, much to our surprise, it was highly sensitive to lysis by nonimmune spleen cells in a ^{51}Cr release assay. NK-mediated lysis shares many of the characteristics of lysis by immune T cells. Thus time kinetic studies show a quick onset of lytic activity, and within 1 hour of incubation a cytolytic effect can be seen. With the YAC-1 as a target, up to 90% lysis in a 12-hr incubation period can be seen, although with other target cells the lytic effects are, in general, considerably lower (10–30% lysis) (Kiessling *et al.*, 1975a). The lytic effect is dose-dependent, although at very high effector target cell ratios (>100:1), a "prozone" with lower lytic activity can be seen (unpublished observation). No evidence of involvement of soluble factors, as measured by adding the supernatant of cocultivated effector and target cells, has been found (Kiessling *et al.*, 1975a). Recently performed time-lapse cinematographic studies seem to strengthen the notion that contact is necessary for lysis to occur (Petrányi *et al.*, unpublished observation). Thus the NK-cell-like cytolytic T lymphocytes (CTL) can lyse tumor target cells efficiently and rapidly after contact. Whether this NK target contact does involve a specific recognition of target antigens, as for CTL, is not yet resolved and will be discussed later.

III. SPECIFICITY OF MOUSE NK CYTOLYTIC ACTIVITY

It is not known whether NK activity is generated as an immune response against some environmental antigen, or whether NK cells gain their activity without previous priming. Moreover, it is not clearly established if this activity involves recognition by a receptor–antigen type of reaction in a manner similar to immune T-cell killing. Nevertheless, several groups of investigators have concluded that mouse NK cells are indeed specific. This specificity has been assessed in two ways. First, direct cytotoxicity tests revealed that certain target cells were highly sensitive to lysis by NK cells while others, although susceptible to alloimmune T-cell killing, showed little or no sensitivity (Kiessling *et al.*, 1975*a*; Herberman *et al.*, 1975*a*). Second, competition assays were performed in which unlabeled competitor cells were added to the reaction mixture of effector and radiolabeled target cells. The ability of competitor cells to inhibit isotope release from the labeled target cells was indicative of common surface structures relevant for NK cytotoxicity. Clearly, cells sensitive to NK lysis proved to be good competitors in such tests (Kiessling *et al.*, 1975*a*; Herberman *et al.*, 1975*a*). Moreover, cells with high sensitivity to NK lysis were generally more efficient competitors than those which exhibited low or no sensitivity (Kiessling *et al.*, 1975*a*; Herberman *et al.*, 1975*a*). In most cases a good positive correlation was found between susceptibility to direct lysis and capacity to inhibit lysis. The specificity pattern detected in direct cytotoxicity seemed therefore to reflect true differences in expression of NK-relevant target structure(s). In our early investigations in a limited number of cell lines, NK specificity appeared to be directed predominantly against mouse Moloney-leukemia-virus-induced lymphomas (Kiessling *et al.*, 1975*a*). Work by other groups, however, favored a less restricted specificity (Herberman *et al.*, 1975*a*; Sendo *et al.*, 1975; Zarling *et al.*, 1975). More recent studies by Becker *et al.* (1977) and our own work in a heterologous system (Haller *et al.*, 1977*b*) showed indeed quite a broad specificity of mouse NK cells.

It is obvious from all available data that mouse NK cells can kill mouse target cells of semisyngeneic and allogeneic origin (Kiessling *et al.*, 1975*a*; Herberman *et al.*, 1975*a*). While T-cell cytotoxicity frequently seems to be H-2-restricted (Zinkernagel and Doherty, 1975; Shearer, 1974), no H-2 homology between target and NK cells is needed for successful lysis to occur. Hence, cell surface structures coded for by the major histocompatibility gene complex seem irrelevant for mouse NK recognition and lysis. This fact is further substantiated by *in vitro* blocking experiments with heteroantibody directed exclusively against the H-2 heavy-chain determinants. Fab fragments of such antibodies were used to block in parallel T-cell killing across H-2 and NK cytotoxicity against the same target cells *in vitro*. T-cell reactivity was inhibited while lysis mediated by NK cells was not affected (Haller, unpublished observation).

There has been considerable discussion whether or not NK reactivity is species-restricted (Nunn *et al.*, 1976; Shellam and Hogg, 1977; Herberman *et al.*, 1976). Heteroreactivity of natural cytotoxicity has been described by Petrányi *et al.* (1974) and Pross and Jondal (1975), showing that human lymphocytes exhibit spontaneous cytotoxicity against mouse target cells. Mouse NK cells were also found capable of specifically lysing certain established human leukemia lines *in vitro* and would therefore seem to be able to act across species barriers (Haller *et al.*, 1977*b*). In the latter assays human T-lymphoma lines and the myeloid leukemia line K562 turned out to be significantly more sensitive targets than the B lymphoma, myeloma, and lymphoblastoid lines tested. Still, our overall ignorance as to what kind of target structure(s) is recognized by NK cells is great. In fact, no distinct target structure for NK activity has so far been defined. Some of the candidate structures which have been suggested as contributors to target-cell susceptibility have recently been reviewed at length by Herberman and Holden (1978). These comprise viral antigenic determinants such as Gross leukemia virus antigens (Zarling *et al.*, 1975) or C-type-virus-associated antigens (Sendo *et al.*, 1975; Herberman *et al.*, 1975*a*). In addition, involvement of nonviral antigenic structures such as embryonic or other antigens expressed after malignant transformation of various cell types has been suggested. The possibility that NK reactivity might be directed against hemopoietic histocompatibility gene (*Hh* gene) products or similar entities must also be considered. Evidence that NK cytotoxicity may be directed against malignant target cells of nonlymphoid origin as well as sometimes also against normal, non-transformed tissue (Herberman and Holden, 1978) adds to the complexity of the picture.

It has been shown for several types of tumors that *in vitro* culture might modulate the expression of some surface antigens. Thus *in vitro*-cultured YAC cells are known to express a higher density of Moloney cell surface antigens (MCSA), but have less *H-2*-determined antigens than the corresponding *in vivo* line (Cikes *et al.*, 1973). With this in mind it is interesting to note that several *in vitro*-cultured MLV tumors consistently show higher lysis susceptibility in the NK system than the ascites lines. Similarly, *in vitro*-cultured lines also have a higher capacity to compete in the above mentioned competition system (Kiessling *et al.*, 1975*a*). Do these differences indicate that *in vitro*-cultured tumor cells express NK target structures which are not present on the ascites cells? *In vitro* as well as *in vivo* experiments suggest that this is not the case. First, a low but selective degree of lysis susceptibility could be seen also with the ascites tumors (Kiessling *et al.*, 1975*a*). Second, we have observed the same relative differences between high- and low-NK-reactive mouse strain cells using YAC ascites or YAC-1 *in vitro* cells as targets (unpublished results). Third, *in vivo* rejection studies show the very same NK-activity-related genotype dependence for the *in vitro* as for the ascites lines. However, 100-fold more YAC-1 cells must be injected into semisyngeneic F_1 hybrids to obtain the same tumor incidence as with YAC ascites cells (Kiessling *et al.*, 1975c). Taken together, these results support a quantitative rather than a qualitative difference between *in vitro*-cultured and ascites tumors with regard to the expression of NK target structures.

We have also considered that *in vitro*-cultured lines may acquire new surface antigens from the constituents of the medium in which they grow. It has been reported that human target cells lost their sensitivity to lysis by autologous non-immune effector cells when they were grown in medium containing human serum instead of fetal calf serum (Sulit *et al.*, 1976). We therefore adapted some of the human cell lines found to be lysable by normal mouse spleen cells for growth in medium supplemented with normal mouse serum. These mouse-serum-grown sublines were found to exhibit the same degree of NK sensitivity in direct or competition assays as the original lines kept in FCS (Haller, unpublished results). Similarly, human-serum-grown hemopoietic cell lines were not less sensitive to lysis by human effector cells than their respective counterparts grown in the presence of FCS. This was even true when the serum source and effector cell donor were from the same individual. We have thus concluded that serum components of the culture medium have no decisive impact on NK reactivity.

Generally, it has to be stated that the precise specificity of NK recognition and lysis is still unclear. This is not totally unexpected if one considers that NK cells might represent a unique and possibly rather complex recognition-surveillance system of quite ancient origin.

IV. EFFECTOR CELL ANALYSIS

When this project started, one main goal was to categorize the mouse natural killer cell within the known groups of effector cells in cell-mediated immunity. As the work proceeded we became gradually aware that this task was impossible; this cell type failed to classify within any previously defined group of lymphocytes or monocyte–macrophages. The notion that we were actually dealing with a "new" type of immunologically active cell was also strengthened by similar reports from other laboratories (Herberman *et al.*, 1975b; Sendo *et al.*, 1975; Zarling *et al.*, 1975). This chapter will briefly review some of the work leading to the conclusion that the NK cell is a non-T non-B type of lymphocyte. The relationship between NK cells and other mechanisms of tumor killing, such as immune T killer cells and antibody-dependent cellular cytotoxicity, will be discussed. Finally, we will review experiments indicating that NK cells probably are one of the most important mechanisms for protection against growth of certain transplantable tumors.

A. NK Cells Lack Characteristics of Mature T Cells

From *in vitro* studies of cellular-immunity immune T cells have been shown to play a major role in tumor resistance (Cerottini and Brunner, 1974). It is therefore natural that much attention has been directed to find a possible relationship between these cells and NK cells. The majority of investigators seem to agree that the NK cell in man and rodents is not a mature T cell (for references, see Herberman and Holden, 1978). In mice, this conclusion is supported by two lines of evidence. First, spleen cells from nude mice on Balb/c background showed even higher NK activity than spleen cells from control (*nu*/+ Balb/c) mice (Kiessling *et al.*, 1975*b*). Similar findings were reported from Herberman's group (Herberman *et al.*, 1975*b*). Second, it has been shown that NK cells are resistant to treatment with anti-theta serum plus complement, while immune T cells in the same set of experiments were killed by this treatment (Kiessling *et al.*, 1975*b*; Kiessling *et al.*, 1976*a*; Herberman *et al.*, 1975*b*). Herberman *et al.*, however, noted a partial reduction in activity after anti-theta treatment of nude spleen, which was interpreted as evidence that some of their NK cells have a low but detectable expression of theta antigen (Herberman *et al.*, 1975*b*).

Another possibility to distinguish NK cells from mature T cells has recently emerged from studies with free-flow electrophoresis. In collaboration with P. Häyry it was found that NK cells seem to have a lower net surface charge than mature T cells, but a higher charge than B cells (Kärre *et al.*, 1978). Thus this intermediate electrophoretic mobility further distinguishes NK cells from T cells as well as B cells.

B. NK Cells Lack Characteristics of B Cells and of Monocyte-Macrophages

Several lines of evidence indicate that NK cells are not B cells. First, when spleen cells from normal or nude mice were passed through a column coated with anti-mouse immunoglobulin, the remaining cells were even more efficient as NK cells than nonpassed (Kiessling *et al.*, 1975*b*). In line with these results, no effect was observed by Herberman *et al.* after pretreatment of NK cells with anti-kappa serum plus complement (Herberman *et al.*, 1975*b*). Therefore, the active killer cell seems to lack detectable immunoglobulin on its surface. It has also been established that the killer cell lacks receptor for C3 (Kiessling *et al.*, 1976*a*; Herberman *et al.*, 1975*b*).

Another point of agreement between different reports on NK cells in the mouse is the low-adherence and nonphagocytic properties of the active cell (Kiessling *et al.*, 1975*b*; Herberman *et al.*, 1975*b*; Sendo *et al.*, 1975; Zarling *et al.*, 1975). This has been measured by column passage of effector cells, and by the iron magnet method. Again, these results are consistent with results from rat as well as human systems (see the review by Herberman and Holden, 1978) similarly showing that the effector cell in natural cell-mediated immunity is low-adherent and nonphagocytic.

The low adherence and nonphagocytic properties of the killer cell would indicate that this cell is not a monocyte–macrophage, and leaves the possibility of the NK cell being a lymphocyte. Results which also support this view were obtained from morphological studies on cells depleted of monocyte–macrophages, T cells, and B cells. Thus spleen cells subjected to such combined fractionation studies as described above were highly efficient as NK cells, and were shown under the light microscope to consist of 90–95% small lymphocytes (Kiessling et al., 1975b). Furthermore, by the use of the 1-g velocity sedimentation method, we have shown that the majority of NK cells seem to sediment as a velocity corresponding to small to medium-size lymphocytes (Kärre et al., 1978). Admittedly, there is yet no direct proof of the NK cell being a small lymphocyte; the evidence for this awaits the isolation of a pure NK-cell population.

C. Relationship between NK Activity and ADCC

The lytic activity of NK cells is highly selective. How do NK cells recognize their target cells? One possibility would be that NK cells, similarly to CTL, have autonomously synthesized receptors. Another possibility is that NK activity is related to ADCC.

It has been shown that many mouse strains produce "natural" antibodies against murine leukemia virus (MuLV) type C viruses or to antigens on tumors induced by or infected with these viruses (Aoki et al., 1966; Ihle et al., 1973; Nowinski and Kaehler, 1974; Aaronson and Stephenson, 1974; Martin and Martin, 1975). The possibility that such natural antibodies serve as specific receptors, passively adsorbed to effector cells in vivo or synthesized in vitro must therefore be considered. Indeed, Blair et al. have shown in microcytotoxicity assays that this mechanism can be of major importance in natural cellular immunity against mouse-mammary-tumor-virus-infected targets (Blair and Lane, 1975).

The NK cell can, however, clearly be distinguished from the K cell mediating ADCC against chicken erythrocyte (CRBC) target cells. Thus K-cell activity was strongly, if not totally, decreased by methods removing high-adherent cell types, in contrast to NK activity (Kiessling et al., 1976a). K-cell activity can also be depleted by passage through an antiimmunoglobulin column or by removal of complement receptor positive cells in contrast to NK cells (Kiessling et al., 1976a). Furthermore, treatment of spleen donors with ^{89}Sr, a "bone marrow"-seeking isotope, strongly suppressed NK activity but had no impact on ADCC to

CRBC (Haller and Wigzell, 1977). Thus a variety of experimental manipulations did clearly distinguish NK cells from K cells functioning in the CRBC system.

It could be argued, and has indeed been shown (Sanderson *et al.*, 1975), that other types of effector cells can be active in ADCC against nucleated mammalian target cells. There are, however, several additional experiments arguing against the concept of antibodies being involved in the present NK system. First, if armed *in vivo* by cytophilic antibodies these Ig-coated cells should be removed by the anti-Ig column, unless only tiny amounts would be enough. Another possibility is that antibodies could be synthesized during the incubation period *in vitro*. If ADCC would be the mechanism behind NK lysis, one would have to anticipate that NK activity should be inhibited by addition of aggregated Ig. This was not the case, since human- as well as mouse-aggregated IgG in concentrations that completely blocked ADCC had no impact on NK activity (Kiessling *et al.*, 1976a). Furthermore, we have demonstrated that the NK activity is trypsin-sensitive (Kiessling *et al.*, 1976a), which contrasts the insensitivity of Fc receptors and ADCC to proteolytic enzyme treatment. A similar trypsin sensitivity of rat NK cells has been demonstrated by Shellam and Hogg (1977). These authors further showed recovery of NK activity after trypsin treatment during consecutive *in vitro* culturing. We have recently confirmed these findings in the mouse NK system (Kärre, unpublished observation). These latter results would seem to indicate that a hypothetical receptor structure on NK cells could actually be resynthesized *in vitro*. It remains to be established, however, if these structures are produced autonomously by the NK cells or are contributed by some other cell population during *in vitro* incubation.

The possibility that NK activity is mediated via ADCC relates directly to the issue of whether the NK cells possess Fc receptors. Initially, Herberman *et al.* concluded that depletion of Fc-receptor-bearing cells had no impact on NK activity (Herberman *et al.*, 1975b). This question was, however, recently reexamined in the same laboratory. By adsorption studies of NK cells from nude or conventional mice on sheep erythrocyte monolayers coated with IgG antibodies, they showed that 50–90% of the total cytotoxic reactivity could be recovered (Herberman and Holden, 1978). We have absolutely no evidence, however, that Fc receptors play any detectable role in the present NK system.

D. NK Cells Possess HP Receptors

NK cells in the mouse system have so far been mainly characterized in negative terms. There has been no clear-cut and unequivocal evidence that mouse NK cells express distinct surface markers comparable to those present on mature cells of the T, B, or monocyte series. In a recent report, however, Glimcher *et al.*

(1977) have shown that pretreatment of normal spleen cells with an anti-Ly-1,2 serum plus complement lead to selective abolishment of NK activity of certain mouse strains. The relevant antibodies in this serum, however, were found not to be directed against Ly-1,2. They were assumed to react with a novel specificity termed "NK," presumably expressed on a tiny subpopulation of spleen cells too small to be detected by trypan blue uptake in conventional cytotoxic tests.

Looking for a simple and reliable NK surface marker we have recently found that, after neuraminidase treatment, mouse NK cells specifically bind to the *Helix pomatia* A hemagglutinin (HP) (Haller *et al.*, 1978*a*). This is a carbohydrate-binding protein with specificity for N-acetyl-D-galactosamine (D-GalNac) and related sugars (Hammarström, 1974). Neuraminidase treatment has previously been shown to uncover HP receptors on certain normal or malignant cell types from various species. In man, receptors for HP are found on a subset of neuraminidase-treated blood lymphocytes mainly representing T cells but are absent on the majority of mature B cells or K cells (Hammarström *et al.*, 1973; Hellström *et al.*, 1976). Monocytes do not express HP receptors. However, cells with surface Ig also expressing receptors for HP are quite frequent in cord blood (Hellström, communication). The possibility thus exists that in the non-T-cell lymphoid series, HP receptors could also be expressed, but predominantly on less differentiated, immature cells. We have therefore fractionated mouse spleen cells on columns containing HP coupled to Sepharose beads. Surface Ig-positive cells passed through such columns. Cytotoxic T lymphocytes (CTL) from alloimmune spleens bound to the beads and could be specifically eluted with D-GalNac. Similarly, NK cells were retained in HP columns. However, the bulk of NK activity could be eluted with a much lower sugar concentration than that necessary for the elution of CTL. Thus, while NK cells possess receptors for HP, their binding properties differ from those of mature T cells. The finding that NK cells express HP receptors may provide a way to obtain "pure" NK-cell populations by combining conventional cell fractionation procedures with affinity chromatography on HP columns. We have planned further characterization of such pure NK-cell populations by specific surface glycoprotein staining and analysis by polyacrylamide gel electrophoresis. Hopefully, this method should allow more precise classification of NK cells.

E. Non-T-Cell Nature of Genetically Controlled Tumor Resistance

The finding that NK cells were non-T cells provided us with yet another possibility to test the *in vivo* relevance of this cell type. Would the *in vivo* resistance to YAC grafts such as NK activity *in vitro* be similarly independent of mature T cells? To test this question, three different systems were applied.

One was the "neutralization text" previously used to demonstrate the importance of immune effector cells (Winn, 1961; Howell *et al.*, 1975). In this "semi-*in vivo*" system, spleen cells were admixed with living YAC cells and inoculated subcutaneously into irradiated syngeneic recipients. The advantage with this method is that the same spleen cell fraction can simultaneously be tested both *in vitro* for NK activity and *in vivo* for protection against tumor growth. The results were clear: spleen cells depleted of T cells, B cells, and monocyte–macrophages were the most efficient fraction both in delaying tumor growth and in the *in vitro* NK assay (Kiessling *et al.*, 1976*b*).

In another experimental series, semisyngeneic A F$_1$ hybrids were thymectomized as adults, then irradiated and reconstituted with fetal liver cells. These mice showed an increased *in vivo* resistance to challenge with small numbers of the YAC cells when compared to the untreated control mice. In contrast, tumor cells histoincompatible with regard to the *H-2* locus showed the expected preferential growth in the thymectomized and reconstituted groups of mice. T-cell depletion of these mice was demonstrated by their inability to produce antibodies to a T-cell-dependent antigen (Kiessling *et al.*, 1976*b*).

Finally, nude mice on Balb/c background used in the same study showed strong resistance to YAC tumor growth. Since these animals were H-2-incompatible with regard to the YAC tumor used, a reaction against *H-2*-determined antigens cannot be excluded. Others, however, have demonstrated high resistance to syngeneic tumors transplanted into nude mice, as will be discussed below.

From these three experimental models, we concluded that *in vivo* protection against YAC cells is independent of mature T cells. Since *in vivo* tumor resistance against tumor growth previously has been attributed mainly to immune T cells (Collavo *et al.*, 1974; Gorczynski and Norbury, 1974; Glaser *et al.*, 1976), the question arises whether the YAC system might be unique in this respect as compared to other tumor host systems. There is, however, an increasing number of reports in the literature showing that this is not the case. Thus, Bonmassar *et al.* observed increased resistance in allogeneic nude mice to the growth of a mouse lymphoma (Bonmassar *et al.*, 1975). This resistance was not abolished by lethal irradiation and was interpreted as being directed against *H-2D–Hh-1* determined specificities expressed on the tumor cells. These findings have important implications with regard to the concept that similar mechanisms may affect resistance to bone marrow grafts and leukemia. There are now several additional reports further indicating T-cell-deficient mice to be quite resistant to growth of certain allogeneic or syngeneic transplantable tumors (Rotter and Trainin, 1975; Giovanella *et al.*, 1974; Skov *et al.*, 1976; Fidler *et al.*, 1976; Greenberg and Greene, 1977). It has also been observed that some human tumors do not grow well in nude mice (Epstein *et al.*, 1976; Schmidt and Good, 1976), a relevant point to bear in mind when considering the lytic effect of mouse NK cells on certain human T-cell lines.

It must be considered, however, that several T-cell-independent mechanisms mediated by, e.g., macrophages or K cells could be active in T-cell-deprived mice. The relative role of NK cells in relation to other non-T-immune mechanisms must therefore be established clearly for each tumor line studied. In two different systems there is now strong evidence in support of the notion that NK cells represent a highly important defense mechanism. Support of this notion comes from recent work by Warner *et al.* Comparing tumor growth in nude and *nu*/+ Balb/c mice, these authors found that the growth rate of the majority of all Balb/c lymphoid tumors tested was significantly lower in the nude animals (Warner *et al.*, 1977). However, only tumors sensitive to lysis by nonimmune effector cells showed this reduced growth rate. Although the exact relationship between the peritoneal exudate cells used as effector cells by these authors and the NK cells used by us has to be further investigated, these results would further stress the decisive role of natural cellular immunity for tumor resistance in nude mice.

In order to analyze the role of NK cells in T-cell-depleted mice, our group has applied a different approach, using bone marrow chimeras. Experiments have shown that NK reactivity in bone marrow chimeras between NK high- and low-reactive strains follows the reactivity of the bone marrow stem cell donor (Haller *et al.*, 1977c). We considered this chimera model to provide a unique change to further prove the role of NK cells in the *in vivo* resistance of T-cell-depleted mice. Therefore, H-2-compatible mice of either high- or low-NK strains were mated with low-reactive A mice syngeneic to the A strain lymphoma YAC. The resulting F_1 hybrid offsprings were again either high- or low-NK-reactive according to the parental haplotype. Furthermore, all offspring F_1 mice were semisyngeneic to YAC and were "identical" at the *H-2* region. Thus, transfers of high- or low-bone-marrow-NK precursor cells into lethally irradiated recipients of low or high NK type were feasible. In order to exclude possible influence of the T-cell system on *in vivo* tumor resistance, the bone marrow recipients were thymectomized prior to reconstitution. For the first time, T-cell-deficient hosts, which expressed either high or low *in vitro* NK activity and yet were genetically identical, with the exception of their hemopoietic tissue, were available for *in vivo* tumor challenge. The results of subcutaneous challenge with small tumor cell doses showed a striking positive correlation between *in vivo* tumor resistance and NK activity *in vitro* (Haller *et al.*, 1977a). Since the *in vivo* manipulations described should help to minimize the complexity of possible effector mechanisms usually involved in *in vivo* phenomena, we consider the positive correlation observed as highly significant, demonstrating a real tumor-protective role of NK cells *in vivo*.

Admittedly, this protective role has so far only been shown for quite a limited number of tumors. Nevertheless, such findings have strong implications on any discussion of the immunosurveillance theory. Based on the concept of T cells as the only relevant cells providing protection against tumors, the failure to find a high incidence of spontaneous tumors in nude mice has been used as a major argument against this theory (Möller and Möller, 1975; Rygaard and Povlsen, 1976). The present demonstration of alternative non-T-cell-dependent mechanisms such as the NK system, and the high probability that these mechanisms may play a major role in protection against tumors, would largely neutralize the preceding argument. The time may thus have come for the opponents of the immunosurveillance theory to modify their criticism and to take the NK cell into consideration as a new and possibly decisive factor.

V. INFLUENCE OF GENETIC AND NONGENETIC FACTORS ON NK ACTIVITY

NK activity is influenced in a positive or negative direction by a number of factors. Some of these factors are genetically determined and an analysis aimed at determining the position of the regulating genes in the mouse genome has been performed. This analysis has, however, been hampered by environmental factors. Thus, even within an inbred strain of mice, a large variation of cytolytic activity could be seen. The nature of this influence is still largely unknown, but some of the nongenetic factors have been more systematically analyzed, as discussed below. The detection of genetic and nongenetic factors with a known influence on NK activity has provided us with excellent tools in analyzing the *in vivo* relevance of NK activity. Knowing that manipulation of NK activity by genetic or nongenetic methods would lead to changes in NK activity, we have tested the outcome of the same treatment on *in vivo* tumor resistance. For this purpose we have used the YAC tumor both as a target cell in the NK assay and as a tumor graft inoculated into semisyngeneic recipients.

A. Age Influence on *in Vitro* NK Activity

A very pronounced age dependence was found by us and other investigators. Fetal liver and spleen cells from newborn mice showed little or no activity. In contrast to immune T cells, which mature during the first week of life in the mouse, the onset of NK activity did not occur until 3 weeks of age, and peak activity was seen when lymphocytes from mice 6–8 weeks old were used. Thereafter a marked decline of activity was seen, and mice 6–12 months old showed very low activity (Kiessling *et al.*, 1975a; Herberman *et al.*, 1975a).

This high NK activity in young mice is suggestive of a sensitization or activation period early in life. According to Herberman *et al.* NK activity might be directed against products of endogenous C-type viruses activated early in life

(Herberman *et al.*, 1975*a*). In addition, other environmental influences, such as hormones, could influence the actual degree of NK activity in an individual. Experiments investigating these possibilities comprised adoptive transfers of marrow cells within the same mouse strain. Thus, bone marrow stem cells from young donors (having high NK activity in their spleens) or old donors (having low NK activity in their spleens) were transplanted into irradiated syngeneic recipients of varying ages. It was found that "old" marrow transplanted into "young" recipients led to low NK activity, whereas transfer of "young" marrow lead to high subsequent NK activity in the spleens of reconstituted old or young recipients (Haller *et al.*, 1977*c*). In conclusion, these experiments would indicate that age-related differences in NK activity are preprogrammed at the level of the transferred bone marrow or fetal liver cells. Some caution must be taken in interpreting these data, however, since a hypothetical agent responsible for activation of NK cells might have been transferred together with the bone marrow or fetal liver cells. Also, transfer of regulatory cells governing NK activity is conceivable. The presence or absence of such regulatory agents could then account for the observed age differences, not necessarily the actual genetic setup of NK precursor cells.

B. Age Influence on *in Vivo* Tumor Resistance

The pronounced influence of age on NK activity prompted us to test whether a similar influence was active on the *in vivo* resistance to transplantable tumors. A positive correlation between *in vitro* NK activity and *in vivo* tumor resistance was observed when mice of different ages were tested in the YAC system. Semisyngeneic F_1 hybrids between high reactive strains and A mice were used for this purpose. The results showed clearly that young mice at "peak" NK age were found to be more resistant to subcutaneous growth of low doses of YAC lymphoma cells than old mice (Haller *et al.*, 1977*a*). It would thus seem clear that the *in vivo* tumor resistance parallels the age-related changes of *in vitro* NK activity. Previous results from Sendo *et al.* using a radiation-induced lymphoma also showed that this was indeed the case (Sendo *et al.*, 1975).

C. Effect of Tumor Induction and of Immunization with Tumor Cells on NK Activity

The classical method of studying tumor immunity has been to use experimental animals bearing tumors induced by oncogeneic agents or immunized with killed syngeneic cells. In most tumor host systems such procedures would lead to the appearance of immune effector cells, as measured, e.g., by cytostatic or cytotoxic effectors *in vitro*. By application of similar methods in the study of

NK cells, several important questions could be analyzed: What changes in NK activity do occur in tumor-bearing mice? Can NK cells be found locally in tumor or in draining lymph nodes? Is it possible to enhance NK activity by immunization?

Several lines of evidence to be discussed later indicate that NK cells are of major importance for rejection of many subcutaneously injected tumor cells. Accordingly, these NK cells can probably migrate from the spleen or peripheral blood, organs known to contain the highest NK activity, into the local site of tumor growth. Alternatively, they could be recruited from cells already present in various organs. Becker and Klein have studied the NK activity against the YAC-1 target in three systems of tumor-bearing animals: (1) in a transplanted methylcholanthrene-induced sarcoma, (2) in a primary MSV-induced sarcoma, and (3) in athymic nude mice carrying grafts of human lymphoblastoid cell lines. In all three systems a pronounced suppression of NK activity in the spleen was found (Becker and Klein, 1976). The authors found no evidence of spleen suppressor cells and concluded that one reason for decreased NK activity in spleens could be that the active killer cell migrated to the tumor. This assumption was supported by experimental data showing that non-T cells, probably NK cells, with considerable cytotoxicity for YAC targets, could be isolated from MSV-induced tumors of CBA mice.

We also have preliminary evidence that inoculation of NK-sensitive target cells into the hind foot pads of semisyngeneic mice led to the rapid increase of NK activity in the draining lymph nodes within less than 24 hours (Haller and Örn, unpublished observations). Similar effects were also exerted by some conventional adjuvants, such as Freund's complete adjuvants. This is to be expected in view of the large number of agents that can induce or augment NK activity.

In conclusion, NK cells can be found locally in the tumor mass or in draining lymph nodes after tumor cell challenge. These findings related to the question of whether or not NK activity can be increased by immunization with the relevant tumor cells. Since it is not yet established if NK activity fullfils the criteria to be classified as a "true" immune reactivity, the existence of specific augmentation of NK activity would add considerable weight to this notion. Herberman *et al.* have recently performed a series of experiments determining the effect of *in vivo* challenge on NK activity (Herberman *et al.*, 1977). They found that reactivity in nude as well as in normal mice of various ages could be augmented by inoculation of tumor cells. The augmented cytotoxicity reached a peak at 3 days after inoculation, and was only seen using tumor cells which appeared to bear target structures recognized by NK cells. Thus it appears that NK activity would increase after immunization, although with different kinetics than seen in the case of immune T cells. The authors concluded that, in most respects, this augmentation of NK reactivity was consistent with the stimulation of specific memory cells by *in vivo* reexposure to the antigen. However, results showing that NK activity could also be increased by agents other than tumor cells, including normal nonmalignant cells, bacteria, and viruses, have been observed by these authors as well as by our group and other groups of investigators. The implication of these findings will be discussed below.

In vivo tumor rejection studies have mostly been performed in animals pre-immunized with the relevant tumor cell. Since NK-cell activity can be augmented by tumor-cell inoculation a question arises as to what extent the increased tumor resistance in immunized mice is due to augmented NK activity. This question has not yet been thoroughly analyzed, but again the YAC system could serve as an example. In semisyngeneic F_1 hybrids immunized with irradiated YAC cells, we have observed an early increase of NK activity, peaking in the spleen at day 2–3, as also described by Herberman *et al.* This augmented activity is followed by pro-longed suppression of NK activity. In hyperimmunized mice NK activity in the spleen is lower than in control mice. Yet, rejection studies have shown increased resistance to subsequent subcutaneous challenge with living YAC cells in pre-immunized mice (Petrányi *et al.*, unpublished observations). Preliminary results indicate that antibodies seem to play the major protective role in these hyper-immune animals (Åsjö, unpublished observations). Thus NK cells seem to con-stitute a major primary barrier against transplantation of YAC cells in nonimmune mice, while other mechanisms are probably dominating in immune animals.

D. Induction of NK Cell Activity by Bacterial Adjuvants

Augmentation of NK reactivity in mice can be achieved by agents other than tumor cells, including normal, nonmalignant cells; bacteria; and viruses (Herber-man *et al.*, 1977). Bacterial immunostimulants such as *Mycobacterium bovis* strain bacillus Calmette–Guérin (BCG) and *Corynebacterium parvum* have been used extensively for cancer immunotherapy in animals and man (Bast *et al.*, 1976; Nathanson, 1974; Halpern *et al.*, 1973). There is general agreement that these adjuvants stimulating the host reticuloendothelial system are effective primarily through "activated" macrophages (Keller, 1976). However, additional effector mechanisms are likely. Recently, Wolfe and collaborators could show that viable BCG organisms given intraperitoneally induced a population of cytotoxic cells in the peritoneal cavity of normal nonimmune mice (1976). These cells appeared within a few days of BCG administration. They clearly dif-fered from macrophages or mature T cells and had many features in common with NK cells. We have observed a similar phenomenon following intraperitoneal inoculation of heat-killed *C. parvum* (Ojo *et al.*, 1978). Induction of NK activity was detectable as early as 12 hours after intraperitoneal administration of bacteria and over a wide dose range. It seemed subject to the genetic regulation observed in the mouse NK system. Thus NK activity generally reached higher levels in high-responder mouse strains than in similarly treated low-responder mice. The peritoneal cavity of the mouse does not usually harbor active NK effector cells. It remains to be elucidated whether the increased NK activity of peritoneal exudate cells after administration of BCG or *C. parvum* is due to a true *de novo* production or rather to migration of NK cells. Alternatively, these bacteria might activate or lead to expansion of a cell population normally residing in the peritoneal cavity. There appeared to be no concomitant decrease of NK re-activity in spleens or blood of animals treated with *C. parvum* by the intraperi-toneal route. On the other hand, the same bacterial preparation injected intra-venously did cause a drastic reduction in splenic NK activity without significant changes in other organs (Ojo *et al.*, 1978). This abolishment of NK reactivity in the spleens was manifested 7–10 days after treatment and remained for more than 3 weeks thereafter. These findings are quite reminiscent of the abrogation of resistance to hemopoietic grafts by intravenous injection of *C. parvum*, a phenomenon that exhibits exactly the same time course (Cudkowicz and Bennet, 1971*a,b*). This common feature would again indicate that possibly a similar effector mechanism is operative in both systems.

It is interesting here to consider some early work on *in vivo* tumor-growth inhibition by killed *C. parvum*. *Corynebacterium parvum* has been shown to con-fer good protection against a Moloney-virus-transformed cell line YCB in syngeneic Balb/c mice (Halpern *et al.*, 1973). Similar increased resistance has been observed in AKR and (AKR × CBA-T6)F_1 hybrid mice against growth of transplanted AKR leukemia cells (Lamensans *et al.*, 1968). Furthermore, a good protection against various tumor cell lines was achieved with Corynebacteria injected intraperitoneally rather than intravenously (Lamensans *et al.*, 1968). It is therefore conceivable that local tumor resistance induced by conventional adjuvants might be effectuated in part by NK cells which would represent a rapid-acting and hitherto unrecognized component of the host response to various immunostimulants.

E. Genetic Analysis of NK Activity

Early in the course of this study it was found that various mouse strains differed in NK activity (Kiessling *et al.*, 1975*a*). Most strains yielded spleen cells with high activity against YAC-1 target, whereas spleen cells from other strains, especially strain A, were low reactors. These intrastrain differences were indica-tive of a genetic control of NK activity, and made a more extensive genetic analysis possible. By analyzing the inheritance of NK activity in various crosses between high- and low-responder strains, the position within the mouse genome of those gene(s) responsible for high NK reactivity was investigated. At first we attempted to determine if high NK activity was inherited as a dominant trait. When the low-reactive A strain was crossed to various other strains, and cells from these F_1 hybrids tested against the semisyngeneic YAC lymphoma of A origin for NK activity, reactivity resembled that of the high-reactive parent (Petrányi et al., 1975). Thus high reactivity was dominant in these crosses.

It is well established that distinct host genes have a marked influence on virus-induced oncogenesis and also on resistance to certain transplantable tumors (Chesebro et al., 1974; Lilly and Pincus, 1973; Mühlbock and Dux, 1974; Williams et al., 1975). Knowing that in many of these models genes mapping in the H-2 locus play a key role in determining susceptibility to a particular neoplasm, it was natural that our interest focused on a possible linkage between H-2 and NK reactivity. To analyze this possibility the offspring from a backcross between the low-reactive A strain and a high-reactive A F_1 hybrid was used.

When spleens from mice of this cross were tested in the NK system, their activities were distributed over a wide range, covering the range of the high- and low-reactive parental strains (Petrányi et al., 1975). A linkage analysis was then performed in the same backcross population to localize the genes controlling NK activity. Spleen cells from mice of this cross were tested individually for NK activity. The same mice were also typed for 10 different markers segregating in this cross; they were typed for H-2 allotype and immunoglobulin heavy-chain allotype (Ig-1 locus), and registered for two coat-color genes, the black–brown locus (B vs. b) and albino-colored locus (c vs. C). Five different tissue isozymes from kidney and liver, together with the C5 serum complement component, were also typed.

Cytolytic activity of heterozygotes was compared to that of homozygotes for each of these markers. The outcome of this linkage analysis can be summarized briefly: highly significant linkage was established only with regard to the H-2 marker.

Thus the importance of genes mapping on mouse chromosome 17 in regulation of NK activity is clearly established. This fact has been confirmed recently in our laboratory in other backcrosses using several different tumor targets (Gunnar Klein, unpublished results). Are the genes controlling high NK reactivity to YAC-1 located within the H-2 complex, as has been shown for H-2-linked immune-response genes? To answer this question, several congeneic resistant (CR) strains have been checked in the NK system (Kiessling et al., unpublished observation). These results reveal that reactivity does not follow the H-2 haplotype in the CR strains tested but rather resembles NK reactivity of the background strain. This is particularly clear when NK activity of both background and H-2 donor is known; e.g., the B.10A strain is highly reactive, similar to the B.10 background strain, but in contrast to the low-reactive A strain. Thus the H-2-linked gene(s) influencing anti-YAC-1 NK reactivity are located on chromosome 17 but probably does (do) not map within the H-2 complex.

There are several possible ways of explaining the genetic influence on the NK activity. It should be stressed that the classification of mouse strains as high or low reactors in this system is more quantitative than qualitative. Sometimes a considerable degree of reactivity could be seen also with mice of low-reactive genotype. Furthermore, NK-cell activity in the low-reactive A strain could be strongly enriched by the appropriate cell fractionation procedure (Kiessling *et al.*, 1975*b*). Also, as shown by Herberman *et al.*, activity could be augmented by boosting with tumor cells or microorganisms (Herberman *et al.*, 1977). It is conceivable that the level of NK reactivity could be determined by the relative number of NK cells rather than the cytolytic potential per cell. However, the finding by others (Herberman *et al.*, 1975*a*) that the same strain could be highly reactive to one tumor target but low-reactive when tested against another would suggest that genetic factors may determine which target-structure NK cells will be recognized rather than the general level of reactivity in each strain. This notion is also strengthened by the results of Herberman *et al.*, demonstrating in competition assay that NK cells can recognize a variety of different specificities (Herberman *et al.*, 1975*a*). Therefore, the possibility exists that NK cells are clonally expressed, with each clone expressing specificity for a distinct antigen.

Thus two levels of genetic regulation of NK reactivity might exist. One might determine the "overall" NK reactivity in a particular strain of mice. The other might more specifically regulate the clonal expression of NK cells with specificity for a certain antigenic determinant. Results favoring the first interpretation as being more important stem from experiments showing that the same genetical influence can be seen when tumors of widely different origin were used as targets. Thus the same differences between high- and low-reactive mouse strains in the NK system were observed against YAC-1 as against certain human T-cell lymphomas (Haller *et al.*, 1977*b*). Also, recent backcross data seem to support this notion. In a (C57BL × DBA) × C57BL backcross, *H-2* heterozygotes were found more reactive than the homozygotes when tested against a variety of syngeneic and allogeneic mouse tumors of different etiological origin (Gunnar Klein, unpublished observations). Since it must be rather unlikely that all these tumors share a common "NK antigen," a more plausible explanation would be an *H-2* influence determining the "general" NK activity.

Taken together, it seems to be clear that NK activity is under genetic influence. Further studies are necessary to analyze the precise position of the "NK genes" and the mechanism by which they confer this influence.

F. Genetic Analysis of Resistance to YAC Cells in Semisyngeneic Mice

Snell was the first to show that a B.10 lymphoma grows more slowly in the F_1 hybrid than in syngeneic mice (Snell, 1958). This observation was later extended by others to several tumor host systems (for a review, see Hellström and

Hellström, 1967). Several immunological as well as nonimmunological interpretations have been suggested to explain this F_1 hybrid resistance effect, but the responsible mechanism is as yet poorly understood. Could NK cells possibly contribute to this increased resistance in F_1 mice?

To assess the participation of the natural killer cell in resistance to tumor cell growth, we therefore compared low- and high-responder strains with regard to their ability to resist small numbers (10^3, 10^4) of living lymphoma cells. The same semisyngeneic A F_1 hybrids were used for both the *in vitro* NK system and the *in vivo* resistance study. There was a high concordance between *in vitro* cytotoxicity and *in vivo* tumor resistance in all genotypes tested (Kiessling *et al.*, 1975c). The *in vitro* low-reactive A and A F_1 hybrids had a shorter tumor latency period and a considerably higher cumulative incidence of tumors than the *in vitro* high-reactive strains.

Resembling the *in vitro* NK system, the *in vivo* resistance test also revealed a difference between the YAC-1 *in vitro* line and the YAC ascites tumor. In order to obtain the same tumor incidence, 100-fold more YAC-1 cells than YAC ascites cells were used; but at this cell dose, the same genotype dependence was noted for the *in vitro* as for the ascites-maintained tumor cells (Kiessling *et al.*, 1975c). This result would be in concert with the view that YAC-1 cells express more of the relevant target structure than do YAC ascites cells, and therefore are more sensitive to *in vitro* NK lysis and *in vivo* tumor resistance, as discussed in Chapter 3.

The relationship between *in vitro* and *in vivo* activity was also studied in an *in vivo* segregation analysis with backcross populations between the low-reactive A strain and two different high-reactive A F_1 hybrids. This was to determine whether the results from the linkage analysis of the NK effect were also valid for *in vivo* resistance to the same MLV lymphoma (YAC). With both backcross populations [(A × C57BL) × A and (A × C57Leaden) × A] we found that *in vivo* resistance to YAC tumor cells was strongly *H-2*-linked, in line with the earlier backcross analysis of the *in vitro* cytotoxicity. No linkage was found with the black–brown locus, with the *Ig-1* locus, or with three different isozyme allotypes (Petrányi *et al.*, 1976).

We also compared the very same backcross mice individually for *in vitro* NK activity and *in vivo* tumor growth resistance. Spleen cells from splenectomized mice were tested for NK activity, and the same mice were then challenged with living YAC tumor cells. These studies revealed that mice with high *in vitro* NK activity generally had better tumor-growth resistance (Petrányi *et al.*, 1976). This positive correlation was not absolute, however, and many mice with high activity displayed low tumor-growth resistance, and vice versa. This probably indicates that several immunological and/or nonimmunological factors other than the NK cells are important in tumor resistance.

In conclusion, *in vitro* NK activity against YAC-1 and *in vivo* resistance to the same tumor would seem to be closely associated. A complete positive correlation between *in vitro* cytotoxicity and *in vivo* tumor resistance was found between various F_1 hybrids, and strong *H-2*-linked influence on NK activity as well as on tumor resistance was revealed. This genetic comparison has therefore proved to be one of the strongest arguments for an *in vivo* relevance of NK cells.

There are several different ways of interpreting the F_1 resistance phenomenon on an immunological basis. One would be that the high reactivity in the F_1 mice is due to introduction of a new set of *Ir* genes from the high reactive parent, thus enabling the F_1 hybrid to recognize tumor-associated transplantation antigens (TATA) expressed on the tumor target, which are not recognized by the poorly reactive parental strain. The X.1 system described by Sato *et al.* would be a candidate for this interpretation (Sato *et al.*, 1973). These authors showed an increased transplantation resistance to a radiation leukemia in certain F_1 hybrids, associated with a gene in the *K* region of the *H-2* complex. Since high resistance in this system was associated with anti-X.1 antibody production, the authors concluded that the responsible gene could be classified as an *Ir* gene. Lately, Sendo *et al.* demonstrated that resistance in this system was also associated with NK activity against the same tumor (Sendo *et al.*, 1975). The possibility therefore exists that NK activity might be partly controlled by *Ir* genes.

Another way of interpreting the increased tumor resistance in *H-2* heterozygote mice would be to assume similar recognition events as in resistance to bone marrow grafts. As will be discussed later, there is good evidence for similar effector mechanism in both natural tumor resistance and resistance to bone marrow grafts. With regard to the genetics, Cudkowicz has shown that heterozygosity at the *H-2D–Hh-1* region is sufficient for the expression of hybrid resistance to two radiation-induced C57BL lymphomas (Cudkowicz, 1968).

Lately, Harmon *et al.* established that heterozygosity within or near the *H-2* region is sufficient to obtain a successful resistance to the EL-4 lymphoma of C57BL origin (Harmon *et al.*, 1977). Interestingly, these authors also confirmed the findings of an *H-2*-linked influence on *in vitro* NK activity by showing that heterozygosity within or near the D-end of the *H-2* complex was necessary for high NK activity against this tumor. The possibility has therefore been considered that the homozygous normal and the tumor cells express antigeneic determinants, analogous to hemopoietic histocompatibility (Hh) antigens, which would be recognized by the F_1 hybrids. This recognition might result in *in vivo* tumor resistance and *in vitro* NK activity. This possibility is of potential interest also in the YAC system, since the mapping of anti-YAC NK activity on chromosome 17 could be explained by the existence of a hypothetical *Hh* locus coding for a surface structure expressed on YAC tumor cells and strain A tissue. However, such structures would be absent in the A F_1 hybrids.

Finally, it must also be pointed out that other immune mechanisms directed against *Hh* gene products of normal and malignant cells are probably active *in vivo*. Also, immune T cells must be considered, as shown by Schmitt-Verhulst and Zats (1977). They demonstrated that normal F_1 responder cells generated Thy-1-positive effector cells specifically cytotoxic for the sensitizing antigens of parental AKR normal or lymphoma cells. It was suggested that resistance to AKR lymphoma cells in an (AKR × DBA) F_1 hybrid was dependent on this mechanism. The relationship between this T-cell-dependent system and resistance to hemopoietic grafts will be discussed in the following chapter.

VI. RELATIONSHIP BETWEEN NK ACTIVITY AND RESISTANCE TO HEMOPOIETIC GRAFTS

The possibility that NK cells might be active also in rejection of nonmalignant hemopoietic grafts has recently been considered. The notion that a similar mechanism might be active in resistance to hemopoietic grafts as in control of leukemogenesis has previously been suggested (Bonmassar *et al.*, 1975; Gallagher *et al.*, 1976). To determine if NK cells might constitute this common mechanism, a collaborative study has been carried out between our laboratory and the laboratory of Dr. Cudkowicz (Kiessling *et al.*, 1977). A similar study was also carried out in collaboration with Dr. Trentin (Trentin *et al.*, 1977).

The resistance to hemopoietic grafts is mediated by a host antigraft reaction which possesses a number of attributes that set it apart from familiar immune mechanisms. In the comparative study the effect of six independent variables known to influence resistance to marrow grafts were investigated in the NK system using YAC-1 lymphoma cells as targets (Kiessling *et al.*, 1977).

Before this study it was already known that both these effector mechanisms shared one important feature: the independence from mature T cells. Thus, resistance to bone marrow grafts is highly active in nude mice (Cudkowicz, 1975), similar to NK activity. This is in contrast to the recently developed *in vitro* system for the generation of cytotoxic F_1 hybrid lymphocytes with specificity against parental *Hh*-gene-determined products (Shearer and Cudkowicz, 1975; Shearer *et al.*, 1976a). This *in vitro* cytotoxic system is generated and affected by Thy-1-positive lymphocytes but, apart from this, seems to share most of the characteristics of *in vivo* resistance to marrow grafts.

The second feature to be considered is the rapid maturation of both of these natural mouse reactivities during the fourth week of life. We found a close correlation in the F_1 hybrid strains studied between the onset at about 22 days of age of NK-cell activity and *in vivo* resistance to bone marrow grafts (Kiessling *et al.*,

1977). It should be mentioned that also the inducibility *in vitro* of Thy-1-positive F_1 cytolytic cells specific for parental targets matures at 23 days of age. In contrast, the competence for most antibody and T-cell-mediated responses to conventional antigens has already matured during the first week of life.

Another feature which is shared by the two natural reactivities is their relative insensitivity to radiation injury. In spleens of irradiated mice, NK activity is enriched in the remaining cells (Kiessling *et al.*, 1977). The interpretation of these results is not easy, however, since spleens of heavily irradiated mice show over 90% reduction of cellularity, and the total NK activity in these mice is probably reduced. This remark is noteworthy since YAC cells grow better in F_1 hybrid mice exposed to 400 rad of X rays than in nonirradiated controls (Kiessling *et al.*, 1976*b*). Hence, the *in vivo* resistance to YAC cells appears to be radiosensitive. Likewise, Cudkowicz *et al.* found that C57BL/10 lymphoma cells grow better in irradiated than in nonirradiated *H-2D-Hh-1* heterozygous F_1 hybrids (Cudkowicz, 1968). Therefore, decrease in total NK cell activity after irradiation could explain this discordance between *in vivo* and *in vitro* data.

A fourth opportunity for comparison was provided for by a heteroantiserum raised in rabbits against mouse bone marrow cells. In previous studies this antiserum depressed resistance to hemopoietic grafts without abrogating antibody formation to sheep erythrocytes or rejection of skin allografts *in vivo* (Till *et al.*, 1970; Shearer *et al.*, 1976*b*). It was found that *in vivo* administration of this antiserum diminished NK-cell activity with dose–response and kinetics analogous to those observed for the abrogation of hybrid resistance.

A fifth comparison was made by determining whether two antimacrophage agents, silica particles and *l*-carrageenan (Allison *et al.*, 1966; Catanzaro *et al.*, 1971) would depress NK-cell activity. Both agents abrogate resistance to hemopoietic grafts *in vivo* and block sensitization *in vitro* of Thy-1-positive F_1 cells against parental targets (Lotzová and Cudkowicz, 1974; Lotzová *et al.*, 1975; Shearer *et al.*, 1976*b*). However, only silica particles were selective *in vitro* by preventing the sensitization of F_1 cells against parental but not against allogeneic targets. *l*-Carrageenan interfered with both *in vitro* responses.

NK-cell activity was reduced after *in vivo* treatment of mice with either silica particles or *l*-carrageenan, but the two agents differed with regard to their suppressive effect on NK cells *in vitro*. Silica particles, which are specifically cytotoxic for macrophages, had no detectable effect *in vitro* on NK function, whereas *l*-carrageenan, which is not as specific an antimacrophage agent, was toxic for NK cells (Kiessling *et al.*, 1977).

The fact that silica does not suppress NK activity when administered *in vitro* supports the previous conclusion that these cells are not macrophages. Yet, silica-sensitive cells seem to be involved in the generation or maturation of NK cells, since NK activity is suppressed by *in vivo* injection of this agent. Likewise, it has been shown that the production of Thy-1-positive F_1 T killer cells with specificity for *Hh* determinants requires silica-sensitive accessory cells during the early stages of sensitization *in vitro* (Shearer *et al.*, 1976*b*). It is then possible that a nonlymphoid cell type, sensitive to heterologous anti-bone-marrow antiserum and to antimacrophage agents, maturing during the fourth week of life in the mouse, serves as an accessory cell for both the anti-Hh and NK host reactivities.

The specificity of F_1 hybrid effectors of marrow graft rejection is directed against *Hh*-gene products. Specific unresponsiveness toward Hh-1-positive cells has been induced in genetically resistant F_1 mice by multiple injections of parental spleen cells (Cudkowicz and Stimpfling, 1964; Shearer and Cudkowicz, 1975). In the present analysis, F_1 mice were given the same pretreatment to establish whether repeated exposure of the F_1 immune system to parental cells would result in loss or reduction of NK-cell activity; and whether splenic NK-cell activity would persist in genetically resistant F_1 hybrids rendered unresponsive to Hh-1-incompatible cells. The experimental results were explicit: pretreatment of AB6F1 mice with A strain spleen cells resulted in significant and consistent reduction of NK-cell activity against YAC-1 target, whereas the pretreatment of these mice with B6 cells resulted in marginal and inconsistent reduction of NK-cell activity (Kiessling *et al.*, 1977). It is to be noted that AB6F1 mice are susceptible to A strain marrow grafts but resistant to B6 grafts, and that pretreatment with B6 spleen cells abrogated such resistance. The independence of NK-cell activity and resistance to B6 marrow grafts (Hh-1-incompatible) was confirmed using the B6C3F1 hybrid, which is resistant to B6 but susceptible to C3H cells. NK-cell activity against YAC-1 targets was not affected by pretreatment with B6 cells, which, in contrast, abrogates resistance to hemopoietic grafts. These data establish that the two natural reactivities investigated are suppressible by multiple injections of parental cells into adult mice, that there are restrictions with respect to the genotype of parental cells to be used, and that the specificities involved are different for YAC-1- and Hh-1-positive targets. Further work is required to clarify the mechanisms and specificities involved.

Yet another similarity between NK-cell activity and resistance to marrow grafting is that both activities are greatly reduced by prolonged exposure of the animals' bone marrow to local irradiation from ^{89}Sr incorporated into bone tissue (Bennet, 1973; Haller and Wigzell, 1977). This similarity will be discussed in the next chapter.

In conclusion, six independent comparisons have given unequivocal results, pointing to an intimate association between NK-cell activity and resistance to hemopoietic grafts. Despite the complexities at the genetic and cellular levels, it appears likely that a common or at the very least a similar mechanism is operative for both reactivities.

VII. GENERATION OF NK CELLS *IN VIVO*

In the young adult mouse, spleen, peripheral blood, and lymph nodes are good sources for NK cells. The bone marrow and peritoneal cavity harbor low NK activity. Thymus cells are consistently inactive (Kiessling *et al.*, 1975*a*; Herberman *et al.*, 1975*a*). The high activity in spleen and peripheral blood has been found subject to drastic changes during the lifetime of an individual. The presence of a functional thymus is unnecessary for NK reactivity. The thymus seems to have, if anything, a suppressive effect on the appearance of NK cells as appears from the high reactivity of nude mice (Kiessling *et al.*, 1975*b*; Herberman *et al.*, 1975*a*). These peculiarities of the NK system prompted us to investigate the generation and maturation of NK function *in vivo* and to try to solve questions as: Are NK cells a cell type of their own, or do they represent cells during a certain stage of differentiation leading to one of the conventional cell types? What is the role of the spleen, which is such a dominating NK organ in young mice? Are there NK-activating hormonal influences present during young adulthood in mice? Does the thymus have an NK-suppressor function?

A. Dependence on Intact Bone Marrow Function

After parenteral administration, radioactive strontium (^{89}Sr) is taken up by bone, where it replaces calcium. This uptake leads to a local irradiation of the entire bone marrow. It is well documented that ^{89}Sr treatment does not affect T- or B-cell function in mice (Bennet, 1973; Kumar *et al.*, 1974; Bennet *et al.*, 1976). However, ^{89}Sr treatment of mice severely impairs marrow-dependent effector cells responsible for rejection of hemopoietic cell grafts (Bennet, 1973). Similarly, such treatment abrogates natural resistance against Friend virus leukemia in mice (Kumar *et al.*, 1974). We were able to show that treatment with ^{89}Sr of young adult mice from NK high-reactive strains resulted in a drastic reduction of spleen NK activity. In contrast, the ability of these treated mice to generate two other kinds of cytotoxic cells, K cells in ADCC against CRBC and killer T cells across H-2 differences, remained largely intact (Haller and Wigzell, 1977). The selective ^{89}Sr sensitivity of NK function was the first hint that NK cells might belong to a similar class of marrow-dependent, immunocompetent cells as the effector cells participating in genetic resistance to hemopoietic grafts and leukemia in mice. Thus the results with ^{89}Sr treatment indicate that, *in vivo*, a functional bone marrow is needed for generation and maintenance of NK activity. Furthermore, these results add to the notion that NK cells are distinct from "conventional" killer cells. Since killer T cells as well as K cells were generated or maintained in the ^{89}Sr-treated mice for prolonged periods of time, it would also seem unlikely that NK cells represent precursor cells to either of these two cell types.

B. NK Function Is Preprogrammed at the Precursor Cell Level

NK activity in the mouse has been shown to be under genetic control. The mechanisms through which NK activity is governed are largely unknown. Thus expression of NK activity in the spleen might depend mainly on host environmental factors. For example, NK cells might be produced as a result of exposure and sensitization to certain antigens. Proposed antigens include structures possibly associated with endogenous C-type viruses (Herberman *et al.*, 1975*a*). On the other hand, differentiation and subsequent activity of NK cells could be preprogrammed genetically at the NK-precursor-cell level. Therefore, it seemed mandatory to determine which factors were decisive in the generation of high or low NK activity *in vivo*. Taking advantage of the fact that *H-2*-compatible mouse strains exist with either high or low NK activity, reciprocal transfers of bone marrow of fetal liver cells were carried out between such mouse pairs. The capacity of the transferred marrow or fetal liver cells to restore NK activity in the spleens of the lethally irradiated recipients was assessed. The main question was whether the resulting high or low NK activity would follow the cell donor or the host genotype. The results were clear: reconstitution of irradiated recipients of either low- or high-NK type with low-NK precursor marrow caused the appearance of low NK activity in the spleens of such animals. Conversely, fetal liver or marrow cells from high NK strains lead to the generation of high splenic NK activity in the recipients, irrespective of their original reactivity. Thus NK activity in the spleen of bone marrow or fetal liver chimeras was found to reflect the reactivity of the hemopoietic cell donor (Haller *et al.*, 1977*c*).

From these experiments we concluded that the generation of NK cells was an inborn and autonomous function of the bone marrow and seemed to depend neither on the genotype nor on other influences of the host environment. It should be mentioned here that the forces by which this host-independent differentiation is driven are still unknown. The possibility that sensitizing agents or NK regulatory cells were transplanted together with the bone marrow inoculum has not been excluded.

C. Role of the Thymus

There is ample evidence that NK-cell activity in nude mice is higher than in their corresponding thymus-bearing littermates (Kiessling *et al.*, 1975*b*; Herberman *et al.*, 1975*a*). It has been reported that grafting of fetal thymuses into histocompatible nude mice resulted in a decrease of NK activity to the level found in nonnude littermates (Herberman and Holden, 1978). Furthermore, neonatal thymectomy of ordinary mice has been claimed to increase NK activity to the high levels detected in athymic nude mice (Herberman and Holden, 1978). It would thus seem that the presence of a thymus exerts a suppressive effect on NK activity.

Using the transfer system between *H-2*-compatible NK-low and NK-high mouse strain combinations already described, a genetic regulatory role of thymus cells on NK generation was investigated. In the preceding paragraph we have shown that transplantation of low bone marrow cells into irradiated high recipients will lead to the appearance of low NK activity in the spleen, and vice versa. However, such experiments do not tell whether NK precursor cells are able to behave in a completely autonomous way or whether their differentiation/maturation, in turn, is regulated by stimulator or suppressor cells of donor origin. Therefore, T lymphocyte control of NK generation was quite conceivable. To explore this matter further, Haller *et al*. thymectomized recipient mice prior to irradiation and reconstitution. The marrow cells used were pretreated with anti-Thy serum and complement to remove contaminating T cells before infusion. Together with the high or low bone marrow inoculum, the lethally irradiated recipients were simultaneously infused with thymocytes from either low or high donors in all four possible combinations. The results showed that NK activity in spleens of the reconstituted mice was generated according to the genetic setup of the bone marrow donor. The thymocyte donor strain or the genotype of the recipient were without influence on and therefore irrelevant to the outcome of the NK reconstitution (Haller *et al*., 1978*b*).

These findings would tend to argue against the idea that T lymphocytes regulate the genetically determined high or low NK reactivity observed among various mouse strains. They do not, however, rule out the role of the thymus as a possible general suppressive organ of NK reactivity in the mouse.

D. Role of the Spleen

The spleen is a prominent organ with regard to NK activity in young adult mice. Although the chimera experiments have shown that the spleen cannot be responsible for the genetically determined level of NK activity in high- or low-reactive mouse strains, it is still possible that NK cells require an intact splenic microenvironment in order to obtain specific cytotoxicity. To investigate this, CBA mice were splenectomized as young adults. NK activity was determined in peripheral blood and lymph nodes and was compared to that of sham-operated littermates. No differences between the two groups were found. A second set of young adult mice was either splenectomized or sham-operated 4 weeks prior to lethal irradiation and reconstitution with syngeneic bone marrow. Again, no differences in NK activity of blood or lymph node cells could be found between these two groups. With regard to NK reactivity, the asplenic mice were reconstituted to the same degree as the control animals (Haller *et al.*, 1978*b*). The spleen is obviously not mandatory for NK generation. In line with these findings is the recent notion that lymph node cells from Lasat mice express high NK activity (Herberman and Holden, 1978). These mice have evolved from crosses between hereditarily asplenic mice with nude mice and therefore lack spleen and thymus (Lozzio *et al.*, 1976).

VIII. CONCLUDING REMARKS

In this review we have attempted to summarize recent developments in the field of naturally occurring cytotoxic cells, known as natural killer (NK) cells. These nonimmune cells exist in healthy, normal mammals and display specific cytolytic activity against various target cells. Although our understanding of these cells is as yet incomplete and many perplexing problems remain, we feel that the data amassed to date warrant the classification of natural killer cells as a new and probably autonomous class of killer cells. Many of the features discussed—surface markers, tissue distribution, age dependence, genetic control, and specificity—would seem to support such an interpretation.

Among the many urgent problems awaiting future clarification are those concerning generation and differentiation of the NK cell. Cooperation of NK cells with other host cells and modification of the activity of these cells by environmental factors await further delineation. Future research should focus attention on some important facts. A genetic analysis with precise mapping of genes related with NK activity has to be further extended. NK cells must be purified. This should hopefully be possible soon using combined fractionation procedures employing classical fractionation procedures and affinity chromatography on HP columns and/or specific rosetting techniques. An important aspect involves the specificity of NK-cell recognition. Target-cell antigeneic determinants must be defined and the NK-cell receptor needs to be characterized. Furthermore, the mode of target-cell recognition and mechanism of killing by these cells must be elucidated.

The most important part of this work should be to better define the *in vivo* role of NK cells. We have summarized here experimental evidence for a protective role of NK cells against transplantation of certain lymphoma cells. This analysis of natural tumor resistance must be extended to involve also other types of tumors. NK cells could conceivably even act as regulators of hemopoiesis and fullfil basic needs for homeostasis of various cell compartments which are subjected to continuous physiological proliferation.

As can be readily appreciated, the questions still far outnumber the answers, and we hope that we have at least put current knowledge of this fascinating system into perspective, while stirring interest in those previously unfamiliar with the importance of the natural killer cell system.

ACKNOWLEDGMENTS

This work was supported by NCI contracts N01-CB-64033 and N01-CB-64023 and the Swedish Cancer Society.

Otto Haller was supported by Stiftung für Biologisch-medizinische Stipendien der Schweizerischen Akademie der Medizinischen Wissenschaften.

Rolf Kiessling is a recipient of a fellowship in cancer immunology from the Cancer Research Institute, New York.

IX. REFERENCES

Aaronson, S. A., and Stephenson, J. R., 1974, *Proc. Natl. Acad. Sci. U.S.* 71:1957.

Allison, A. C., Harington, J. S., and Birbeck, M. 1966, *J. Exp. Med.* 124:141.

Aoki, T., Boyse, E. A., and Old, L. J., 1966, *Cancer Res.* 26:1415.

Bast, R. C., Bast, B. S., and Rapp, H. J., 1976, *Ann. N.Y. Acad. Sci.* 277:60.

Becker, S., and Klein, E., 1976, *Eur. J. Immunol.* 6:892.

Becker, S., Fenyö, E. M., and Klein, E., 1977, *Eur. J. Immunol.* 6:882.

Bennet, M., 1973, *J. Immunol.* 110:510.

Bennet, M., Baker, E. E., Eastcott, J. W., Kumar, V., and Yonkosky, D., 1976, *J. Reticuloendothel. Soc.* 20:71.

Blair, P. B., and Lane, M. A., 1975, *J. Immunol.* 115:184.

Bonmassar, E., Campanile, F., Houchens, D., Crino, L., and Goldin, A., 1975, *Transplantation* 20:343.

Catanzaro, P. J., Schwartz, H. J., and Graham, R. C., 1971, *Amer. J. Pathol.* 64:387.

Cerottini, J.-C., and Brunner, K. T., 1974, *Adv. Immunol.* 18:67.

Chesebro, B., Wehrly, K., and Stimpfling, J., 1974, *J. Exp. Med.* 140:1457.

Cikes, M., Friberg, S., Jr., and Klein, G., 1973, *J. Natl. Cancer Inst.* 50:347.

Collavo, D., Colombatti, A., Chieco-Bianchi, L., and Davies, A. J. S., 1974, *Nature* 249:169.

Cudkowicz, G., 1968, in: *The Proliferation and Spread of Neoplastic Cells* (Twenty-third Annual M.D. Anderson Symposium on Fundamental Cancer Research), pp. 661–691, Williams & Wilkins, Baltimore.

Cudkowicz, G., 1975, *Proc. Amer. Assoc. Cancer Res.* 16:170 (Abstract).

Cudkowicz, G., and Bennet, M., 1971a, *J. Exp. Med.* 134:83.

Cudkowicz, G., and Bennet, M., 1971b, *J. Exp. Med.* 134:1513.

Cudkowicz, G., and Stimpfling, J. H., 1964, *Nature* 204:450.

Epstein, A. L., and Herman, M. M., Kim, H., Dorfman, R. F., and Kaplan, H. S., 1976, *Cancer* 37:2158.

Fidler, I. J., Caines, S., and Dolan, Z., 1976, *Transplantation* 22:208.

Gallagher, M. T., Lotzova, E., and Trentin, J. J., 1976, *Biomedicine* 25:1.

Giovanella, B. C., Stehlin, J. S., and Williams, L. J., Jr., 1974, *J. Natl. Cancer Inst.* 52:921.

Glaser, M., Lavrin, D. H., and Herberman, R. B., 1976, *J. Immunol.* 116:1507.

Glimcher, L., Shen, F. W., and Cantor, H., 1977, *J. Exp. Med.* 145:1.

Gorczynski, R. M., and Norbury, C., 1974, *Brit. J. Cancer* 30:118.

Greenberg, A. H., and Greene, M., 1977, *Nature* 264:356.

Haller, O., and Wigzell, H., 1977, *J. Immunol.* 118:1503.

Haller, O., Hansson, M., Kiessling, R., and Wigzell, H., 1977a, *Nature* 270:609.

Haller, O., Kiessling, R., Örn, A., Kärre, K., Nilsson, K., and Wigzell, H., 1977b, *Int. J. Cancer* 20:93.

Haller, O., Kiessling, R., Örn, A., and Wigzell, H., 1977c, *J. Exp. Med.* 145:1411.

Haller, O., Gidlund, M., Hellström, U., Hammarström, S., and Wigzell, H., 1978a, submitted for publication.

Haller, O., Gidlund, M., Kurnik, J., and Wigzell, H., 1978b, submitted for publication.

Halpern, B., Fray, A., Crepin, J., Platica, O., Lorinet, A. M., Rabourdin, A., Sparros, L., and Isac, R., 1973, in: *Immunopotentiation* (Ciba Foundation Symposium), pp. 217–236, Elsevier, Excerpta Medica, North-Holland, Amsterdam.

Hammarström, S., 1974, *Ann. N.Y. Acad. Sci.* 234:183.

Hammarström, S., Hellström, U., Perlmann, P., and Dillner, M-L., 1973, *J. Exp. Med.* 138:1270.

Harmon, R. C., Clark, E., O'Toole, C., and Wicker, L., 1977, *Immunogenetics* 4:601.

Hellström, K. E., and Hellström, I., 1967, *Progr. Exp. Tumor Res.* 9:40.

Hellström, U., Hammarström, S., Dillner, M.-L., Perlmann, H., and Perlmann, P., 1976, *Scand. J. Immunol.* (Suppl. 5): 45.

Herberman, R. B., and Holden, H. T., 1978, *Advances in Cancer Research* (G. Klein and S. Weinhouse, eds.), Academic Press, New York (in press).

Herberman, R. B., Nunn, M. E., and Lavrin, D. H., 1975a, *Int. J. Cancer* 16:216.

Herberman, R. B., Nunn, M. E., Holden, H. T., and Lavrin, D. H., 1975b, *Int. J. Cancer* 16:230.

Herberman, R. B., Nunn, M. E., Holden, H. T., Staal, S., and Djeu, J. Y., 1977, *Int. J. Cancer* 19:555.

Herberman, R. B., West, W. H., Holden, H. T., Kay, H. D., Djeu, J. Y., and Bonnard, G. D., 1976, in: *Proc. 16th Int. Cong. Hematology*.

Howell, S., Dean, J., and Law, L., 1975, *Int. J. Cancer* 15:152.

Ihle, J. N., Yurconic, M., Jr., and Hanna M. G., Jr., 1973, *J. Exp. Med.* 138:194.

Kärre, K., Häyry, P., Becker, S., Haller, O., and Kiessling, R., 1978, submitted for publication.

Keller, R., 1976, in: *Immunobiology of the Macrophage* (D. S. Nelsson, ed.), p. 487, Academic Press, New York.

Kiessling, R., Klein, E., and Wigzell, H., 1975a, *Eur. J. Immunol.* 5:112.

Kiessling, R., Klein, E., Pross, H., and Wigzell, H., 1975b, *Eur. J. Immunol.* 5:117.

Kiessling, R., Petrányi, G., Klein, G., and Wigzell, H., 1975c, *Int. J. Cancer* 15:933.

Kiessling, R., Petrányi, G., Kärre, K., Jondal, M., Tracey, D., and Wigzell, H., 1976a, *J. Exp. Med.* 143:772.

Kiessling, R., Petrányi, G., Klein, G., and Wigzell, H., 1976b, *Int. J. Cancer* 17:275.

Kiessling, R., Hochman, P., Haller, O., Shearer, G., Wigzell, H., and Cudkowicz, G., 1977, *Eur. J. Immunol.* 7:655.

Kumar, V., Bennet, M., and Eckner, R. J., 1974, *J. Exp. Med.* 139:1093.

Lamensans, A., Stiffel, C., Mollier, M. F., Canrent, M., Mouton, D., and Biozzi, G., 1968, *Rev. Fr. Étud. Clin. Biol.* 13:733.

Lilly, F., and Pincus, T., 1973, *Adv. Cancer Res.* **17**:231.
Lotzová, E., and Cudkowicz, G., 1974, *J. Immunol.* **113**:798.
Lotzová, E., Gallagher, M. T., and Trentin, J. J., 1975, *Biomedicine* **22**:387.
Lozzio, B. B., Machado, E. A., Lozzio, C. B., and Lair, S., 1976, *J. Exp. Med.* **143**:225.
Martin, S., and Martin, J., 1975, *Nature* **256**:498.
Möller, G., and Möller, E., 1975, *J. Natl. Cancer Inst.* **55**:755.
Mühlbock, O., and Dux, A., 1974, *J. Natl. Cancer Inst.* **53**: 993.
Nathanson, L., 1974, *Semin. Oncol.* **1**:337.
Nowinski, R. C., and Kaehler, S. L., 1974, *Science* **185**:869.
Nunn, M. E., Djeu, J. Y., Glaser, M., Lavrin, D. H., and Herberman, R. B., 1976, *J. Natl. Cancer Inst.* **56**:393.
Ojo, E., Haller, O., and Wigzell, H., 1978, submitted for publication.
Perlmann, P., Perlmann, H., and Biberfeld, P., 1972, *J. Immunol.* **108**:558.
Petrányi, G. G., Benczur, M., Onody, C. E., and Holland, S. R., 1974, *Lancet* **1**:736.
Petrányi, G. G., Kiessling, R ., and Klein, G., 1975, *Immunogenetics* **2**:53.
Petrányi, G. G., Kiessling, R., Povey, S., Klein, G., Herzenberg, L., and Wigzell, H., 1976, *Immunogenetics* **3**:15.
Pross, H. F., and Jondal, M., 1975, *Clin. Exp. Immunol.* **21**:226.
Rotter, V., and Trainin, N., 1975, *Transplantation* **20**:68.
Rygaard, J., and Povlsen, C. O., 1976, *Transplant. Rev.* **28**:43.
Sanderson, C. J., Clark, I. A., and Taylor, G. A., 1975, *Nature* **253**:376.
Sato, H., Boyse, E. A., Aoki, T., Iritani, C., and Old, L. J., 1973, *J. Exp. Med.* **138**:593.
Schmidt, M., and Good, R. A., 1976, *Lancet* **1**:39.
Schmitt-Verhulst, A., and Zats, M., 1977, *J. Immunol.* **1**:330.
Sendo, F., Aoki, T., Boyse, E. A., and Buofo, C. K., 1975, *J. Natl. Cancer Inst.* **55**:603.
Shearer, G. M., 1974, *Eur. J. Immunol.* **4**:527.
Shearer, G. M., and Cudkowicz, G., 1975, *Science* **190**:890.
Shearer, G. M., Garbarino, C. A., and Cudkowicz, G., 1976*a*, *J. Immunol.* **117**:754.
Shearer, G. M., Waksal, H., and Cudkowicz, G., 1976*b*, *Transplant. Proc.* **8**:469.
Shellam, G. R., and Hogg, N., 1977, *Int. J. Cancer* **19**:212.
Skov, C. B., Holland, J. M., and Perkins. E. H., 1976, *J. Natl. Cancer Inst.* **56**:193.
Snell, G. D., 1958, *J. Natl. Cancer Inst.* **21**:843.
Sulit, H. L., Golub, S. H., Irie, R. S., Gupta, R. K., Grooms, G. A., and Morton, D. L., 1976, *Int. J. Cancer* **17**:461.
Svedmyr, E., and Jondal, M., 1975, *Proc. Natl. Acad. Sci. U.S.* **72**:1622.
Till, J. E., Wilson, S., and McCulloch, E. A., 1970, *Science* **169**:1327.
Trentin, J., Kiessling, R., Wigzell, H., Gallagher, M., Datta, S., and Kulkarni, S., 1977, in: *Experimental Hematology Today* (S. Baum and D. Ledney, eds.), Springer Verlag, New York.
Warner, N. L., Wodruff, M. F., and Burton, R. C., 1977, *Int. J. Cancer* **20**:146.
Williams, R. M., Dorf, M. E., and Benacerraf, B., 1975, *Cancer Res.* **35**:1586.
Winn, H. J., 1961, *J. Immunol.* **86**:228.
Wolfe, S. A., Tracey, D. E., and Henney, C. S., 1976, *Nature* **262**:584.
Zarling, J. M., Nowinski, R. C., and Bach, F. H., 1975, *Proc. Natl. Acad. Sci. U.S.* **72**:2780.
Zinkernagel, R. M., and Doherty, P. C., 1975, *J. Exp. Med.* **141**:1427.

Chapter 7

Allotypes of IgM and IgD Receptors in the Mouse: A Probe for Lymphocyte Differentiation

James W. Goding*

The Walter and Eliza Hall Institute of Medical Research
The Royal Melbourne Hospital
Melbourne, Victoria 3050, Australia

I. LYMPHOCYTE SURFACE IMMUNOGLOBULIN

A. Use of Antiimmunoglobulin Sera to Study Lymphocyte Receptors

In 1899, Metchnikoff proposed that macrophages might be studied using antimacrophage serum. The farsighted nature of this idea is indicated by the fact that virtually all the current methods for the study of lymphocyte surface receptors for antigen involve the use of antireceptor antisera. This somewhat circular approach (i.e., the use of antibodies to study antibodies) may be regarded as an example of the value of those methods of analysis which exploit biochemical affinities rather than classical chemistry.

If antibodies are to be used successfully as a biological probe, it is self-evident that the investigator must understand the specificity of the antisera. Especially important in this regard are (1) the *purity of the antigen* used to elicit the antibodies, (2) *cross-reaction* of the antigen with shared determinants on other molecules (e.g., immunoglobulin light chains), and (3) *genetic differences* between individuals in a species, or between species, in their immune responsiveness. In addition, the specificity of antisera may be intentionally modified by *absorption* (to remove unwanted antibody populations) and/or by *elution* from immobilized antigen to produce "purified" antibodies to that antigen.

*Present address: Department of Genetics, Stanford University School of Medicine, Stanford, California.

203

The most common approach to the serological study of the immuno-globulins has involved the immunization of one species with highly purified immunoglobulin from another species (xenoantisera). The specificity of such antisera depends largely on the purity of the antigen used and the phylogenetic distance between the two species.

An alternative approach utilizes allelic forms (allotypes) of immunoglobulins *within a species*. Individuals (or inbred strains) within a species are immunized against products of other individuals which possess different allelic forms of that product. Such an approach may enable the generation of specific *alloantisera*, even if the antigen is not extremely pure.

There are no known myelomas of the IgD class in the mouse, and IgD is not present in detectable levels in mouse serum. The problem of obtaining highly purified IgD from lymphocyte membranes is formidable. In later sections of this chapter it will be shown that allotypes of murine IgD may be used to generate highly specific antisera to this molecule, in the absence of any purification at all.

The demonstration of allelic forms also allows mapping of genes. In the mouse, this approach led to the demonstration that the genes coding for the γ2a, α, γ2b, and γ1 heavy chains (*Ig-1*, *Ig-2*, *Ig-3*, and *Ig-4*, respectively) are very closely linked to each other in a "heavy-chain cluster" (Herzenberg and Warner, 1968). More recently, the discovery of serologically detectable allelic forms of murine δ chains (Goding *et al.*, 1976, 1977) and μ chains (Herzenberg *et al.*, 1976; Warner *et al.*, 1977) has allowed the definition of two new heavy-chain loci. These genes (*Ig-5* and *Ig-6*, respectively) also map in the heavy-chain region.

IgM and IgD are now thought to constitute the major receptor types on the surface of B cells. Alloantisera to these molecules will thus provide a powerful new tool for the study of B-cell differentiation, and may also allow improved understanding of the immunoglobulin heavy-chain gene cluster.

B. What Classes of Immunoglobulin Are Present on the Surface of Lymphocytes?

A minimal theory of antigen recognition involving clonal selection might envisage that surface receptors are identical to the antibody product which an individual lymphocyte is destined to secrete upon activation. This notion, of "receptor equals product," has received qualified support from most workers (see Wigzell, 1973). However, following the first demonstrations of surface immunoglobulin on lymphocytes, two rather contradictory streams of data on the *classes* of surface immunoglobulin appeared. Current work has shown that neither was completely correct.

On the one hand, studies using fluorescein or ^{125}I-labeled antiimmuno-globulin reagents indicated that *all* classes of immunoglobulin were represented on the surface of B cells. Large numbers of B cells were found to possess surface IgM, IgG, and IgA (e.g., Nossal *et al.*, 1972). There was general agreement, however, that IgM was the dominant class (Warner, 1974).

On the other hand, early studies involving biochemical characterization of surface immunoglobulin revealed only μ chains and light chains, or at the most only traces of γ chains (Marchalonis and Cone, 1973; Vitetta and Uhr, 1973).

The notion of "receptor equals product" was especially difficult to accommodate within the framework of these results, since while the predominant surface immunoglobulin on B cells was generally agreed to be IgM, by far the major serum immunoglobulin is IgG. Confusion was compounded by the finding (van Boxel *et al.*, 1972; Rowe *et al.*, 1973a,b) that IgD (which is only present in trace amounts in serum) was present on a large percentage of B cells. The wide range of reported percentages of cells bearing classes other than IgM was considered by Warner (1974) to be suggestive of differences in technique rather than real biological differences.

As workers in the field gained experience, there was a gradual increase in the level of sophistication in the study of surface immunoglobulins. Increasing attention was paid to the need for avoidance of binding of antisera to the Fc receptor on B cells, and liquid-phase absorptions of antisera gave way to solid-phase absorptions, with consequent reduction in the problems due to soluble antigen–antibody complexes. Manipulations to achieve chain-specific antisera became increasingly sophisticated (Vitetta and Uhr, 1975). The paradox concerning the detection of surface IgG by antiglobulin binding gradually became explicable in terms of technical problems including (1) inadequate specificity of antisera, (2) natural antibodies to membrane components, (3) the presence of aggregates and complexes in sera, and (4) cytophilic antibodies (Vitetta and Uhr, 1975; Winchester *et al.*, 1975a).

The last of these has proven particularly important, especially for peripheral blood cells, many of which may possess cytophilic IgG. It is now essential that experiments on surface immunoglobulin control for cytophilic immunoglobulins. The simple expedient of incubating the cells for a few hours at 37°C is often sufficient to allow shedding of cytophilic IgG, and may radically alter results and their interpretation. Experiments which purport to show surface IgG, or lack of allelic exclusion of receptors (see later), are quite meaningless unless controls for cytophilic IgG are included.

In parallel with a gradual decline in the accepted figures for cells bearing γ chains, the presence of a new immunoglobulin class, which was poorly (if at all) represented in serum, came into prominence.

IgD was first described by Rowe and Fahey (1965) on the basis of an unusual myeloma protein. It soon became clear that although IgD was present in only minute amounts in serum, this class was very prominent on the surface of lymphocytes (van Boxel *et al.*, 1972; Rowe *et al.*, 1973a,b). The biological function of this class could then be ascribed to a role as a lymphocyte receptor (Rowe *et al.*, 1973*a*).

Initial reports on the presence of IgD on lymphocyte surfaces stressed the prominence of this class on cells from neonates (van Boxel *et al.*, 1972; Rowe *et al.*, 1973*b*). However, close examination of the data presented in these early papers does not fully support this conclusion. The published data were quite consistent with the notion that the percentage of cells with surface immuno-globulin of *any* class was considerably higher in cord blood than in adult blood. Cells bearing IgM only or IgD only were present, but the most common cells with surface immunoglobulin bore both chains, as was the case for adult per-ipheral blood lymphocytes. It is now clear that IgD follows IgM in ontogeny rather than preceding it (Gupta *et al.*, 1976; Gathings *et al.*, 1976). The great majority of human blood lymphocytes (Winchester *et al.*, 1975*a*) and tonsil lymphocytes (Ferrarini *et al.*, 1976*a*) in adults bear both IgM and IgD.

For several years following the discovery of IgD in humans, there was no evidence for an homologous product in other species. The situation underwent a dramatic change, however, when improved biochemical techniques revealed a new immunoglobulin class on murine B lymphocytes, which was not represented in serum (Melcher *et al.*, 1974; Abney and Parkhouse, 1974). This molecule, which migrated a little faster than μ chain in SDS–polyacrylamide gel electro-phoresis, was precipitable by antisera to light chains but not by antisera to any of the known heavy-chain classes. It was shown to appear after IgM in ontogeny (Vitetta *et al.*, 1974). In view of its predominant expression on the surface of B lymphocytes, its lack of reactivity with antisera to known heavy-chain deter-minants, and its apparent susceptibility to proteolysis, it was postulated that this molecule was the murine homologue of human IgD (Vitetta and Uhr, 1975; Abney and Parkhouse, 1974).

The question of whether an IgD homologue exists in other species is open. There are some strong indications that such a molecule is present in certain monkeys and in rabbits (Pernis *et al.*, 1975; Martin *et al.*, 1976) and rats (Ruddick and Leslie, 1977). It seems very likely that a counterpart to IgD will be found in all mammalian species, and possibly in birds. If such a molecule is found in birds, this would suggest that IgD is a universal component of the immune system in all species.

II. PREPARATION OF ANTISERA TO MURINE IgD

A. Antigen Purification by Affinity Chromatography

A fundamental requirement for the production of specific xenoantisera is the *purity of the antigen*. So far, there is only one report of the successful prep-aration of specific xenoantisera to murine IgD (Abney *et al.*, 1976). The antigen used was prepared by detergent solubilization of the spleen cell membranes of some 2000 mice. IgM receptors were depleted from the mixture by passage over an anti-μ-Sepharose column, and the remaining receptors were adsorbed to anti-κ-Sepharose. These columns were then used to immunize rabbits. No attempt was made to elute the antigen. After absorption of the resulting antisera against immobilized myeloma immunoglobulins of all other classes, the remaining antibodies were shown to be specific for IgD.

B. Antibodies to IgD in Murine Alloantisera

In the course of studies on the structure of H-2 and Ia antigens, the author set up a method for the isolation of these antigens, based on a technique originally developed by Kessler (1975). The plasma membranes of lymphocytes were labeled with ^{125}I by the lactoperoxidase technique, and then solubilized by the nonionic detergent Nonidet P-40 (NP-40). Antisera to the membrane proteins of interest were then added, and the resulting antigen–antibody complexes isolated by binding to protein A containing staphylococci (protein A binds specifically and with high affinity to γ chains of most mammalian species; see Goding, 1978). After the bacteria were washed, complexes were dissociated and the radioactive components analyzed by polyacrylamide gel electrophoresis (PAGE) in the presence of sodium dodecyl sulfate (SDS).

Some difficulty was experienced in obtaining satisfactory gel patterns using congenic antisera against the *H-2K* or *H-2D* products, and in one experiment an extra group, using a noncongenic "anti-H-2" serum, was included. This antiserum was made in C57Bl/6 (*H-2^b*, *Ig^b*) mice against the spleen cells of CBA (*H-2^k*, *Ig^a*) mice (see Table I for the details of mouse strains). Since these strains are unrelated, it was expected that this serum would reveal a very complex gel pattern consisting of both H-2 and non-H-2 antigens.

In contrast to these expectations, the gel pattern from this serum was surprisingly simple (Fig. 1). Even more surprisingly, a plausible explanation for most of the peaks could be offered (Goding *et al.*, 1976). The central two peaks possessed the mobilities expected for H-2 and Ia antigens, while the outer two peaks coincided exactly with immunoglobulin light chains and δ chains.

Indirect immunofluorescence experiments were performed in an attempt to test the hypothesis that the outer peaks were indeed δ chains and light chains. Spleen and thymus cells from C3H.SW (*H-2^b*, *Ig^a*) were used as targets for the C57B1/6 anti-CBA serum. These mice possess the same H-2 type as C57B1/6 mice, and hence will not reveal anti-H-2 antibodies in an H-2^b anti-H-2^k serum, yet they resemble CBA in heavy-chain genes. Cells were treated with C57Bl/6 anti-CBA serum followed by fluorescein-conjugated antisera to mouse γ chains. About one-third of spleen cells, but no thymocytes, were stained. Control C57B1/6 (*H-2^b*, *Ig^b*) cells showed only 1–2% positive.

The availability of an allotype congenic partner strain to C57B1/6 (C57B1/

Table I. IgD Allotypic Specificities in Inbred Strains

Strain	H-2 type	Ig-1 type	Ig-5 specificity[a]		
CBA	k	a	1	–	–
C3H	k	a	1	–	–
C3H.SW	b	a	1	–	–
Balb/c	d	a	1	–	–
SJL.Ig^a (SJA)	s	a	1	–	–
NZB	d	e	1	–	3
C57Bl/6.Ig^e	b	e	1	–	3
A/J	a	e	1	–	3
C57Bl/6	b	b	–	2	3
B10.BR	k	b	–	2	3
SJL	s	b	–	2	3
Balb/c.Ig^b (BAB)	d	b	–	2	3

[a]A myeloma cell hybrid secreting homogeneous anti-Ig-5^b has recently been described (Pearson *et al.*, 1977). This antibody reacts with cells of A/J (Ig-5^e) mice (Pearson, T., Ziegler, A., and Milstein, C., unpublished), indicating a shared determinant between Ig-5^b and Ig-5^e (specificity 3).

6.Ig^e; Goding *et al.*, 1976) provided a convenient way of testing for linkage of the δ-like antigen to the heavy-chain cluster. This strain is identical to C57Bl/6 (Ig^b) except for the heavy-chain genes, which were derived from NZB (Ig^e) by repeated backcrossing with selection for NZB heavy-chain allotypes. The NZB and CBA γ and α allotypes cross-react extensively, and it was hoped that a similar cross-reaction might pertain with the δ allotypes. When tested on C57Bl/6.Ig^e, identical results to those seen with C3H.SW were obtained, indicating linkage of the IgD-like antigen to the heavy-chain cluster. On the other hand, virtually all the spleen and thymus cells from B10.BR (H-2^k) mice were stained, indicating the presence of antibodies to products of the *H-2* complex. The allotype-linked antigen detected on C57Bl/6.Ig^e cells was removed by "capping off" surface immunoglobulin with anti-light-chain serum but not with anti-μ-chain serum (Goding *et al.*, 1976).

In a parallel set of experiments, it was shown that the gel peaks corresponding in mobility to δ and light chains could be removed by passage of the detergent lysate over anti-light-chain-Sepharose (Fig. 2). When the C57Bl/6 anti-CBA serum was tested on C57Bl/6.Ig^e cells, only the δ and light-chain peaks were visible (Fig. 3). In contrast, when tested on B10.BR (which is identical to C57Bl/6 except for the H-2 segment, which resembles that of CBA), only H-2 and Ia antigens were detected (Fig. 3).

The C57B1/6 anti-CBA serum (abbreviated DA-1) failed to show precipi-tating activity against the following radioiodinated myeloma proteins: HPC-76 (μ, K), HPC-77 (γ1, K), HPC-82 (γ2a, K), HPC-84 (γ2b, K), J-606 (γ3, K) and HPC-14 (α, K). It was thus unlikely that the allotype-linked gene product was any of the presently known serum immunoglobulins. Moreover, there was no detectable precipitin line when the serum was tested against CBA serum in immunoelectrophoresis. These findings indicated that the antigen was not present in large amounts in serum.

It was concluded from these data that certain murine alloantisera contain

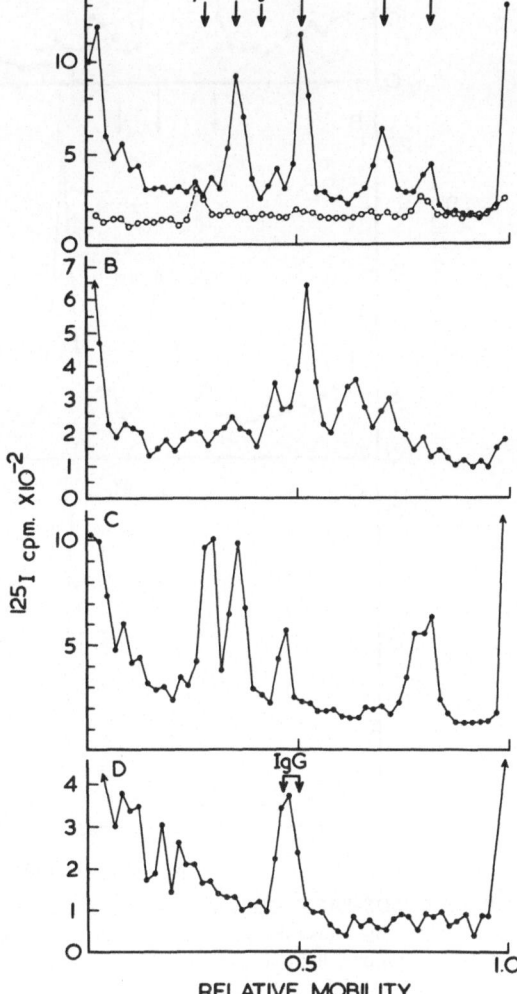

Figure 1. SDS–PAGE analysis of ^{125}I-labeled CBA membrane pro-teins recognized by alloantiserum. (A and D) CBA splenocyte membrane proteins bound by C57Bl anti-CBA spleen-1 serum (●---●), or by staphylococci alone (○---○). (B) CBA thymo-cyte membrane proteins bound by C57Bl anti-CBA serum. (C) CBA splenocyte membrane pro-teins bound by rabbit anti-mouse light-chain serum. Gels A–C were of 10% acrylamide, 0.25% bis-acrylamide concentration, and samples were reduced with 2-mercaptoethanol. Gel D was of 5% acrylamide, 0.12% bisacryla-mide concentration, and samples were not reduced.

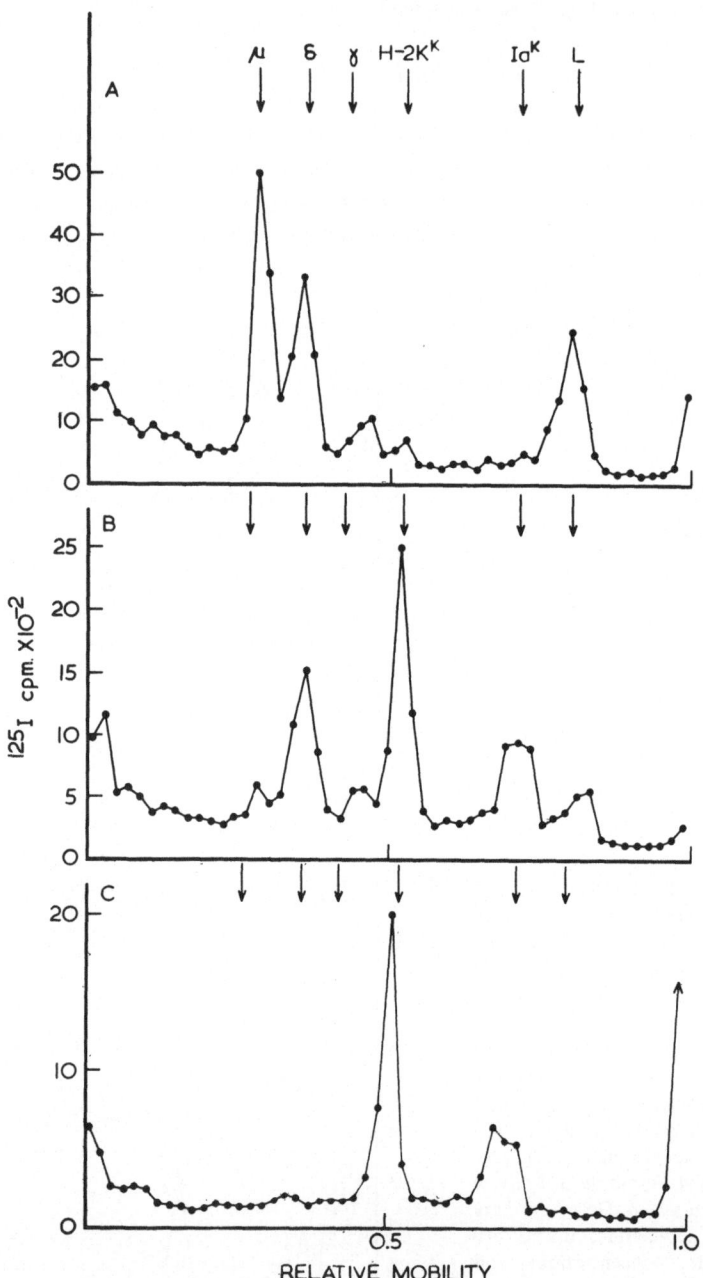

Figure 2. SDS–PAGE analysis ^{125}I-labeled CBA splenocyte membrane proteins recognized by alloantiserum. (A) CBA splenocyte membrane proteins bound by rabbit anti-mouse light-chain serum. (B) CBA splenocyte membrane proteins bound by C57Bl anti-CBA serum. (C) Immunoglobulin-depleted CBA splenocyte membrane proteins bound by C57Bl anti-CBA serum. All gels were of 10% acrylamide, 0.25% bisacrylamide concentration. All samples were reduced with mercaptoethanol.

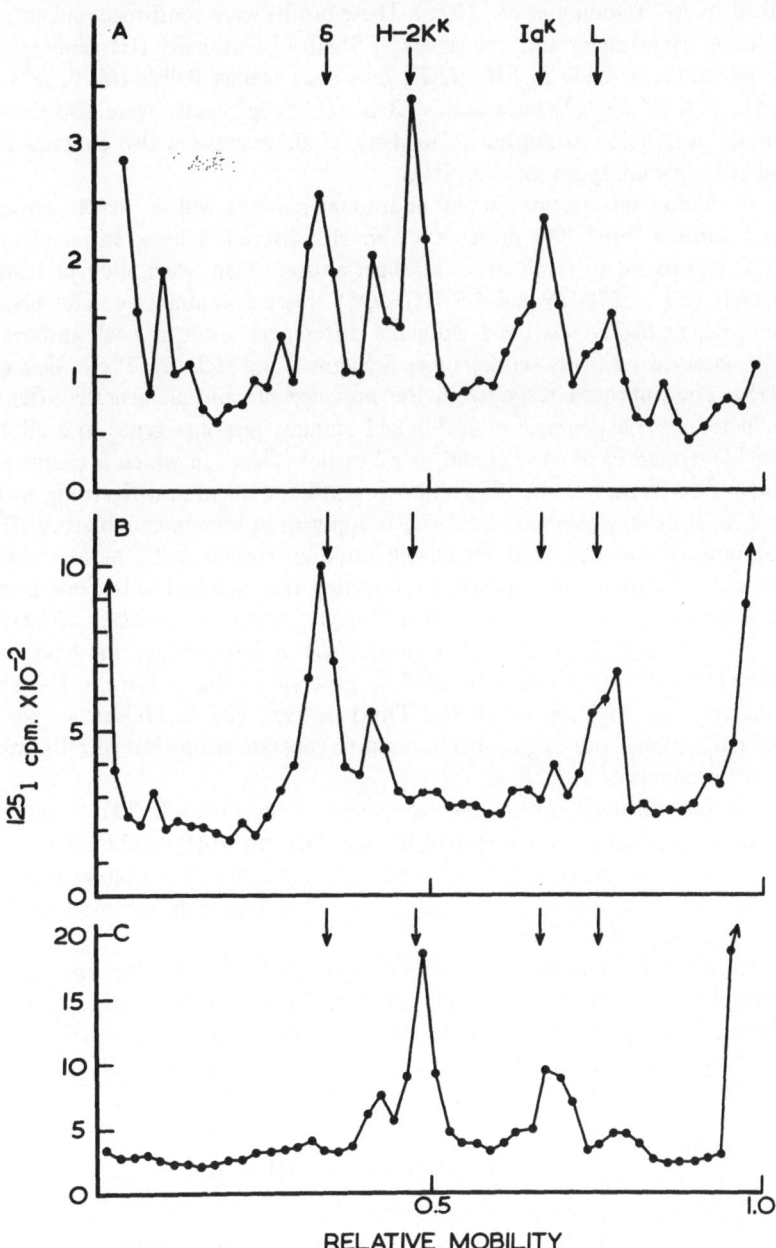

Figure 3. SDS–PAGE analysis of ^{125}I-labeled splenocyte membrane proteins from congenic mice recognized by C57Bl/6 anti-CBA serum. (A) CBA cells. (B) C57Bl/6. Ig^e cells. (C) B10.BR cells. All conditions as for Fig. 2.

antibodies to allotypes of murine IgD, and the locus (*Ig-5*) coding for δ chains is linked to *Ig-1* (Goding *et al.*, 1976). These results were confirmed and extended by L. A. Herzenberg and colleagues at Stanford University (Herzenberg *et al.*, 1976). Antisera made in SJL (*H-2^s*, *Ig^b*) mice against Balb/c (*H-2^d*, *Ig^a*) cells, and in SJA (*H-2^s*, *Ig^a*) mice against BAB (*H-2^d*, *Ig^b*) cells, were also shown to contain antibodies to murine IgD. Many of these antisera also contained antibodies to IgM allotypes (Section III).

In closing this section, a few additional remarks will be made concerning these antisera. First, the presence of an H-2 difference between recipient and donor was found to result in far stronger antisera than when allotype congenic partners (e.g., C57B1/6 and C57B1/6.*Ig^e*) are cross-immunized. This phenomenon, where highly restricted antigenic differences result in weak antisera, has been observed by many workers (see Schierman and McBride, 1969; Shen *et al.*, 1975). The improved response in the presence of multiple genetic differences could reflect the presence of *H-2*-linked immune response genes to δ allotypes (see Lieberman *et al.*, 1972) and/or a "carrier effect" in which δ chains act as hapten (see Wernet *et al.*, 1976). Concurrent immunization with strong antigens (such as H-2) may also have nonspecific adjuvant or immunostimulatory effects.

Second, the strategy used for raising anti-δ antibodies is of general usefulness. The anti-δ antisera were raised by injecting the recipient with cells from an unrelated donor, and were tested on a congenic partner strain which differs from the recipient only in the genetic characteristic of interest (i.e., the heavy-chain cluster). This approach may be used to generate strong antisera to H-2 and Ia antigens (e.g., Fig. 3), or to the Thy-1 antigen (I.F.C. McKenzie, personal communication), and might also be used to generate strong but specific antisera against products of other loci.

So far, anti-IgD antibodies have been detected in C57B1/6 anti-CBA, C57B1/6 anti-Balb/c, SJL anti-Balb/c, and SJA anti-BAB combinations. These antibodies (and antibodies to IgM allotypes) are almost certainly present in many other antisera, and constitute a potential hazard in interpreting results using noncongenic alloantisera.

Murine IgD thus exists in at least two allelic forms. The known strain distribution of δ allotypes is summarized in Table I. By the choice of suitable inbred and congenic strains of mice (e.g., C57B1/6 anti-CBA serum tested on C57B1/*Ig^e* cells), operationally monospecific anti-IgD sera are easily generated.

III. ALLOTYPES OF MURINE IgM

A. Antibodies to IgM in "Conventional" Antiallotype Sera

In the course of work on the δ-chain allotypes, control sera in radioimmunoassays included conventional antiallotype reagents made by cross-immunization with pertussis–anti-pertussis complexes. While none of these sera precipitated IgD, occasional sera showed strain-specific precipitation of serum IgM. These results were the first indications of genetic polymorphisms of IgM, and led to the identification of the Ig-6 locus coding for μ chains (Warner et al., 1977).

These sera were also capable of precipitating IgM receptors from detergent lysates of ^{125}I-labeled spleen cells (Figs. 4 and 5). The radioimmunoassay analyses of these "conventional" sera are described in Section IIIC. It should be emphasized that only a minority (approximately 5%) of conventional antiallotype sera showed reactivity against IgM.

In each case, the conventional antiallotype sera were made in C57B1/6 mice against immunoglobulins from CBA mice. The sera were capable of staining splenic B cells from Balb/c (Ig^a) mice by indirect immunofluorescence using fluorescein-conjugated anti-γ-chain serum as a sandwich reagent. They also stained the Balb/c IgM-bearing B-cell lymphoma WEHI-231. Staining was inhibited by pretreatment of the cells with heterologous anti-μ serum. The sera did not, however, stain spleen cells from Balb/c.Ig^b mice (see also Section IIIC). Since these strains differ only at the heavy-chain cluster, it was concluded that the locus coding for μ chains (Ig-6) was closely linked to Ig-1 (Warner et al., 1977).

B. Antibodies to IgM in Antilymphocyte Alloantisera

Following the discovery of the IgD allotypes (Goding et al., 1976), a collaborative project was set up between the Stanford and Melbourne groups. The Stanford group employed a strategy identical (except for differing mouse strains) to that already described (Section IIB). Mice of strain SJL.Ig^a (SJA) were immunized with spleen cells from C3H.SW.Ig^b (CWB) or Balb/c.Ig^b (BAB) mice. It was expected that this immunization protocol would elicit antibodies to the Ig-$5b$ allele. However, the activity of many of these antisera could be abolished by absorption with serum globulins of appropriate strain, and their reactions in indirect immunofluorescence was inhibitable by pretreatment of the cells with heterologous anti-μ (Herzenberg et al., 1976). In addition, these sera were shown to be capable of precipitating IgM receptors from splenic B cells of appropriate allotype (Figs. 6 and 7).

In a proportion of cases, however, not all the staining activity could be abolished by exhaustive absorption with serum immunoglobulins. These sera (but not those in which the staining was completely abolished by absorption) were found to have precipitating activity against δ chains in addition to μ chains (e.g., Fig. 7). Similarly, later bleeds of C57B1/6 anti-CBA spleen cell antisera were often found to contain antibodies to μ chains as well as δ chains. The gradual change in specificity of one such immunization is shown in Fig. 8. By the third bleed, definite anti-μ activity was seen in gel patterns and was con-

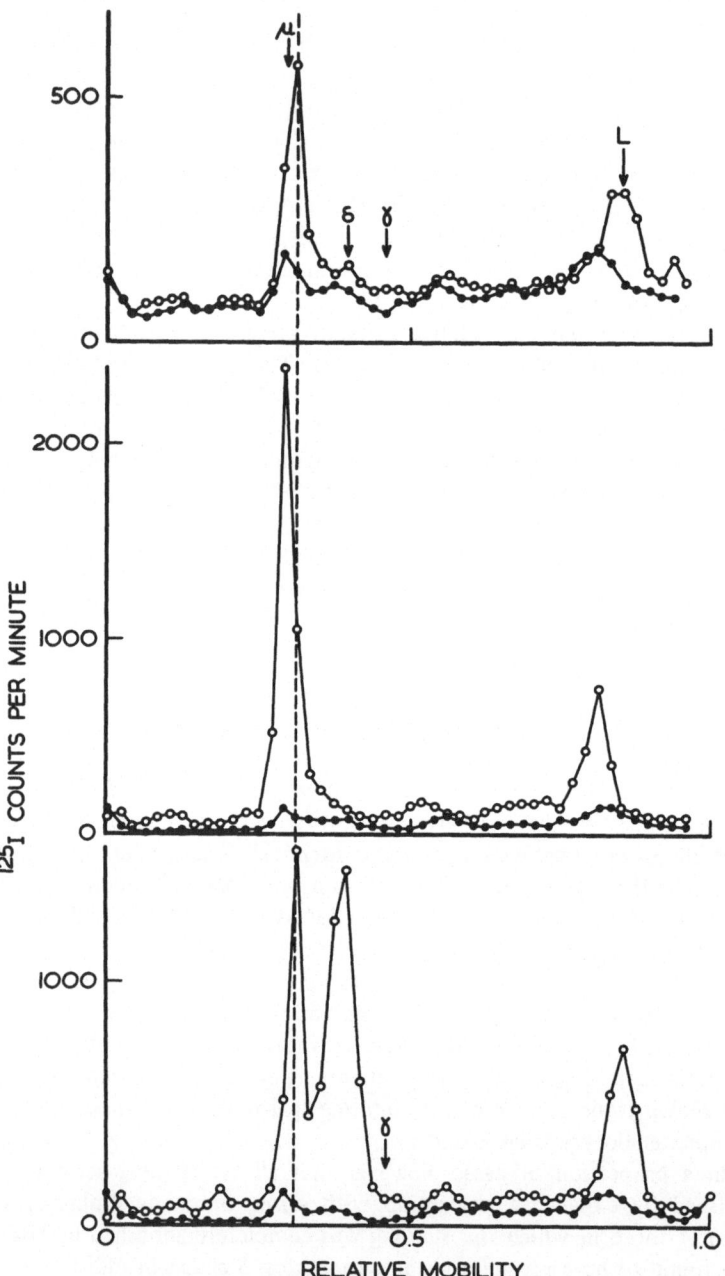

Figure 4. SDS–PAGE analysis of ^{125}I-labeled CBA splenocyte membrane proteins recognized by: (A) conventional antiallotype serum G1A2 (C57Bl/6 anti-CBA); (B) rabbit anti-mouse μ chain; (C) rabbit anti-mouse light chain and μ chain. All gels were 10% acrylamide, and all samples were reduced with mercaptoethanol. ○——○, experimental; ●——●, control (no serum).

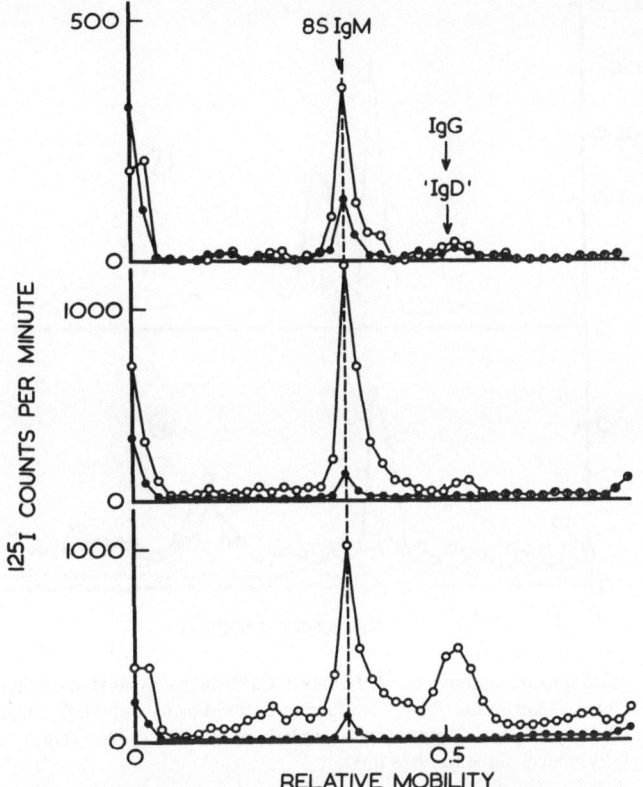

Figure 5. SDS–PAGE analysis of ^{125}I-labeled CBA splenocyte membrane proteins recognized by: (A) conventional antiallotype serum G1A2 (see Fig. 9); (B) rabbit anti-mouse μ chain; (C) rabbit anti-mouse light chain and μ chain. All gels 5% acrylamide; samples were *not* reduced. ○——○, experimental; ●——●, control (no serum).

firmed by radioimmunoassay (Section IIIC). Thus, it may be concluded that some anti-spleen cell sera contain antibodies to IgM, some to IgD, and some to both (Table II).

C. Specificity Analysis by Radioimmunoassay

Much of our current knowledge concerning immunoglobulin allotypes comes from radioimmunoassay (RIA) analysis using radioiodinated myeloma proteins as antigen. This form of analysis is potentially far more sensitive than gel diffusion in agar, and many sera which are negative by Ouchterlony analysis have high titers in RIA. For optimal precipitation, it is important to observe the require-

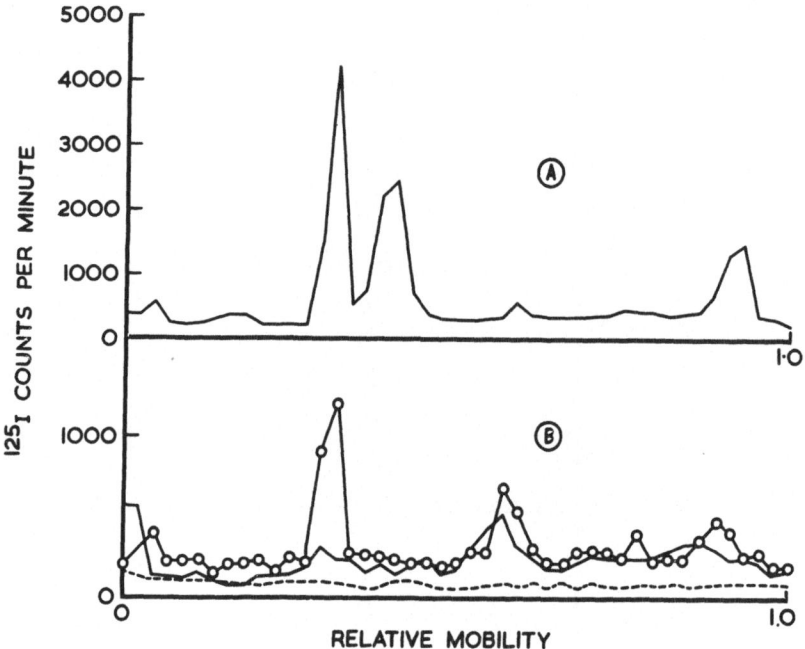

Figure 6. SDS–PAGE analysis of ^{125}I-labeled C57Bl/6 splenocyte membrane proteins recognized by (A) antiserum R640 (containing antibodies to μ and light chains) and (B) SJA anti-CWB splenocyte serum (open circles) or normal mouse serum (continuous line) or staphylococci alone (dashed line).

ments for *low-ionic-strength buffers* and *traces of C1q* (Herzenberg and Warner, 1968; Herzenberg and Herzenberg, 1978). Most mouse myelomas are of Balb/c (Ig^a), NZB (Ig^e), or (Balb/c × NZB) F_1 origin (Warner, 1975), although some myelomas induced in Balb/c.Ig^b mice are now available. Table III summarizes the strains of the IgM myelomas used in the allotype studies. The lack of availability of highly purified murine IgD has prevented the use of RIA for analysis of IgD specificities.

Analysis of IgM allotypic specificities by RIA is complicated by several other considerations. The μ-chain allotypic determinants are very labile and are destroyed by excessive concentrations of chloramine-T during iodination, which may account for the previous failures to detect IgM allotypes. The determinants are also destroyed by acid and low concentrations of thiocyanate. In some cases, precipitation is rather poor in single antibody systems, but the detection of antibodies (especially Ig-6b) is greatly facilitated by the addition of heterologous anti-mouse-γ-chain serum as a "second antibody."

Figure 9 shows the RIA analysis of several sera tested against IgM or IgG_{2a} myelomas. Both the conventional antiallotype sera (GA-20 and GA-26) were capable of precipitating IgG_{2a}, but only GA-20 precipitated IgM. Conversely, serum MA3 (late bleed of C57/Bl/6 anti-CBA spleen serum) precipitated IgM but not IgG2a.

Normal serum from Ig^a mice was capable of inhibiting the precipitation of HPC-76 (Ig-6^a) by serum MA3, while serum from Ig^b and Ig^e mice was not (Fig. 10). These results suggest that, unlike the δ-chain allotypes, Ig-6a and Ig-6e do not cross-react greatly. Of particular interest was the failure of any of the anti-Ig-6a sera to precipitate HPC-208, an IgM myeloma which arose in a (Balb/c X NZB) F_1 hybrid mouse. This myeloma protein was readily precipitable by a

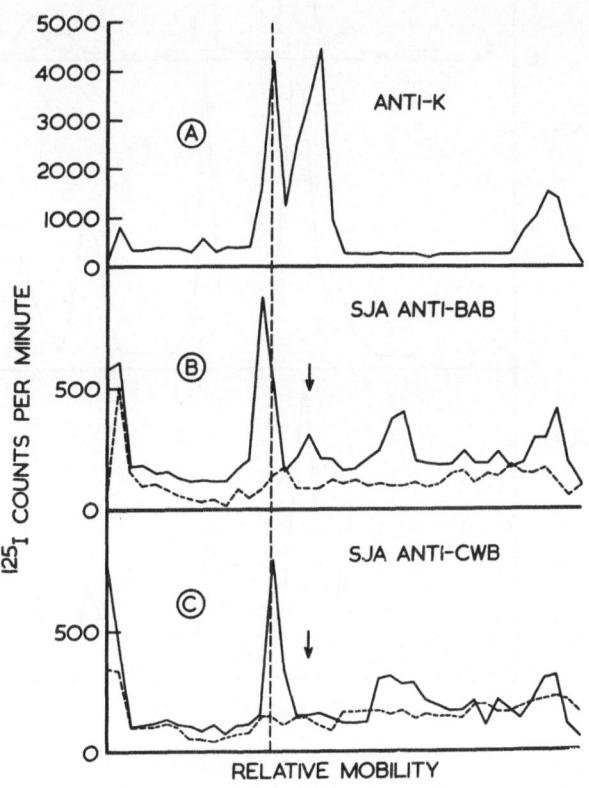

Figure 7. SDS–PAGE analysis of ^{125}I-labeled C57Bl/6 spleno-cyte membrane proteins recognized by antisera to kappa light chains (A), SJA anti-BAB/14 serum (B), and SJA anti-CWB serum (C). Dashed lines: no serum added.

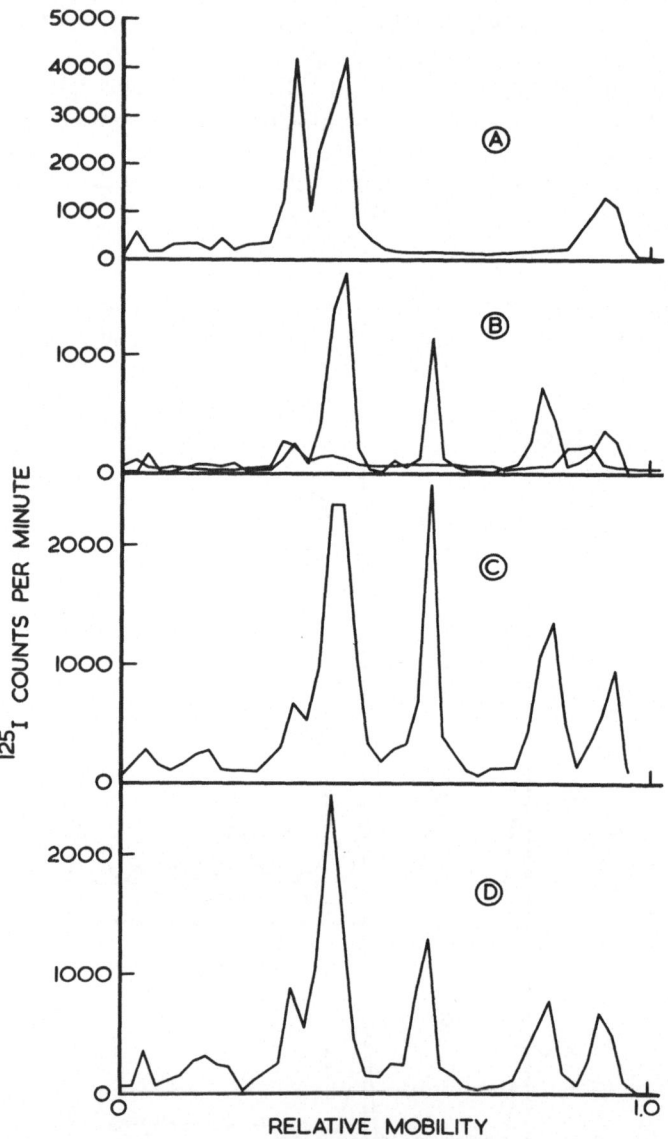

Figure 8. SDS–PAGE analysis of ^{125}I-labeled CBA splenocyte membrane proteins recognized by: (A) antibodies to light chains and μ chains. (B) C57Bl/6 anti-CBA spleen serum (bleed 1); lower line, no serum. (C) C57Bl/6 anti-CBA spleen serum (bled 2 weeks later). (D) C57Bl/6 anti-CBA spleen serum MA-3 (bled 4 weeks after bleed 2); two boosts of 30×10^6 cells were given between bleeds 2 and 3.

Table II. Precipitation of Various Immunoglobulin Classes by Alloantisera

Serum	Precipitation of ^{125}I IgG2a (HPC-149) (Ig-1a)	Precipitation of ^{125}I IgM		Heavy chain isolated from spleen cells on PAGE
		Ig-6a HPC-76	Ig-6b CBPC.112	
G1A2[a]	+	+	−	μ
GA20[a]	+	+	−	μ
GA26[a]	+	−	−	Nil
DA1[b]	−	−	−	δ
MA3[c]	−	+	−	$\mu + \delta$
MB3[d]	−	−	+	μ

[a]C57Bl/6 anti-CBA anti-pertussis serum/pertussis complex.
[b]C57Bl/6 anti-CBA spleen cell (early bleed).
[c]C57Bl/6 anti-CBA spleen cell (late bleed).
[d]SJL.Ig^{a} anti-C3H.SW.Ig^{b} spleen cell.

Table III. Allotypic Specificities of IgM Myelomas

Myeloma	Strain of origin	Ig-6 allele
MOPC-104 (μ, λ)	Balb/c	a
HPC-76 (μ, K)	Balb/c	a
HPC-208 (IgM)	Balb/c × NZB F$_1$	e
CBPC.112 (IgM)	Balb/c.Ig^{b}	b

heterologous anti-μ serum. Furthermore, HPC-208 was not capable of inhibiting precipitation of HPC-76 (Ig^{a}) by serum MA3. It may thus be concluded that HPC-208 inherited the *Ig-6e* allele of the NZB parent.

On the other hand, the precipitation of HPC-76 (Ig-6a) by serum GA-20 (made against serum IgM) was *partially* inhibited by HPC-208, indicating the sharing of *some* specificities between Ig-6a and Ig-6e. It is an intriguing possibility that the discrepancy between the results using sera against cells versus serum IgM reflects a portion of the μ chain which is "buried" in the lymphocyte membrane but is accessible in serum IgM (see Fu and Kunkel, 1974; Jones *et al.*, 1974; Williams, 1975).

The *Ig-6e* and *Ig-6b* alleles are *not identical*, however, since an antiserum made

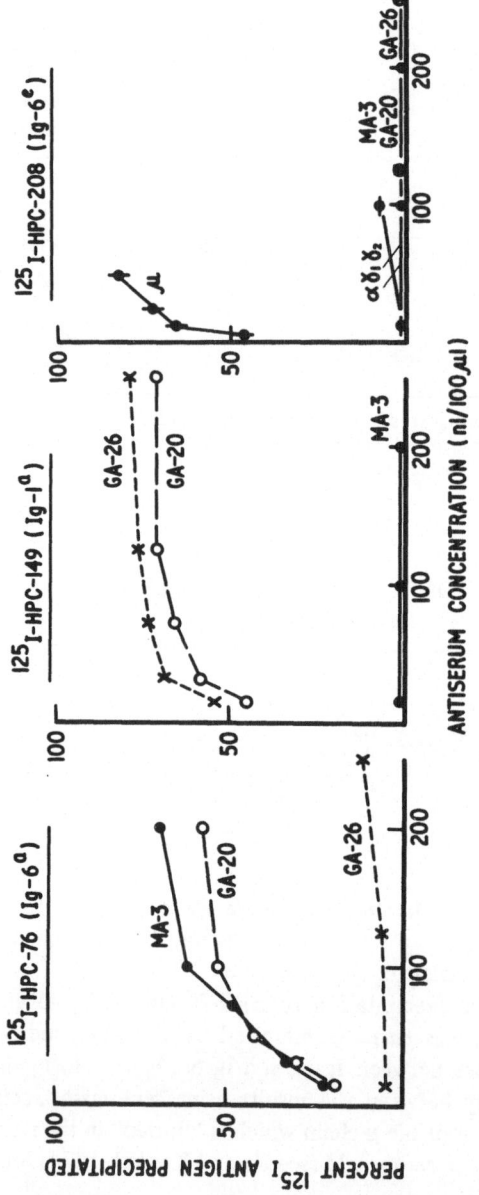

Figure 9. Radioimmunoassay analysis of various antisera. *Left panel:* Comparison of "conventional" antiallotype sera GA-20 and GA-26 with anti-spleen cell serum MA-3 tested against IgM derived from BALB/c (Ig^a). *Middle panel:* Comparison of "conventional" antiallotype sera GA-20 and GA-26 with anti-spleen cell serum MA-3 tested against IgG2a derived from BALB/c (Ig^a). *Right panel:* Comparison of "conventional" antiallotype sera as above, goat anti-γ and rabbit anti-μ sera, tested against IgM derived from NZB mice (Ig^e). Sera GA-20 and GA-26 were made in C57Bl/6 mice against CBA immunoglobulin complexed to pertussis organisms.

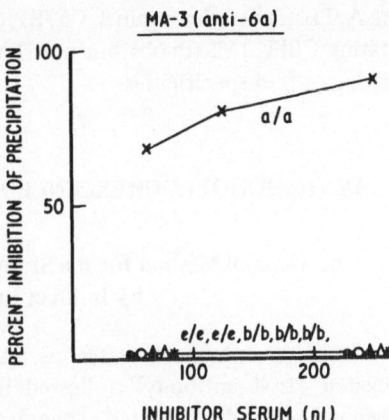

Figure 10. Inhibition of precipitation of ^{125}I HPC-76 (Ig-6a) by serum from mice of various allotypes. All inhibition sera were derived from 8-week-old mice of the following allotype congenic strains: Balb/c (Ig^a), Balb/c.Ig^b, NZB (Ig^e), and NZB.Ig-1^b. Serum MA3 is a late bleed of C57Bl/6 anti-CBA spleen cell serum.

Table IV. IgM Allotypic Specificities in Inbred Strains

Strain	Ig-1 type	Ig-6 specificity[a]			
CBA	a	1	2	–	–
Balb/c	a	1	2	–	–
SJL.Ig^a (SJA)	a	1	2	–	–
C3H	a	1	2	–	–
C3H.SW	a	1	2	–	–
C57Bl/6	b	–	–	3	4
SJL	b	–	–	3	4
Balb/c.Ig^b (BAB)	b	–	–	3	4
C3H.SW.Ig^b (CWB)	b	–	–	3	4
NZB	e	–	2	–	4
C57Bl/6.Ig^e	e	–	2	–	4

[a]Specificity 1 is defined by precipitation of HPC-76 (Ig-6a) by antibodies in C57Bl/6 anti-CBA "conventional" anti-allotype serum (GA20). Precipitation is *not* inhibited by IgM from mice (Ig-6e). Specificity 2 is defined by *partial* inhibition by Ig-6e of precipitation of HPC-76 by the above antiserum, indicating a shared specificity between Ig-6a and Ig-6e. Specificity 3 is defined by precipitation of CBPC-112 (Ig-6b) by A.TL (Ig^e) anti-C57Bl/6 (Ig^b) serum, which is not inhibited by IgM of A.TL (Ig^e) or CBA (Ig^a). Specificity 4 is defined by the precipitation of CBPC-112 by serum MB3 (SJA anti-CWB spleen), which is inhibited by IgM from NZB (Ig-6e) but not CBA (Ig-6a).

in A.TL (Ig^e) mice against C57B1/6 (Ig^b) spleen cells was capable of precipitating CBPC.112 (Ig-6b) but not HPC-208 (Ig-6e). Table IV shows a provisional listing of *Ig-6* specificities.

IV. IMMUNOFLUORESCENCE STUDIES OF SURFACE IgM AND IgD

A. General Method for the Study of Lymphocyte Surface Alloantigens by Indirect Immunofluorescence

Indirect immunofluorescence, in which cells are treated with an unconjugated "first antibody" followed by a fluorescein or rhodamine-conjugated "second antibody" directed at the first, has found widespread acceptance for the study of tissue antigens. Two advantages of indirect immunofluorescence over direct immunofluorescence are the following:

1. Increased sensitivity due to "amplification" (each IgG molecule of "first antibody" is capable of binding several "second antibody" molecules); directly conjugated mouse antisera are frequently rather weak.

2. One fluorescein-conjugated antibody will suffice to examine the properties of many "first antibodies"; it is not necessary to prepare IgG fractions or fluorescein conjugates of each individual antiserum to be tested. However, the technique has been of rather limited usefulness in the study of lymphocyte alloantigens, because the second antibody (fluorescein-conjugated anti-mouse immunoglobulin) usually stains all B cells, even in the absence of first antibody.

The current realization that very few B cells bear surface IgG has allowed a reappraisal of the indirect immunofluorescence technique for the study of lymphocyte alloantigens. Most strong alloantibodies are predominantly of the IgG class, and only a small minority of B cells bear surface IgG. Thus, if a lymphocyte suspension is treated with alloantiserum and then washed, the presence of membrane-bound alloantibodies may be "revealed" by fluorescent antisera which are specific for γ chains. This technique should be useful for the study of virtually any alloantigen (e.g., H-2, Ia, or Thy-1 antigens), provided that the population bearing the antigen in question is larger than 1–2% of the total cells. For such a technique to be usable, the fluorescent anti-γ serum must be impeccable in its specificity and must not contain aggregates or complexes which might bind nonspecifically to Fc receptors on B (and T) cells. The use of $F(ab)_2$ fragments, as recommended by Winchester *et al.* (1975*a,b*) has not proven essential, provided that the sera are very carefully prepared (Goding and Layton, 1976; see also Goding, 1976). In this context, it may be pointed out that Winchester and colleagues use $F(ab)_2$ fragments for the second antibody but *not* for the first antibody.

Table V. Allelic Exclusion at the *Ig-5* Locus (Coding
for an IgD-like Cell Surface Immunoglobulin
in the Mouse)[a]

	C57Bl/6 (Ig^{bb}) (control)	C57Bl/6.Ig^{ee} (homozygote)	C57Bl/6.Ig^{be} (heterozygote)
% labeled	0.5	43	22
Grains/cell in labeled cells	–	53 ± 11.7	56 ± 12.9

[a]Five million homozygous (C57Bl/6.Ig^{ee} N14F5), heterozygous (C57Bl/6.Ig^{be} N19), or control (C57Bl/6) spleen cells were held with C57Bl/6 anti-CBA/H antiserum (1:10 dilution in 200 µl), washed, held with ^{125}I-labeled protein A (1.0 µg/ml in 200 µl; 40 µCi/µg), washed again, and processed for autoradiography. Exposure time: 1 day. In each case, cells were pools from three animals (J. W. Goding, unpublished data).

Anti-γ sandwich reagents have also been used successfully by the author in autoradiographic experiments. A very convenient and sensitive technique involves ^{125}I-labeled staphylococcal protein A (see Section IIB) as a sandwich layer. Since this molecule is not an immunoglobulin, it cannot bind to Fc receptors. Cells are treated with alloantiserum, washed, held with ^{125}I-labeled protein A, washed again, and processed for autoradiography. For most strong alloantisera, adequate numbers of grains develop after 24 hours of exposure. The technique has a very low background and is capable of extreme sensitivity. In the absence of alloantibody, approximately 1% of spleen cells are labeled. Table V shows an example of the application of this technique in the study of allelic exclusion of murine IgD.

B. Organ Distribution of Surface IgM and IgD

The use of anti-γ as a fluorescent sandwich reagent allowed the development of a double-fluorescence technique, in which red and green fluorochromes are used to reveal the simultaneous presence of IgM and IgD receptors on individual cells (Goding and Layton, 1976). In passing, it may be mentioned that while most of the data in this review concern surface immunoglobulin, the technique has also been used by the author to study the simultaneous presence immunoglobulin and Ia antigens on B cells.

Cells from 11-week-old C57Bl/6.Ig^e (experimental) or C57Bl/6 (control) mice were treated with C57Bl/6 anti-CBA serum, washed, treated with rhodamine conjugated anti-γ-chain serum, washed again, and finally treated with fluorescein conjugated anti-µ-chain serum. After a final wash, cells were examined by fluorescence microscopy using appropriate filters. (There is probably no need to add the anti-μ and anti-γ in separate sequential steps; preliminary experiments indicate that specific staining can be achieved by adding a mixture of both in the one step.)

The results of an organ survey of the distribution of cells bearing surface IgM and IgD are summarized in Fig. 11. The great majority of B cells (i.e., those cells bearing surface immunoglobulin) in spleen, lymph node, and Peyer's patches bore both μ and δ chains on their surface (Table V), although there was a very considerable heterogeneity in the relative intensities of each receptor type on individual cells. There was no obvious direct or inverse correlation between the relative intensities of staining of the two classes. The majority of B cells in thoracic duct lymph also bore both chains (Goding and Layton, 1976).

In spleen, but not in lymph nodes, Peyer's patches, or thoracic duct, there was a distinct but minor subpopulation of cells bearing IgM but not IgD. This population accounted for 60–70% of the B cells in bone marrow, the remainder of which bore both chains.

On the other hand, very few cells bearing IgD but not IgM were detected (Fig. 11). This result differs significantly from those obtained by Abney *et al.* (1976) and Vitetta and Uhr (1976), who published data indicating that a substantial proportion of B cells bear IgD only. Recent studies using the fluorescence-activated cell sorter (which provides an objective and sensitive assessment of the fluorescence intensity on individual cells) have added support to our contention that cells bearing only IgD are uncommon (Herzenberg *et al.*, 1976; Scher *et al.*, 1976a,b). They have also confirmed the visual impression of marked heterogeneity in brightness of staining of individual cells. It is thus likely that the discrepancy between our results (Goding and Layton, 1976) and those of Abney *et al.* (1976) reflect differences in sensitivity, optical systems, and the threshold of brightness above which a cell is scored as positive.

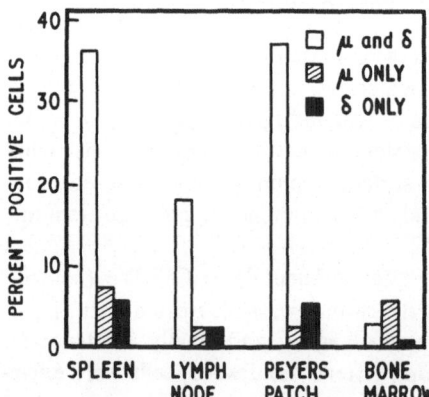

Figure 11. Organ distribution of surface IgM and IgD in the mouse.

It is now clear that most human B cells possess both IgM and IgD. Cells bearing only IgM probably represent a real subpopulation, especially in bone marrow, but cells bearing only IgD are uncommon in humans (Preud'homme *et al.*, 1975; Ferrarini *et al.*, 1976*a*). There is thus a very close parallel between the results obtained in mice and men.

C. Ontogeny of IgM and IgD Receptors

The availability of specific antisera to murine IgD has allowed studies on the ontogeny of surface immunoglobulin on individual cells. The results are summarized in Fig. 12. In newborn mice, IgM is the major surface immunoglobulin. Following birth, the percentage of cells bearing surface IgM rises steadily. By day 9, a few cells bearing both IgM and IgD are visible in lymph node, but virtually none are present in spleen. Over the next few weeks, the fraction of B cells bearing both chains steadily increases, and by 4-6 weeks, the majority of B cells in spleen, lymph node, Peyer's patches, thoracic duct, and peripheral blood bear

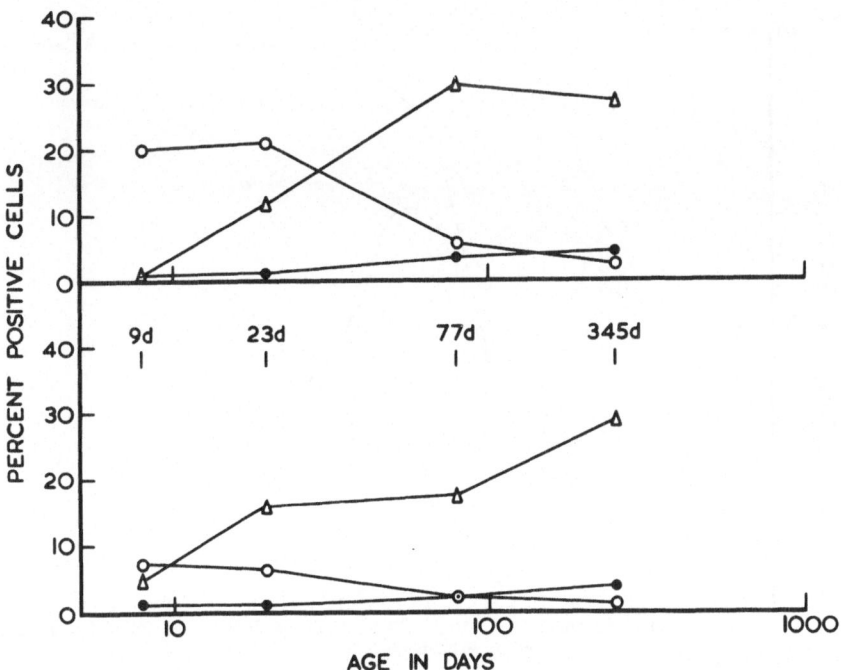

Figure 12. Ontogeny of surface immunoglobulin in the mouse. o——o, IgM only. △——△, IgM plus IgD. ●——●, IgD only. Upper panel, spleen; lower panel, lymph node.

both chains. Even at one year, the great majority of B cells in these organs are "doubles."

The finding that cells bearing only IgM are the first to appear in ontogeny suggests that these cells may be relatively immature. It may thus be significant that 10-20% of splenic B cells, and about 60% of bone marrow B cells bear IgM only. For a given age, the fraction of doubles is consistently greater in lymph node than in spleen. After 4-6 weeks, cells bearing only IgM are uncommon in lymph node.

These results are consistent with the view that newly arising B lymphocytes in bone marrow and spleen initially bear only IgM, but later acquire IgD in addition. At about the time of acquisition of IgD, they may migrate to lymph nodes.

This concept of B-cell maturation is also supported by two additional lines of evidence:

1. When lethally irradiated mice are reconstituted with stem cells, the first newly emerging B cells bear IgM only. Cells bearing both IgM and IgD are first seen a few days after the "IgM only" cells (Fig. 13).

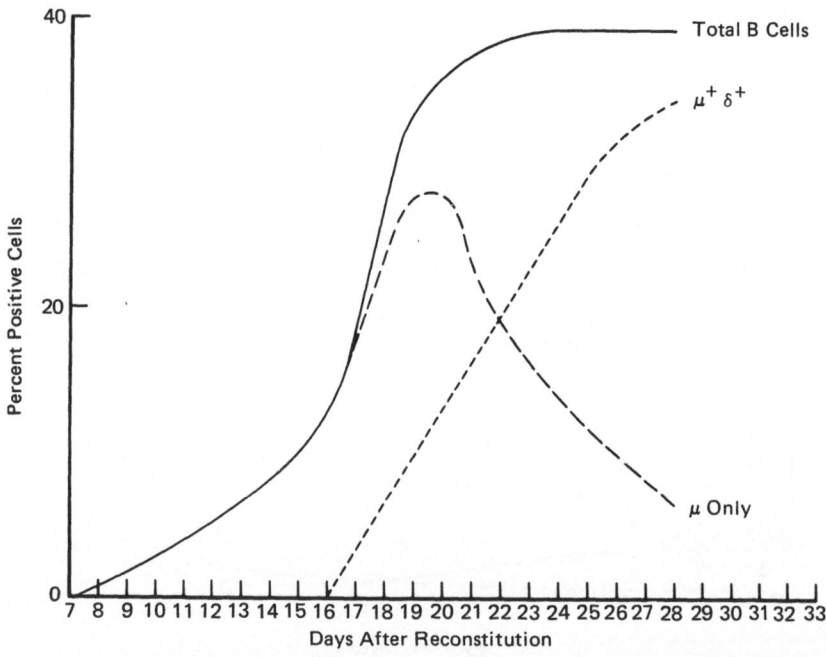

Figure 13. Development of B cells after reconstitution of lethally irradiated mice with stem cells (schematic). C57Bl/6 mice were irradiated (850 R) and reconstituted with 5×10^6 cells from the livers of newborn C57Bl/6.Ig^e mice (J. W. Goding, unpublished data).

2. Mice treated with anti-μ antibodies from birth totally lack all immunoglobulin-bearing cells.

Taken together, these results argue against the possibility that the $\mu^+ \delta$-cells and the $\mu^+ \delta^+$-cells represent separate but parallel lines of development.

The sequence following antigenic stimulation is still unclear, although recent work from several laboratories suggests that B cells *lose* IgD following activation by bacterial lipopolysaccharide (Bourgois *et al.*, 1977), pokeweed mitogen (Preud'homme, 1977), or sheep red blood cells (J. Layton, unpublished). Thus it seems likely that there is a second category of "IgM only" cells, which are B cells that have been recently activated by antigen. These cells may have blast morphology.

Some reports suggest that all the "IgG memory" in secondary responses is contained in the very small subpopulation of B cells bearing surface IgG (Mason, 1976; Okumura *et al.*, 1976). These studies should be regarded as preliminary, since the time course of the response following adoptive transfer was not studied in detail. The "adoptive transfer" assay is very complex, and results obtained at only one time point may be misleading (Stocker *et al.*, 1974). Recent data suggest that some IgG memory can be shown to reside in cells which do not bear surface IgG, if the assay is 10–12 days after transfer rather than the customary 7 days (S. Strober, personal communication).

D. Surface Immunoglobulin on Antibody-Containing Cells

Information on the surface immunoglobulins of antibody-containing cells is still rather scanty. The most complete published studies are those of Ferrarini *et al.* (1976*a,b*). These authors made a detailed study of the surface immunoglobulins of antibody-containing cells in human tonsils. Their results may be summarized as follows:

1. Nearly all cells containing IgM, IgD, or IgA had detectable amounts of the cytoplasmic immunoglobulin type on their surface, while only about half of the cells containing IgG bore detectable surface IgG.

2. None of the cells containing IgG or IgA had significant amounts of other classes on their surface.

3. About half of the IgM-containing cells had surface IgD, but only about 7% of IgD-containing cells had surface IgM.

Early in the murine immune response, most plaque-forming cells possess detectable amounts of surface IgD. With the passage of time, there is a gradual loss of IgD, and late in the immune response, most plaque-forming cells do not possess detectable IgD (S. Black, personal communication). These results are consistent with those obtained in human tonsils.

So far, there is only evidence for IgD-secreting cells in man. A careful search failed to reveal any IgD-containing cells in mice (Parkhouse *et al.*, 1977) or in monkeys (Corte *et al.*, 1978).

E. Capping of Surface IgM and IgD

All the available evidence indicates that IgM and IgD receptors behave as independent entities on the cell membrane. Capping of IgM receptors by anti-μ serum does not induce redistribution of IgD, and each receptor type may be independently precipitated from detergent lysates of surface radioiodinated lymphocytes (Abney et al., 1976; Goding et al., 1976; Goding and Layton, 1976). When capping is induced by binding of antigen to receptors, however, both receptor types are almost always found in the cap (Goding and Layton, 1976). The simplest interpretation of these results is that on any individual cell, the two receptor types share the same variable region (see also Section VB).

F. Allelic Exclusion and Haplotype Exclusion

An unusual feature of immunoglobulin gene expression is that of *allelic exclusion*, which is the process whereby individual cells express the product of only one chromosome at a given locus. The only other genetic system in which allelic exclusion is known to occur is that involving the random inactivation of one X chromosome in females (Lyon, 1961; Nesbitt and Gartler, 1971).

Allelic exclusion, which may be regarded as a logical outcome of clonal selection, has been amply demonstrated for immunoglobulin-containing and immunoglobulin-secreting cells (Pernis et al., 1965; Cebra et al., 1966). These cells represent the end result of antigenic stimulation, and the question of whether or not the receptors on B cells (prior to stimulation) show allelic exclusion has been controversial (Greaves, 1971; Wolf et al., 1971; Anderson, 1972; Warner, 1974; Linthicum and Sell, 1976; Sell, 1977). A good deal of this controversy may be explained by the same reasons which caused uncertainty regarding the presence of IgG on the surface of B cells (i.e., inadequate specificity of antisera, binding of antisera to Fc receptors, and the presence of cytophilic immunoglobulin on cell surfaces; see Section IB). All these factors cause errors in the direction of a failure to demonstrate allelic exclusion. The presence of allotypic markers on both major B cell receptors has allowed the demonstration that both are subject to allelic exclusion (Goding et al., 1976; Herzenberg et al., 1976).

When the fraction of B cells staining for IgD (*Ig-5e* allotype) in heterozygous (*Ig-5be*) mice was compared to that obtained in homozygous (*Ig-5ee*) mice, it was found that about half of all B cells were stained in the former case, while virtually all B cells were stained in the latter (Goding et al., 1976). Since the visual assessment of fluorescence assessment is subjective, this experiment was repeated using autoradiography (Table V). In heterozygotes, about half the number of cells were labeled when compared to homozygotes, yet the number of grains per labeled cell was similar in each case. Taking the reasonable assumption that heterozygotes and homozygotes possess similar amounts of total IgD on individual cells, it may be concluded that in heterozygotes each individual cell expresses only one IgD allele.

In addition, simultaneous staining of heterozygotes for both *Ig-5a* and *Ig-6a* allotypes did not significantly increase the proportion of stained cells above that obtained with either reagent alone. Since nearly all B cells have both IgM and IgD receptors, it would appear that a given cell expresses only one heavy-chain chromosomal region for all immunoglobulin classes. This remarkable phenomenon has been termed "haplotype exclusion" (Herzenberg *et al.*, 1976). Its significance will be discussed in more detail in Section V.

V. IMPLICATIONS FOR ORGANIZATION OF IMMUNOGLOBULIN HEAVY-CHAIN GENES

A. The Heavy-Chain Linkage Group

Antibody genes in mammalian cells consist of at least three families, encoding for K light chain, λ light chains, and heavy chains, each of which is apparently on a different autosome (reviewed by Gally and Edelman, 1972; Hood *et al.*, 1975). In all species in which data are available, the heavy-chain genes form a very tightly linked cluster (Gally and Edelman, 1972; Herzenberg and Warner, 1968; Herzenberg *et al.*, 1968). No recombinations between mouse heavy-chain constant-region loci were found in some 3000 segregants tested (Weigert *et al.*, 1975). Even in wild mice, only a limited number of linkage groups have been found, although the presence in some wild mice of allotypic combinations not present in inbred strains suggests that recombination can occur (Lieberman and Potter, 1969).

Many lines of evidence indicate that the genes coding for the variable and constant regions of light or heavy chains are separate but very closely linked (Gally and Edelman 1972; Eichmann, 1975; Weigert *et al.*, 1975). A recombination frequency of 0.3% was found between rabbit variable- and constant-region genes, as assessed by allotypic markers (Weigert *et al.*, 1975). Similarly, it has been estimated that the recombination frequency in the mouse between variable-region genes (as assessed by idiotypic polymorphisms) and constant-region genes (as assessed by constant-region polymorphisms) is of the order of 0.4% (Eichmann, 1975).

Previous studies (Potter and Lieberman, 1967; Herzenberg and Warner, 1968; Herzenberg *et al.*, 1968) have documented the existence of genetic polymorphisms for γ2a, α, γ2b, and γ1 heavy chains, defining the *Ig-1, Ig-2, Ig-3*, and *Ig-4* loci, respectively. Now, some 10 years after the identification of the

Ig-4 locus, it is possible to add the *Ig-5* locus (controlling expression of δ chains) and the *Ig-6* locus (controlling expression of μ chains). These new loci are shown schematically in Fig. 14. The exact order of genes is unknown, and the numerical order reflects the order of discovery rather than the actual gene order. So far, there is no evidence for allelic forms of IgG_3 and IgE in the mouse, but it may be assumed that the genes for the γ3 and ε chains are contained in the heavy-chain cluster.

Very close linkage of the *Ig-5* and *Ig-6* loci to *Ig-1* is indicated by the following data (Sections II and III):

1. In immunofluorescence experiments involving C57Bl/6, Balb/c, and SJL mice and their appropriate allotype congenic strains (involving 15–20 backcross generations per strain), staining only occurred when the targets cells possessed the appropriate allotype.

2. Antisera to Ig-6a precipitated the IgM myeloma HPC-76 of Balb/c. (*Ig^a*) origin but not CPC.112 of Balb/c.*Ig^b* origin; antisera to Ig-6b showed the opposite pattern.

3. Precipitation of HPC-76 by anti-Ig-6a was inhibited by normal serum from Balb/c mice but not by serum from Balb/c.*Ig^b* mice (Fig. 10).

4. In the F_2 generation, the *Ig-6* locus was always inherited with the *Ig-1* locus (N. L. Warner, unpublished data).

The finding that (unlike the γ, α, and δ allotypes) Ig-6e appears to be more closely related to Ig-6b than Ig-6a suggested that the *Ig^e* haplotype may have resulted from recombination between the *Ig^a* and *Ig^b* haplotypes, with a crossover between *Ig-6* and the other loci. The detection of antibodies to the *Ig-6* specificity 2 in C57Bl/6 anti-CBA "conventional" antiallotype serum (made

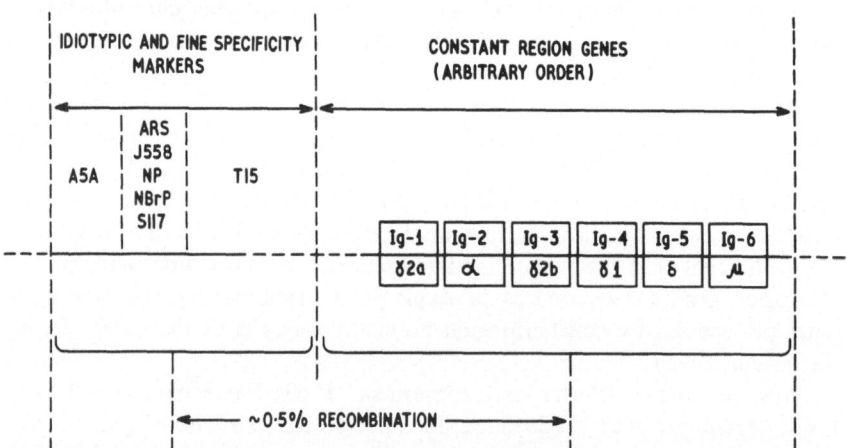

Figure 14. The heavy-chain linkage group in the mouse. Note that the order of constant-region genes is arbitrary. It is likely, but unproved, that the idiotypic markers represent distinct structural genes. (Adapted from Eichmann, 1975.)

against serum IgM) but not in the corresponding anti-spleen antiserum, might suggest that this portion of the molecule is "buried" or inaccessible in the cell membrane (see Section IIIC). It may be speculated that the similarity of the Ig-6b and Ig-6e allotypes reflects an early intracistronic recombination event which occurred toward the carboxy terminal end of the μ chain (W. Van der Loo, personal communication). Such a notion would imply that the μ chain gene is at one end of the heavy-chain constant-region gene cluster, which is consistent with its early evolutionary origin. However, the complex serological patterns indicate that such an interpretation may be too simple.

One word of caution should be expressed at this point. In many cases, it is not easy to establish whether genetic polymorphisms represent *structural* or *regulatory* genes. Genetic polymorphisms of two types may exist. Certain genetic polymorphisms represent single amino acid substitutions, and can often be accounted for by single base changes in DNA. These are known as "simple" allotypes, and are represented by certain globin and immunoglobulin light chain polymorphisms in humans (Kitchen and Boyer, 1974; Gally and Edelman, 1972). Simple allotypes probably reflect structural genes. Other polymorphisms, notably those of rat light chains (Gutman *et al.*, 1975), histocompatibility antigens (Silver and Hood, 1976), and possibly rabbit heavy-chain variable-region genes (Gally and Edelman, 1972) consist of multiple amino acid substitutions. These are difficult to explain in evolutionary terms (Hood *et al.*, 1975; Silver and Hood, 1976; Gutman *et al.*, 1975) and it has been suggested that they reflect *regulatory* genes determining *which of several structural genes are expressed* (Bodmer, 1973; Gutman *et al.*, 1975). The mouse γ and α chain allotypes are serologically complex and may involve multiple amino acid substitutions. So far, nothing is known of the structural basis of the μ-chain and δ-chain allotypes. Nonetheless, the concept that the mouse heavy-chain gene polymorphisms represent structural genes remains a useful working hypothesis.

Since genetic polymorphisms have been demonstrated for six out of eight known immunoglobulin heavy chains in the mouse, it is not unreasonable to suppose that the remaining heavy-chain genes will eventually be shown to have allelic forms. There is now much evidence in favor of the idea that the genes controlling the variable region of the T-cell receptor are linked to the heavy-chain cluster (see Raff, 1976). The finding of allotypes of the T-cell-receptor constant region would have enormous importance. A search for heavy-chain-linked allelic forms of T-cell surface structures is under way in our laboratory.

B. Shared V Regions, Class Switches, Haplotype Exclusion, and Clonal Restriction

Many lines of evidence indicate that IgM and IgD receptors on individual cells possess the same variable region. It has been shown that IgM and IgD on chronic lymphatic leukemia cells bear the same idiotype (Salsano *et al.*, 1974; Fu *et al.*, 1975). In a case of macroglobulinemia, in which the antibody was directed against IgG, Pernis *et al.* (1974) showed that the surface IgM and IgD on the tumor cells also had specificity for IgG.

Similar evidence is available for normal B cells. Raff and colleagues (1973) showed that all the membrane immunoglobulin detected by a polyvalent serum on individual cells binding polymerized flagellin could be capped by this antigen, suggesting homogeneity of combining sites. Although these authors did not use chain-specific antisera, it is likely that many of the cells examined bore both IgM and IgD receptors. More recently, we have examined the question using heterologous anti-μ and anti-δ allotype sera in double-fluorescence experiments (Goding and Layton, 1976). Cells binding the hapten NIP (4-hydroxy-3-iodo-5-nitrophenylacetic acid) were isolated by binding to NIP-gelatin using a technique developed by Haas and Layton (1975). The great majority of antigen-binding B cells bore both IgM and IgD. When the receptors on antigen-binding cells were capped with antigen, both receptors were almost always found in the cap, indicating that they bore similar or identical binding sites. Control experiments showed that the receptors capped independently when capping was induced by chain-specific sera. Similar results were reported by Stern and McConnell (1976), who studied antigen-binding cells from human tonsils using a rosetting technique.

Taken as a whole, the data provide compelling evidence that individual lymphocytes express the same V region attached to two different constant regions. It seems very likely that IgM and IgD are synthesized simultaneously, since their half-life is of the order of 4 hours (Ferrarini *et al.*, 1976*a*), while normal and neoplastic B cells can survive for at least 6 weeks (Sprent and Miller, 1972).

The joining of the variable and constant regions of immunoglobulin chains almost certainly occurs prior to messenger RNA (mRNA) synthesis (Milstein *et al.*, 1974). Unless the half-life of heavy-chain mRNA is very long (and there is very little information on the turnover of mRNA in mammalian cells), it would appear that both messages must be transcribed simultaneously, creating considerable problems for models of immunoglobulin genes. The models which are best able to explain the data are those which involve multiple copies of the same V gene or a "copy-choice" mechanism (Williamson and Fitzmaurice, 1976) for V-C gene integration. This type of model is not unprecedented in biology (Delbrück and Stent, 1957).

According to this model, one copy of a (randomly?) selected V gene is made for each heavy-chain gene, and the individual copies are simultaneously inserted adjacent to each heavy-chain gene. The current data on V-gene counting by DNA/RNA hybridization of heavy-chain genes are not yet sufficiently advanced to confirm or refute this notion (see Williamson, 1976, for a discussion on the limitations of this technique). Such a model would allow the simultaneous expression of two or more V genes, and "switches" of class of immunoglobulin synthesis by individual cells (Gearhart *et al.*, 1975; Sledge *et al.*, 1976) would simply involve differential gene activation.

The evidence for allelic exclusion of IgM and IgD receptors has already been given (Section IVF). Of particular interest is the finding (Herzenberg *et al.*, 1976) that, on individual cells, IgM and IgD receptors always come from the same chromosome ("haplotype exclusion"). Similarly, the V and C regions on individual IgG and IgA molecules almost always come from the same chromosome (Gally and Edelman, 1972). The discovery of haplotype exclusion raises the question of whether a given lymphocyte remains committed to a given chromosome throughout its life (and that of its progeny). This idea has not yet been examined, but the availability of antiallotype sera renders it eminently testable. One may predict quite confidently that the answer will be in the affirmative.

The relatively high frequency of recombination between V and C gene markers (Section VA) indicates that V and C genes are not contiguous in the germ line. Recent work using restriction enzyme fragments suggests that a *rearrangement* of immunoglobulin genes occurs during B-cell development, bringing these genes into closer proximity (Hozumi and Tonegawa, 1976; Tonegawa *et al.*, 1977). There is now strong evidence for nucleotide sequence rearrangements in many other systems, including adenovirus (Chow *et al.*, 1977), SV40 (Aloni *et al.*, 1977; Hsu and Ford, 1977), *E. coli* (Nevers and Saedler, 1977), and *Drosophila* (Glover, 1977). Very recently, the gene for ovalbumin in chickens has also been shown to be split (Breathnach *et al.*, 1977). One may speculate that very early in B-cell development, each cell makes a commitment to a given chromosome containing a given V gene, and that clonal restriction, haplotype exclusion, and V-C joining are all implemented during this process (see Goding *et al.*, 1977, for further details).

VI. FUNCTIONAL ROLE OF B-CELL RECEPTORS

A. Immature Cells

The mechanism of self–nonself discrimination is one of the central issues in immunology. The simplest and most elegant hypothesis to explain this discrimination is the "clonal abortion" theory (Lederberg, 1959; Nossal, 1957; Burnet, 1959; Nossal and Pike, 1975*a,b*; Stocker and Nossal, 1976). The theory states that the newly emerging B cell passes through a phase in which encounter with antigen results in permanent inactivation. Just as the first person encountered by a newborn babe is its mother, so the first antigen encountered by a newborn lymphocyte is likely to be "self." If the cell survives this "refereeing" process, it matures into a phase in which contact with antigen induces division and antibody synthesis.

There is now a large body of evidence to support the theory. Immature B cells in bone marrow (Nossal and Pike, 1975b), spleen from neonatal mice (Cambier et al., 1976; Metcalf and Klinman, 1976; Bruyns et al., 1976; Stocker, 1977), and B cells maturing from fetal liver cells (Nossal and Pike, 1975a; Elson, 1977) are exquisitely sensitive to tolerance induction (reviewed by Nossal et al., 1976). In addition, and in contrast to mature lymphocytes, B cells in bone marrow or neonatal spleen do not resynthesize their receptors following modulation by antiimmunoglobulin antisera (Raff et al., 1975; Sidman and Unanue, 1975).

The orderly sequence of acquisition of IgM and IgD receptors, which is independent of antigenic stimulation and T cells (Vitetta and Uhr, 1975), is undoubtedly of profound importance in lymphocyte function. The presence of these two major receptor types suggests that they transmit *different messages* to the cell. Since it seems very unlikely that any of the surface immunoglobulins span the membrane, one may speculate that surface IgM and IgD are attached to different "anchor" molecules in the membrane, possibly associated with different intracellular enzyme systems.

The simplest (and therefore most attractive) formulation is that the immature B cells bearing only IgM receptors are tolerized by antigen, while the cells bearing both IgM and IgD receptors are activated by antigen. However, the verification or refutation of this idea may encounter many difficulties.

The presence of considerable numbers of cells bearing both IgM and IgD in adult bone marrow (Fig. 11) indicates the presence of a population of relatively mature B cells in addition to the immature population bearing only IgM receptors. Thus neonatal spleen (Fig. 12) or fetal liver (Fig. 13) probably represent much more suitable populations for the study of clonal abortion tolerogenesis. Moreover, the probable existence of two distinct "IgM only" B-cell subsets (i.e., immature and activated) will complicate the interpretation of experiments designed to test B-cell function by selecting for subsets bearing particular receptor classes. The most suitable cell sources for such experiments will probably be those which contain relatively large numbers of immature "IgM only" cells and relatively few activated "IgM only" cells.

In addition, the assay of B-cell tolerance may well yield different results, depending on the various combinations of thymus-dependent or thymus-independent antigens used in tolerance induction and challenge (Metcalf and Klinman, 1976; Elson, 1977; Cambier et al., 1977).

The functional capacity of the "IgM only" immature B cells is not yet clear. There is some (albeit rather weak) evidence that these cells are capable of responding to T-independent antigens. The precursor frequency of cells responding *in vitro* (3 days) to haptenated polymerized flagellin (POL) is not greatly different in 7-day-old mice and adult mice (B. Pike and G. J. V. Nossal, unpublished observations). When lethally irradiated mice are repopulated with fetal liver, the first IgD-bearing cells do not begin to appear until around day 16 (Fig. 13), yet these mice are capable of good responses to haptenated POL 5 days after challenge on day 14 (Nossal and Pike, 1973).

Finally, one of the major problems in assessing the functional capacity of B-cell subpopulations is the problem of *nonlinear readout systems* (Stocker *et al.*, 1974; Stocker and Nossal, 1976). The powerful negative feedback effects of antigen–antibody complexes often "damp down" large responses, and very small numbers of responding cells may dramatically outperform large numbers on a cell-for-cell basis (Stocker and Nossal, 1976). These effects will often tend to minimize differences between separated B-cell subsets unless care is taken to use linear systems, such as analysis by limit dilution (e.g., Stocker and Nossal, 1976; Metcalf and Klinman, 1976).

B. Mature Cells

The marked susceptibility of IgD to proteolysis raises the possibility that B-cell activation involves proteolytic cleavage (Vitetta and Uhr, 1975) possibly via enzymes secreted by T cells or macrophages. In this regard, it is noteworthy that trypsin is a very effective B-cell mitogen (Vischer 1974). The optimal mitogenic concentrations of trypsin are in the order of 1.0 μg/ml, while even 100 times this concentration does not remove all the IgD from intact B cells (J. W. Goding, unpublished observations). However, it is clear that the optimal concentrations of antigen for B-cell function do not saturate the receptors (Nossal and Layton, 1975), and the concentration of polypeptide hormones needed for maximum biological effect is also much less than is required to saturate the available receptors (Catt and Dufau, 1973).

It now seems clear that the "typical mature B cell" bears both IgM and IgD receptors. It is probable that the percentage of cells bearing only IgD is small, and these cells may simply represent the "tail end" of a population of doubles, which do not have enough IgM for detection by visual fluorescence. On the other hand, the populations bearing only IgM are certainly real. Thus it now seems very unlikely that the IgM–IgD doubles represent cells in a transitional state between IgM and IgD.

A sequence of B-cell maturation is proposed in Fig. 15. Immature B cells possess IgM only. At this stage they are very susceptible to tolerance induction. If they are not tolerized by encounter with antigen, they mature into B cells bearing both IgM and IgD. After encounter with antigen, these cells lose IgD,

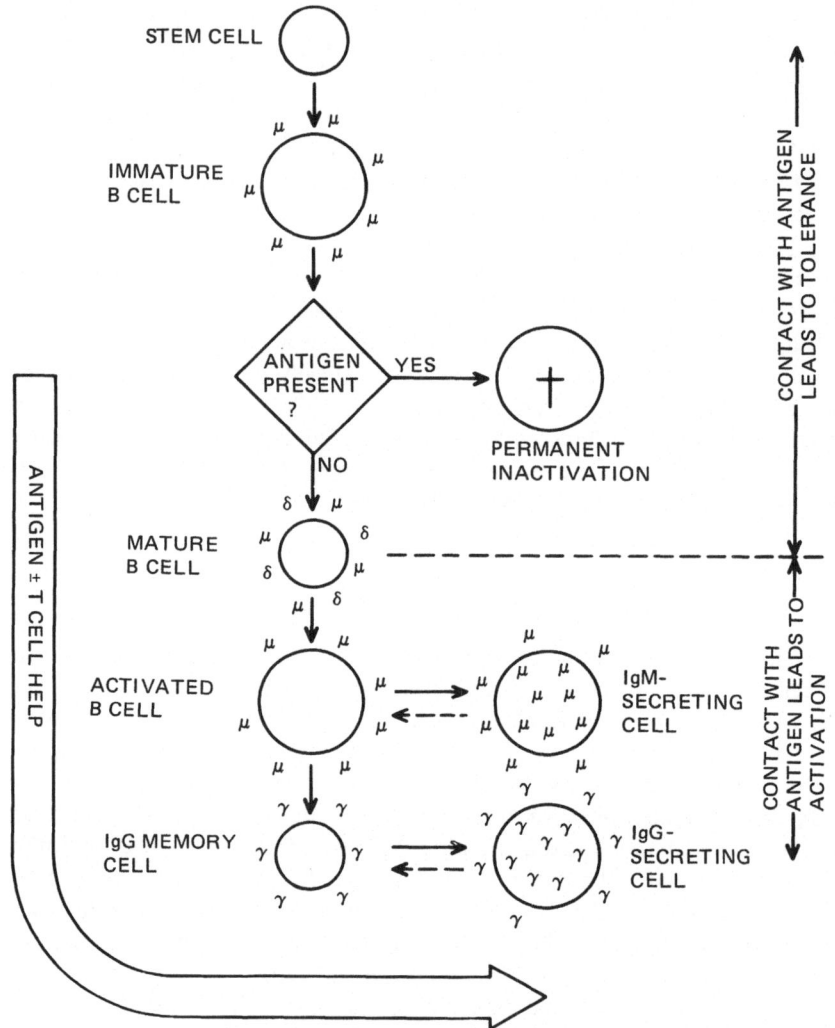

Figure 15. Proposed scheme for B-cell differentiation.

and begin division and differentiation into IgM-secreting cells (Bourgois *et al.*, 1977; Preud'homme, 1977). Some of these mature into IgG-secreting cells or IgG memory cells, which bear IgG on their surface.

Whatever models are proposed for B-cell activation, they must take into account the new findings concerning receptors. The predominance of cells bearing both IgM and IgD receptors argues against those models which ascribe a mere "antigen-focusing" role to surface immunoglobulin. It seems clear that activation of the B cell involves more than just binding of antigen to receptor, and probably involves additional signals from T cells and macrophages (see Möller, 1975). The function of surface immunoglobulin receptors thus remains a major challenge.

VII. SUMMARY

Antibodies to IgD and IgM are present in many mouse alloantisera made against lymphocytes. Antibodies to IgM are also present in a small minority of conventional antiallotype sera made against pertussis/anti-pertussis complexes. These antibodies reflect different allelic forms of IgD and IgM in different mouse strains, and allowed the mapping of the δ- and μ-chain genes (*Ig-5* and *Ig-6*, respectively) to the heavy-chain complex.

The variable portions of IgM and IgD receptors on individual cells bearing both chains are similar or identical. Both receptors show allelic exclusion and come from the same chromosome on individual cells (haplotype exclusion). It is suggested that very early in B lymphocyte differentiation there is a commitment to a given chromosome, and translocation of one copy of a given variable region gene to each heavy-chain gene. Subsequent switches of immunoglobulin class then involve differential gene activation.

Immature B cells possess IgM receptors only and mature into cells bearing both IgM and IgD receptors. After activation with antigen, IgD is probably lost. These findings are discussed within the framework of the clonal abortion theory of B-lymphocyte tolerance.

ACKNOWLEDGMENTS

This work was supported by the National Health and Medical Research Council, Canberra, Australia, by grant AI-O-3958 and contract NIH-NCI-G-7-3889 from the National Institutes of Health, U.S. Public Health Service, Bethesda, Md.

I am especially grateful to the many colleagues who contributed to this work, particularly to N. Warner, J. Layton, G. Warr, L. Herzenberg, W. van der Loo, S. Black, M. Loken, and B. Osborne.

VIII. REFERENCES

Abney, E. R., and Parkhouse, R. M. E., 1974, Candidate for immunoglobulin D present on murine B lymphocytes, *Nature* 252:600.

Abney, E. R., Hunter, I. R., and Parkhouse, R. M. E., 1976, Preparation and characterisation of an antiserum to the mouse candidate for immunoglobulin D, *Nature* 259:404.

Aloni, Y., Dhar, R., Laub, O., Horowitz, M., and Khoury, G., 1977, Novel mechanism for RNA maturation: The leader sequences of simian virus 40 mRNA are not transcribed adjacent to the coding structures, *Proc. Natl. Acad. Sci. U.S.* 74:3686–3690.

Anderson, H. R., 1972, Allotype suppression of adult mouse spleen cells: Cell differentiation, class restriction and allotypic exclusion, *Eur. J. Immunol.* 2:11.

Bodmer, W. F., 1973, A new genetic model for allelism at histocompatibility and other complex loci; polymorphism for control of gene expression, *Transplant. Proc.* 5:1471.

Bourgois, A., Kitajima, K., Hunter, I. R., and Askonas, B. A., 1977, Surface immunoglobulins of lipopolysaccharide-stimulated cells. The behaviour of IgM, IgD and IgG, *Eur. J. Immunol.* 7:151.

Breathnach, R., Mandel, J. L., and Chambon, P., 1977, Ovalbumin gene is split in chicken DNA, *Nature* 270:314–319.

Bruyns, C., Urbain-Vansanten, G., Planard, C., De Vos-Cloetens, C., and Urbain, J., 1976, Ontogeny of mouse B lymphocytes and inactivation by antigen of early B lymphocytes, *Proc. Natl. Acad. Sci. U.S.* 73:2462.

Burnet, F. M., 1959, *The Clonal Selection Theory of Acquired Immunity*, Cambridge University Press, New York.

Cambier, J. C., Kettman, J. R., Vitetta, E. S., and Uhr, J. W., 1976, Differential susceptibility of neonatal and adult murine spleen cells to *in vitro* induction of B-cell tolerance, *J. Exp. Med.* 144:293.

Cambier, J. C., Vitetta, E. S., Uhr, J. W., and Kettman, J. R., 1977, B cell tolerance. II. TNP_{17} HgG induced tolerance in adult and neonatal murine B cells responsive to T dependent and independent forms of the same hapten, *J. Exp. Med.* 145:778.

Catt, K. J., and Dufau, M. L., 1973, Interactions of LH and hCG with testicular gonadotrophin receptors, *Adv. Exp. Med. Biol.* 36:379.

Cebra, J. J., Colberg, J. E., and Dray, S., 1966, Rabbit lymphoid cells differentiated with respect to α-, γ-, and μ-heavy polypeptide chains and to allotypic markers Aa1 and Aa2, *J. Exp. Med.* 123:547.

Chow, L. T., Gelinas, R. E., Broker, T. R., and Roberts, R. J., 1977, An amazing sequence arrangement at the 5' end of adenovirus 2 messenger RNA, *Cell* 12:1–8.

Corte, G., Ferrarini, M., Tonda, P., Bargellesi, A., and Pernis, B., 1978, Membrane IgD on monkey lymphocytes, *Eur. J. Immunol* (in press).

Delbrück, M., and Stent, G. S., 1957, On the mechanism of DNA replication, in: *Chemical Basis of Heredity* (W. D. McElroy and B. Glass, eds.), pp. 699–736, Johns Hopkins Press, Baltimore.

Eichmann, K., 1975, Genetic control of antibody specificity in the mouse, *Immunogenetics* 2:491.

Elson, C. J., 1977, Tolerance in differentiating B lymphocytes, *Eur. J. Immunol.* 7:6.

Ferrarini, M., Corte, G., Viale, G., Durante, M. L., and Bargellesi, A., 1976a, Membrane Ig on human lymphocytes: Rate of turnover of IgD and IgM on the surface of human tonsil cells, *Eur. J. Immunol.* 6:372.

Ferrarini, M., Viale, G., Risso, A., and Pernis, B., 1976b, A study of the immunoglobulin classes present on the membrane and in the cytoplasm of human tonsil plasma cells, *Eur. J. Immunol.* 6:562.

Fu, S. M., and Kunkel, H. G., 1974, Membrane immunoglobulins of B lymphocytes. Inability to detect certain characteristic IgM and IgD antigens, *J. Exp. Med.* 140:895.

Fu, S. M., Winchester, R. J., and Kunkel, H. G., 1975, Similar idiotypic specificity for the membrane IgD and IgM of human B lymphocytes, *J. Immunol.* 114:250.

Gally, J. A., and Edelman, G. M., 1972, The genetic control of immunoglobulin synthesis, *Ann. Rev. Genet.* **6**:1.

Gathings, W. E., Cooper, M. D., Lawton, A. W., and Alford, C. A., 1976, B cell ontogeny in humans, *Fed. Proc.* **35**:276 (Abstract).

Gearhart, P. J., Sigal, N. H., and Klinman, N. R., 1975, Production of antibodies of identical idiotype but diverse immunoglobulin classes by cells derived from a single stimulated B cell, *Proc. Natl. Acad. Sci. U.S.* **72**:1707.

Glover, D. M., 1977, Cloned segment of *Drosophila melanogaster* rDNA containing new types of sequence insertion, *Proc. Natl. Acad. Sci. U.S.* **74**:4932–4936.

Goding, J. W., 1976, Conjugation of antibodies with fluorochromes: Modifications to the standard methods, *J. Immunol. Methods* **13**:215–226.

Goding, J. W., 1978, Use of staphylococcal protein A as an immunological reagent, *J. Immunol. Methods* (in press).

Goding, J. W., and Layton, J. E., 1976, Antigen-induced co-capping of IgM and IgD-like receptors on murine B cells, *J. Exp. Med.* **144**:852.

Goding, J. W., Warr, G. W., and Warner, N. L., 1976, Genetic polymorphism of IgD-like cell surface immunoglobulin in the mouse, *Proc. Natl. Acad. Sci. U.S.* **73**:1305.

Goding, J. W., Scott, D. W., and Layton, J. E., 1977, Genetics, cellular expression and function of IgD and IgM receptors, *Immunol. Rev.* **37**:152.

Greaves, M. F., 1971, The expression of immunoglobulin determinants on the surface of antigen-binding lymphoid cells in mice. II. Allotypes of the Ig-1 locus, *Eur. J. Immunol.* **1**:195.

Gupta, S., Pahwa, R., O'Reilly, R., Good, R. A., and Siegal, F., 1976, Ontogeny of lymphocyte subpopulations in human fetal liver, *Proc. Natl. Acad. Sci. U.S.* **73**:919.

Gutman, G. A., Loh, E., and Hood, L., 1975, Structure and regulation of immunoglobulins: Kappa allotypes in the rat have multiple amino-acid differences in the constant region, *Proc. Natl. Acad. Sci. U.S.* **72**:5046.

Haas, W., and Layton, J. E., 1975, Separation of antigen-specific lymphocytes. I. Enrichment of antigen-binding cells, *J. Exp. Med.* **141**:1004.

Herzenberg, L. A., and Herzenberg, L. A., 1978, Mouse immunoglobulin allotypes: Description and special methodology, in: *Handbook of Experimental Immunology* (D. M. Weir, ed.), 3rd ed., Chap. 12, Blackwell, Oxford (in press).

Herzenberg, L. A., and Warner, N. L., 1968, Genetic control of mouse immunoglobulins, in: *Regulation of the Antibody Response* (B. Cinader, ed.), p. 322, Charles C Thomas, Springfield, Ill.

Herzenberg, L. A., McDevitt, H. O., and Herzenberg, L. A., 1968, Genetics of antibodies, *Ann. Rev. Genet.* **2**:209.

Herzenberg, L. A., Herzenberg, L. A., Black, S. J., Loken, M. R., Okumura, K., van der Loo, W., Osborne, B. A., Hewgill, D., Goding, J. W., Gutman, G., and Warner, N. L., 1976, Surface markers and functional relationships of cells involved in murine B lymphocyte differentiation (including the description of IgM and IgD allotypes), *Cold Spring Harbor Symp. Quant. Biol.* **16**:33–45.

Hood, L., Campbell, J. H., and Elgin, S. C. R., 1975, The organisation, expression, and evolution of antibody genes and other multigene families, *Ann. Rev. Genet.* **9**:305.

Hozumi, N., and Tonegawa, S., 1976, Evidence for somatic rearrangement of immunoglobulin genes coding for variable and constant regions, *Proc. Natl. Acad. Sci. U.S.* **73**:3628.

Hsu, M., and Ford, J., 1977, Sequence arrangements of the 5′ ends of simian virus 40 16S and 19S mRNAs, *Proc. Natl. Acad. Sci. U.S.* **74**:4982–4985.

Jones, P., Craig, S. W., Cebra, J. J., and Herzenberg, L. A., 1974, Restriction of gene expression in B lymphocytes and their progeny. II. Committment to immunoglobulin heavy chain isotype, *J. Exp. Med.* **140**:452.

Kessler, S. W., 1975, Rapid isolation of antigens from cells with a staphylococcal protein A-antibody adsorbent: Parameters of the interaction of antibody–antigen complexes with protein A, *J. Immunol.* **115**:1617.

Kitchen, H., and Boyer, S. (eds.), 1974, Hemoglobin: Comparative molecular biology models for the study of disease, *Ann. N.Y. Acad. Sci.* **241**.

Lederberg, J., 1959, Genes and antibodies, *Science* **129**:1649.

Lieberman, R., and Potter, M., 1969, Crossing over between genes in the immunoglobulin heavy chain linkage group of the mouse, *J. Exp. Med.* **130**:519.

Lieberman, R., Paul, W. E., Humphrey, W., and Stimpfling, J. H., 1972, *H-2*-linked immune response (*Ir*) genes. Independent loci for *Ir-IgG* and *Ir-IgA* genes, *J. Exp. Med.* **136**:1231.

Linthicum, D. S., and Sell, S., 1976, Surface immunoglobulin on rabbit lymphoid cells. III. Double expression and separate endocytosis of surface immunoglobulin allotypes on heterozygous lymphocytes demonstrated by immunoelectron microscopic labeling, *Cell. Immunol.* **27**:240.

Lyon, M. F., 1961, Gene action in the X chromosome of the mouse (*Mus musculus* L.), *Nature* **190**:270.

Marchalonis, J. J., and Cone, R. E., 1973, Biochemical and biological characteristics of lymphocyte surface immunoglobulin, *Transplant. Rev.* **14**:3.

Martin, L. N., Leslie, G. A., and Hindes, R., 1976, Lymphocyte surface IgD and IgD and IgM in non-human primates, *Int. Arch. Allergy Appl. Immunol.* **51**:320.

Mason, S. W., 1976, The class of surface immunoglobulin carrying IgG memory in rat thoracic duct lymph; the size of the subpopulation mediating IgG memory, *J. Exp. Med.* **143**:1122.

Melcher, U., Vitetta, E. S., McWilliams, M., Lamm, M. E., Phillips-Quagliata, J. M., and Uhr, J. W., 1974, Cell surface immunoglobulins. X. Identification of an IgD-like molecule on the surface of murine splenocytes, *J. Exp. Med.* **140**:1427.

Metcalf, E. S., and Klinman, N. R., 1976, *In vitro* tolerance induction of neonatal murine spleen cells, *J. Exp. Med.* **143**:1327.

Metchnikoff, E., 1899, Etudes sur la résorption des cellules, *Ann. Inst. Pasteur* **13**:737.

Milstein, C., Brownlee, G. G., Cartwright, E. M., and Jarvis, J. M., 1974, Sequence analysis of immunoglobulin light chain messenger RNA, *Nature* **252**:354.

Möller, G. (ed.), 1975, Concepts of B lymphocyte activation, *Transplant Rev.* **23**.

Nesbitt, M. N., and Gartler, S. M., 1971, The applications of genetic mosaicism to developmental problems, *Ann. Rev. Genet.* **5**:143.

Nossal, G. J. V., 1957, The immunological response of foetal mice to influenza virus, *Aust. J. Exp. Biol.* **35**:549.

Nossal, G. J. V., and Layton, J. E., 1975, Antigen-induced aggregation and modulation of receptors on hapten-specific B lymphocytes, *J. Exp. Med.* **143**:511.

Nossal, G. J. V., and Pike, B. L., 1973, Studies on the differentiation of B lymphocytes in the mouse, *Immunology* **25**:33.

Nossal, G. J. V., and Pike, B. L., 1975*a*, New concepts in immunological tolerance, in: *Immunological Aspects of Neoplasia* (Proceedings of the 26th Annual Symposium on Fundamental Cancer Research of the University of Texas), (E. M. Hersh and M. Schlamowitz, eds.), M. D. Anderson Hospital and Tumor Institute, Houston.

Nossal, G. J. V., and Pike, B. L., 1975*b*, Evidence for the clonal abortion theory of B-lymphocyte tolerance, *J. Exp. Med.* **141**:904.

Nossal, G. J. V., Warner, N. L., Lewis, H., and Sprent, J., 1972, Quantitative features of a sandwich radioimmunolabeling technique for lymphocyte surface receptors, *J. Exp. Med.* **135**:405.

Nossal, G. J. V., Pike, B. L., Stocker, J. W., Layton, J. E., and Goding, J. W., 1976, Hapten-specific B lymphocytes: enrichment, cloning, receptor analysis and tolerance induction, *Cold Spring Harbor Symp. Quant. Biol.* 16:237-243.

Okumura, K., Julius, M. H., Tsu, T., Herzenberg, L. A., and Herzenberg, L. A., 1976, Demonstration that IgG memory is carried by IgG-bearing cells, *Eur. J. Immunol.* 6:467.

Parkhouse, R. M. E., Abney, E. R., Bourgois, A., and Willcox, H. N. A., 1977, Functional and structural characterisation of immunoglobulin on murine B-lymphocytes, *Cold Spring Harbor Symp. Quant. Biol.* 41:698.

Pearson, T., Galfrè, G., Ziegler, A., and Milstein, C., 1977, A myeloma-hybrid producing antibody specific for an allotypic determinant on IgD-like molecules in the mouse, *Eur. J. Immunol.* 7:684.

Pernis, B., Chiappino, G., Kelus, A. S., and Gell, P. G. H., 1965, Cellular localization of immunoglobulins with different allotypic specificities in rabbit lymphoid tissues, *J. Exp. Med.* 122:853.

Pernis, B., Brouet, J. C., and Seligmann, M., 1974, IgD and IgM on the membrane of lymphoid cells in macroglobulinemia. Evidence for identity of membrane IgD and IgM antibody activity in a case with anti-IgG receptors, *Eur. J. Immunol.* 4:776.

Pernis, B., Forni, L., and Knight, K. L., 1975, The problem of an IgD equivalent in non-primates, in: *Membrane Receptors of Lymphocytes* (M. Seligmann, J. L. Preud'homme, and F. Kourilsky, eds.), p. 57, North-Holland/Elsevier, Amsterdam.

Potter, M., and Lieberman, R., 1967, Genetics of immunoglobulin in the mouse, *Adv. Immunol.* 7:92.

Preud'homme, J. L., 1977, Loss of surface IgD by human B lymphocytes during polyclonal activation, *Eur. J. Immunol.* 7:191.

Preud'homme, J. L., Clauvel, J., Seligmann, M., 1975, Immunoglobulin D-bearing lymphocytes in primary immunodeficiencies, *J. Immunol.* 114:481.

Raff, M. C., 1976, T cell recognition at Cold Spring Harbor (editorial), *Nature* 263:10.

Raff, M. C., Feldmann, M., and de Petris, S., 1973, Monospecificity of B lymphocytes, *J. Exp. Med.* 137:1024.

Raff, M. C., Owen, J. J. T., Cooper, M. D., Lawton, A. R., Megson, M., and Gathings, W. E., 1975, Differences in susceptibility of mature and immature mouse B lymphocytes to anti-immunoglobulin induced immunoglobulin suppression *in vitro:* possible implications for B cell tolerance to self, *J. Exp. Med.* 142:1052.

Rowe, D. S., and Fahey, J. L., 1965, A new class of human immunoglobulin. I. A unique myeloma protein, *J. Exp. Med.* 121:171.

Rowe, D. S., Hug, K., Forni, L., and Pernis, B., 1973a, Immunoglobulin D as a lymphocyte receptor, *J. Exp. Med.* 138:965.

Rowe, D. S., Hug, K., Fault, W. P., McCormick, J. N., and Gerber, H., 1973b, IgD on the surface of peripheral blood lymphocytes of the human newborn, *Nature New Biol.* 242:155.

Ruddick, J. H., and Leslie, G. A., 1977, Structure and biologic functions of human IgD. XI. Identification and ontogeny of a rat lymphocyte immunoglobulin having antigenic cross-reactivity with human IgD, *J. Immunol.* 118:1025-1031.

Salsano, P., Froland, S. S., Natvig, J. B., and Michaelsen, T. E., 1974, Same idiotype of B-lymphocyte membrane IgD and IgM. Formal evidence for monoclonality of chronic lymphocytic leukemia cells, *Scand. J. Immunol.* 3:841.

Scher, I., Wistar, R., Asofsky, R., and Paul, W. E., 1976a, B-lymphocyte heterogeneity: Ontogenetic development and organ distribution of B lymphocyte populations defined by their density of surface immunoglobulin, *J. Exp. Med.* 144:494.

Scher, I., Sharrow, S. O., and Paul, W. E., 1976b, X-linked B-lymphocyte defect in CBA/N mice. III. Abnormal development of B-lymphocyte populations defined by their densities of surface immunoglobulin, *J. Exp. Med.* **144**:507.

Schierman, L. W., and McBride, R. A., 1969, Adjuvant activity of erythrocyte isoantigens, *Science* **156**:658.

Sell, S., 1977, Demonstration of double allelic expression (allelic inclusion) of rabbit K light chain allotypes on heterozygous lymphocytes by double allotype sequential stimulation, *Cell. Immunol.* **28**:133.

Shen, F. W., Boyse, E. A., and Cantor, H., 1975, Preparation and use of Ly antisera, *Immunogenetics* **2**:591.

Sidman, C. L., and Unanue, E. R., 1975, Receptor-mediated inactivation of early B lymphocytes, *Nature* **257**:149.

Silver, J., and Hood, L., 1976, Preliminary amino acid sequences of transplantation antigens: Genetic and evolutionary implications, in: *Contemporary Topics in Molecular Immunology*, Vol. 5 (H. N. Eisen and R. A. Reisfeld, eds.), p. 35, Plenum Press, New York.

Sledge, C., Fair, D. S., Black, B., Krueger, R. G., and Hood, L., 1976, Antibody differentiation: Apparent sequence identity between variable sequences shared by IgA and IgG immunoglobulins, *Proc. Natl. Acad. Sci., U.S.* **73**:923.

Sprent, J., and Miller, J. F. A. P., 1972, Thoracic duct lymphocytes from nude mice: Migratory properties and life span, *Eur. J. Immunol.* **2**:384.

Stern, C., and McConnell, I., 1976, Immunoglobulins M and D as antigen-binding receptors on the same cell, with shared specificity, *Eur. J. Immunol.* **6**:225.

Stocker, J. W., 1977, Tolerance induction in maturing B cells, *Immunology* **32**:283.

Stocker, J. W., and Nossal, G. J. V., 1976, Pathways to immunological tolerance: An approach through the study of maturing B lymphocytes, in: *Contemporary Topics in Immunobiology*, Vol. 5 (W. O. Weigle, ed.), p. 191, Plenum Press, New York.

Stocker, J. W., Osmond, D. G., and Nossal, G. J. V., 1974, Differentiation of lymphocytes in the mouse bone marrow. III. The adoptive response of bone marrow cells to a thymus cell-independent antigen, *Immunology* **27**:795.

Tonegawa, S., Brack, C., Hozumi, N., and Schuller, R., 1977, Cloning of an immunoglobulin variable region gene from mouse embryo, *Proc. Natl. Acad. Sci. U.S.* **74**:3518–3522.

van Boxel, J. A., Paul, W. E., Terry, W. D., and Green, I., 1972, IgD-bearing human lymphocytes, *J. Immunol.* **109**:648.

Vischer, T. L., 1974, Stimulation of mouse B lymphocytes by trypsin, *J. Immunol.* **113**:58.

Vitetta, E. S., and Uhr, J. W., 1973, Synthesis, transport, dynamics and fate of cell surface Ig and alloantigens in murine lymphocytes, *Transplant. Rev.* **14**:50.

Vitetta, E. S., and Uhr, J. W., 1975, Immunoglobulin-receptors revisited, *Science* **189**:964.

Vitetta, E. S., and Uhr, J. W., 1976, Cell surface immunoglobulin. XV. The presence of IgM and an IgD-like molecule on the same cell in murine lymphoid tissue, *Eur. J. Immunol.* **6**:140.

Vitetta, E. S., Melcher, U., McWilliams, M., Lamm, M. E., Phillips-Quagliata, J. M., and Uhr, J. W., 1974, Cell surface immunoglobulin. XI. The appearance of an IgD-like molecule on murine lymphoid cells during ontogeny, *J. Exp. Med.* **141**:206.

Warner, N. L., 1974, Membrane immunoglobulins and antigen receptors on B and T lymphocytes, *Adv. Immunol.* **19**:67.

Warner, N. L., 1975, Autoimmunity and the pathogenesis of plasma cell tumor induction in NZB inbred and hybrid mice, *Immunogenetics* **2**:1.

Warner, N. L., Goding, J. W., Gutman, G. A., Warr, G. W., Herzenberg, L. A., Osborne, B. A., van der Loo, W., Black, S. J., and Loken, M. R., 1977, Allotypes of mouse IgM immunoglobulin, *Nature* **265**:447.

Weigert, M., Potter, M., and Sachs, D., 1975, Genetics of the immunoglobulin variable region, *Immunogenetics* **1**:511.

Wernet, D., Shafran, H., and Lilly, F., 1976, Genetic regulation of the antibody response to H-2D^b alloantigens in mice. III. Inhibition of the IgG response to noncongenic cells by preimmunisation with congenic cells, *J. Exp. Med.* **144**:654.

Wigzell, H., 1973, On the relationship between cellular and humoral antibodies, *Contemporary Topics in Immunobiology*, Vol. 3 (M. D. Cooper, ed.), p. 77, Plenum Press, New York.

Williams, A. F., 1975, IgG2 and other immunoglobulin classes on the cell surface of rat lymphoid cells, *Eur. J. Immunol.* **5**:883.

Williamson, A. R., 1976, The biological origin of antibody diversity, *Ann. Rev. Biochem.* **45**:467.

Williamson, A. R., and Fitzmaurice, L. C., 1976, Arrangement and rearrangement of antibody genes, in: *The Generation of Antibody Diversity: A New Look* (A. J. Cunningham, ed.), Academic Press, New York.

Winchester, R. J., Fu, S. M., Hoffman, T., and Kunkel, H. G., 1975a, IgG on lymphocyte surfaces: Technical problems and the significance of a third cell population, *J. Immunol.* **114**:1210.

Winchester, R. J., Fu, S. M., Wernet, P., Kunkel, H. G., Dupont, B., and Jersild, C., 1975b, Recognition by pregnancy serums of non-HL-A alloantigens selectively expressed on B lymphocytes, *J. Exp. Med.* **141**:924.

Wolf, B., Janeway, C. A., Coombs, R. R. A., Catty, D., Gell, P. G. H., and Kelus, A. S., 1971, Immunoglobulin determinants on the lymphocytes of normal rabbits. III. As4 and As6 determinants on individual lymphocytes and the concept of allelic exclusion, *Immunology* **20**:931.

Chapter 8

Immunoglobulin Isotype Expression

John F. Kearney

*Department of Microbiology
and the Comprehensive Cancer Center
University of Alabama Medical Center
Birmingham, Alabama 35294*

and

Erika R. Abney

*Department of Zoology
University College London
London, England*

I. INTRODUCTION*

Many different kinds of observations suggest that during development of the B cell line, individual V_H genes determining the antibody specificity of an immunoglobulin molecule can be expressed with multiple C_H genes. Thus each clone of B cells, defined by expression of a variable-region gene for the light and heavy chains of the immunoglobulin molecule, ultimately contains plasma cells synthesizing immunoglobulins of all classes. The most convincing observations to support this concept include (1) shared light chains and V-region sequences by biclonal myeloma proteins of different heavy-chain isotypes (Wang *et al.*, 1969, 1970), and (2) production of antibodies of different heavy-chain classes but with identical idiotype by the progeny of single precursor cells in clonal assays (Press and Klinman, 1973).

*Abbreviations used in this paper: Ig, immunoglobulin; sIg, surface immunoglobulin; cIg, cytoplasmic immunoglobulin; LPS, bacterial lipopolysaccharide; FITC, fluorescein isothiocyanate; RITC, rhodamine isothiocyanate.

Two different models have been proposed to explain association of V regions to different C regions, both of which suggest that precursors of cells synthesizing IgG or IgA are derived from IgM-bearing lymphocytes by a genetic switch mechanism. One model, derived largely from ontogenetic studies in chickens, holds that this intraclonal switch is antigen-independent and occurs under the influence of the inductive microenvironment for B-cell differentiation (Kincade *et al.*, 1970; Cooper *et al.*, 1972.) During this phase of differentiation clonal sublines of B lymphocytes, with the potential to synthesize different immunoglobulin isotypes, are generated and seeded to peripheral lymphoid organs. The alternative model, proposed in slightly different forms by several different workers, holds that the switch of IgM-bearing lymphocytes to synthesis of IgG or IgA is antigen-driven in conjunction with factors provided by auxiliary cells (Pierce *et al.*, 1972; Warner, 1974; Vitetta and Uhr, 1975).

There is convincing evidence to suggest that the precursor for cells secreting IgG, IgA, or IgE initially expresses surface IgM at some developmental stage. Suppression of all immunoglobulin isotypes results after neonatal treatment with anti-μ-chain antibodies (reviewed in Lawton *et al.*, 1975; Manning *et al.*, 1976). The development of cells secreting IgG and IgA antibodies to sheep erythrocytes *in vitro* is inhibited by inclusion of anti-μ in cultures (Pierce *et al.*, 1972). More direct evidence, such as (1) the presence of IgG-secreting plasma cells with IgM on their surface membrane in rabbits (Pernis *et al.*, 1971), and (2) the detection of a low number of antibody-forming cells simultaneously secreting IgG and IgM isotypes (Nossal *et al.*, 1971), suggested that such a switch could be manifested by the simultaneous expression of more than one immunoglobulin isotype by one B cell. It was subsequently shown that IgD was expressed simultaneously with IgM on the surface of most B cells in humans (Lobo *et al.*, 1975; van Boxel *et al.*, 1972; Kubo *et al.*, 1974; Rowe *et al.*, 1973; Knapp *et al.*, 1973) and in mice (Abney and Parkhouse, 1974; Melcher *et al.*, 1974). Furthermore, it was shown that when a lymphocyte simultaneously expresses multiple classes of surface Ig, those classes share the same idiotype or antigen specificity (at least for sIgM and sIgD) (Salsano *et al.*, 1974; Fu *et al.*, 1975; Goding and Layton, 1976). With these findings came the realization that at least two immunoglobulin classes can be synthesized and expressed on the surface of a B lymphocyte and that variable regions are shared by these two molecules. In contrast to these observations, many earlier investigations showed that the terminally differentiated progeny of lymphocytes, the plasma cells, were generally restricted to the synthesis of a single species of immunoglobulin molecule (Mellors and Korngold, 1963; Bernier and Cebra, 1964; Cebra *et al.*, 1966).

We have approached the problem of development of isotype diversity within the B cell line in two ways. First, the simultaneous expression of IgD with IgM on many B cells prompted us to carry out a systematic study of the interrelationships of other isotypes, IgG and IgA, on normal B cells during ontogeny and in various lymphoid organs of adult mice. Second, as an approach to the problem of regulation of immunoglobulin isotype expression, an *in vitro* system has been used in which the polyclonal mitogen LPS stimulates murine B lymphocytes to differentiate to plasma cells synthesizing various classes of mouse immunoglobulins (IgM, IgG$_1$, IgG$_2$, IgG$_3$, and IgA). Attempts to obtain information at the single-cell level on changes in immunoglobulin class expression, immunoglobulin secretion, and other aspects of B-cell function during pauciclonal antigen-driven responses are limited by the small numbers of cells that respond. However, the polyclonal responses of LPS-stimulated B lymphocytes provides large numbers of activated cells which appear similar, if not identical, to antigen-triggered cells in their fundamental physiological responses. Using this system we have been able to (1) determine some of the cellular mechanisms for the LPS-induced expression of other immunoglobulin isotypes on IgM-bearing cells, (2) examine the regulatory mechanisms involved in the LPS-dependent maturation of IgM-bearing precursors into plasma cells restricted to synthesis of IgG or IgA isotypes, and (3) relate findings in this system to our observations on expression of different isotypes *in vivo*.

II. ONTOGENY OF IMMUNOGLOBULIN ISOTYPES

The details of methods used in these studies are contained in the following references: Abney *et al.* (1975), Kearney and Lawton (1975*a*, *b*), and Kearney *et al.* (1976*a*, *b*), and will only be mentioned briefly.

Lymphocyte suspensions from different tissues of mice at various stages of development were stained with various combinations of purified, fluorochrome-coupled, and isotype-specific (IgM, IgG, IgA) antibodies. Each suspension was first stained with antibody to one class of Ig, then counterstained with a contrasting labeled antibody to another class. The cells were examined for the presence of one or both labeled antibodies. In these studies it is crucial to exclude potential problems arising from staining artifacts. Controls done to ensure specificity included the following:

1. Two sets of antiisotype reagents were prepared, which, when cross-tested, stained totally overlapping subpopulations of cells.

2. The specificity of the antibody reagents was checked by a sensitive radioimmunoassay using high-specific-activity ^{125}I-labeled mouse myeloma proteins as antigens.

3. The antibodies were checked by fluorescent microscopy against a panel of mouse myeloma tumor cells representative of each of the major isotypes (IgM, IgA, IgG$_1$, IgG$_2$, and IgG$_3$).

4. The rabbit anti-mouse δ chain used in those studies was checked in a co-

staining experiment with the recently described anti-δ allotype antibody (Goding et al., 1976) on splenic lymphocytes. Here, the anti-δ antibody was revealed by indirect fluorescence using fluorescent-labeled goat antibodies to mouse IgG_1; again the concordance was excellent. A further indication of the monospecificity of the rabbit anti-mouse δ chain was its failure to stain lymphocytes of mice rendered deficient in B lymphocytes by chronic treatment with anti-mouse μ-chain antibody.

5. A systematic search for IgD-positive plasma cells in the lymphoid tissue of mice (and in cultures of LPS-activated cells) proved negative. The latter observation, apart from stressing the monospecificity of the antiserum, also suggests that in the mouse, IgD functions only as a receptor antibody.

A more difficult problem is to ensure that the presence of labeled antibody on the cell surface represents detection of Ig endogenously synthesized by the cells that show staining rather than mouse immunoglobulins or labeled goat antibody taken up via Fc receptors. That the latter did not occur to any significant extent is indicated by the rarity of doubles when cells were stained with combinations of antibodies to IgG subclasses or to IgG and IgA. The lack of cytophilic binding of our reagents is probably due to the fact that they were made in goats, as it has been recently shown that goat IgG antibodies do not bind efficiently to Fc receptors on B cells (Alexander and Sanders, 1977).

A summary of the results obtained by membrane immunofluorescence is presented in Table I (Abney et al., 1978). Analysis of surface immunoglobulin on lymphocytes from fetal liver and neonatal spleen showed that the only isotype detected was IgM. This was true not only for pre-B cells, which first appear in fetal liver at day 10–13 (Melchers et al., 1975a; Raff et al., 1976), but for the first surface immunoglobulin-positive cells, which appear at day 16 or 17 of gestation (Nossal and Pike, 1973; Owen et al., 1974). The first definitive indication of total isotype diversity was in spleens from 3-day-old mice (Table I, column 1). Although the main Ig class represented is clearly IgM (6.2% total nucleated cells), all other known isotypes were detected. (IgE was not studied because of the lack of a suitable antiserum.) At this stage, cells bearing other isotypes invariably expressed sIgM as well. The detection of only infrequent doubles by staining simultaneously for sIgD and for sIgG or sIgA at this stage suggests that each of these isotypes is initially expressed singly on separate populations of sIgM-bearing cells. However, this situation changes rapidly, so that in 7-day-old mice (Table I, columns 2 and 3), large numbers of B cells expressing sIgG or sIgA, have sIgM and have acquired sIgD. Thus, B cells may simultaneously bear at least three different isotypes. We shall refer to these as trebles and on the basis of the developmental order of appearance, we conclude that they arise by a sequential expression of sIgD by the $sIgM^+.sIgG^+$ (or $sIgA^+$) doubles.

The most frequent incidence of trebles is in the 7-day lymph node, where

Table I. Ontogeny and Tissue Distribution of BALB/c Lymphocytes
Bearing Different Combinations of Immunoglobulin Isotypes

Stained with:	3-day spleen	7-day spleen	7-day PLN[a]	Adult spleen	Adult TDL[b]	Adult BM
IgM						
% total[c]	6.2	6.4	25.8	39	16.3	4.7
% sIgD[d]	4	47	90	83	96	34
IgD						
% total	0.2	3.4	25.0	40	13.8	1.2
% sIgM[d]	100	95	90	91	83	100
IgG$_1$						
% total	0.02	0.05	0.6	0.5	0.4	–
% sIgM	100.0	100	100	44	0	–
% sIgD	0	–	100	53	0	–
IgG$_2$						
% total	0.4	0.2	0.8	2.2	03	0.2
% sIgM	100	100	98	69	81	76
% sIgD	0	30	96	50	36	33
IgG$_3$						
% total	0.9	1.1	1.3	0.8	1.1	0.3
% sIgM	100	100	100	83	86	91
% sIgD	3	20	95	46	75	0
IgA						
% total	0.05	0.05	0.06	0.6	1.7	0.8
% sIgM	100	100	100	8	0	20
% sIgD	0	29	100	12	0	13

[a]PLN, peripheral lymph node suspensions were made from pooled axillary, inguinal, and cervical lymph nodes.
[b]TDL, thoracic duct lymphocytes separated from a 0- to 24-hr collection of thoracic duct lymph.
[c]These figures represent the total percentage of cells in cell suspensions which express a particular isotype.
[d]% sIgM or sIgD under each class or subclass heading represents the percentage of cells of this particular isotype which also expresses sIgM or sIgD.

essentially all sIgG$^+$ and sIgA$^+$ cells also have sIgM and sIgD (Table I, column 3). As an example, consider the data for sIgG$_2$$^+$ cells: 98% of all sIgG$_2$$^+$ cells also had sIgM. Although triple-staining experiments were not performed, since 96% of the parallel preparation of sIgG$_2$$^+$ cells also stained for sIgD, we are forced to conclude that by this time in ontogeny the majority of sIgG$_2$$^+$ cells also express sIgM and sIgD. Similar arguments apply to the results in the same tissue for cells expressing sIgA and other sIgG subclasses. By comparison, trebles, although present, are relatively less numerous in the spleen of the 7-day mouse

(Table I, column 2). For example, although 100% of $sIgG_2^+$ lymphocytes bear IgM, only 30% have, in addition, sIgD. In the spleen, 30% of the $sIgG_2^+$ cells must be trebles and the remaining 70% are of the phenotype $sIgM^+.sIgG_2^+.sIgD^-$, and therefore probably less mature than the trebles. These observations also suggest that the lymph node, at this stage of development, may be a site for the further differentiation, or homing, of more mature B cells than the spleen. This conclusion is supported by the observation of preferential splenic homing of young B cells from the bone marrow (Ryser and Vassalli, 1974).

Examination of lymphocytes from adult mice reveals that many lymphocytes bearing IgG or IgA may have lost sIgM and sIgD (Table I, columns 4 and 5). This trend is especially obvious for adult thoracic duct lymphocytes with IgA or IgG_1 which are mostly devoid of any other isotype (see particularly the data of Table I, column 5). At the other extreme, even in adult mice, $sIgG_3^+$ lymphocytes are frequently found to have $sIgM^+$ and $sIgD^+$, whereas an intermediate situation is seen in the $sIgG_2^+$ populations.

Our interpretation of these observations is that subsequent to exposure to antigen and during development to isotype-restricted plasma cells, there is a loss of sIgM and sIgD from the triple cells. Therefore, the conversion of trebles to cells expressing only sIgG, for example, is probably via an $IgM^+.IgG^+.IgD^-$ intermediate. Adult bone marrow, as might be expected for a site of B-cell generation, contains a relatively large proportion of $sIgM^+.sIgD^-$ lymphocytes (Table I, column 6).

III. *IN VITRO* ACTIVATION OF MOUSE B CELLS

Previously, LPS had been shown to induce only a polyclonal IgM response (Andersson *et al.*, 1972) which limited its usefulness in the study of switching of immunoglobulin isotypes during the differentiation of B cells to plasma cells *in vitro*. Improvements in techniques subsequently enabled us and others to obtain differentiation of IgG- and IgA-synthesizing plasma cells in this system (Kearney and Lawton, 1975a; Melchers *et al.*, 1975a; Pernis *et al.*, 1977; Askonas and North, 1977). In our studies cytoplasmic or surface immunoglobulins synthesized by LPS-activated cells were detected by fluorescence microscopy using the reagents described above.

It was first shown that the LPS-dependent differentiation of IgG- and IgA-synthesizing plasma cells is apparently independent of T cells, since lymphocytes from congenitally athymic mice and from fetal liver, which lack T cells, behave similarly to conventional mice (Kearney and Lawton, 1975b; Andersson *et al.*, 1976). This model was then used to investigate the possibility of "switching" in expression of immunoglobulin isotypes by B cells differentiating *in vitro*.

Because the first immunoglobulin class expressed by pre-B cells and surface Ig-positive B cells is IgM, it was of interest to investigate the potential of these early B cells to differentiate to plasma cells synthesizing other Ig classes *in vitro*. In an ontogenetic study it was shown that as soon as sIgM$^+$ B cells were detectable in fetal liver at 16–17 days of gestation, they could be stimulated by LPS to differentiate to mature cells synthesizing IgM and IgG$_2$ isotypes. Later in spleen and liver cultures at day 19–20 of gestation, IgG$_1$- and IgA-synthesizing cells were detected (Kearney and Lawton, 1975b). The proportions of plasma cells containing the various immunoglobulin classes in cultures of newborn spleen were similar to those in adult spleen cells, suggesting that the relative inability of neonatal mice to make antibody responses may not reside in functional immaturity of young B cells, but may be related to slow maturation of auxiliary cells such as T cells and macrophages (Mosier and Johnson, 1975; Blaese and Lawrence, 1977). An important finding in these experiments was that a B cell bearing only IgM and no other isotype, and which was also probably devoid of other B-lymphocyte receptors (i.e., C3, Fc, IgD; Kearney *et al.*, 1977a), could act as the precursor for cells synthesizing all immunoglobulin isotypes if triggered to terminal differentiation by an appropriate signal. That these sIgM$^+$ cells could be found at an early stage of fetal life (16–17 days) before any prior exposure to exogenous antigens indicates that the genetic potential to switch to other classes of immunoglobulin is present in the earliest members of the B-cell line and develops independently of exogenous antigen and auxiliary cells.

The LPS-induced differentiation of isotype-restricted plasma cells was then used to study the mechanisms whereby cells expressing one or more isotypes eventually became plasma cells restricted to synthesis of only one isotype. We had previously shown that anti-mouse IgM (μ-chain-specific) (Lawton and Cooper, 1974), when added to cultures of newborn and adult spleen cells, produced a dose-related suppression of differentiation of IgG as well as IgM synthesizing cells, with newborn cells being much more susceptible to suppression (Kearney *et al.*, 1976b). Our results (Kearney *et al.*, 1975a) and those of Pernis *et al.* (1977), therefore, confirmed indirectly that the LPS-inducible precursors for IgG-synthesizing cells expressed IgM receptors in the newborn and in the adult.

To investigate the cellular events involved in the apparent isotype switch after LPS stimulation, the early expression of other surface immunoglobulin isotypes on developing B cells was studied *in vitro*. A population of cells highly enriched for μ-bearing B lymphocytes was prepared by culturing <12-hr CBA neonatal liver and spleen cells for 5–7 days. The resulting population of cells was harvested and cleared of nonviable cells by centrifugation over a Ficoll-Hypaque gradient. Ninety percent of these cells, which had the morphology of large or medium lymphocytes, were brightly stained for sIgM. These cells were then exposed to LPS (50 μg/ml) in the presence or absence of metabolic inhibi-

tors and stained for surface immunoglobulin with various combinations of
purified fluorescent antibodies to mouse immunoglobulin isotypes. Within 6-12
hr, LPS induced an increase in the proportion of surface IgM-positive cells,
which expressed another isotype (Fig. 1). This increase occurred even when
cellular proliferation was blocked by cytosine arabinoside and hydroxyurea.

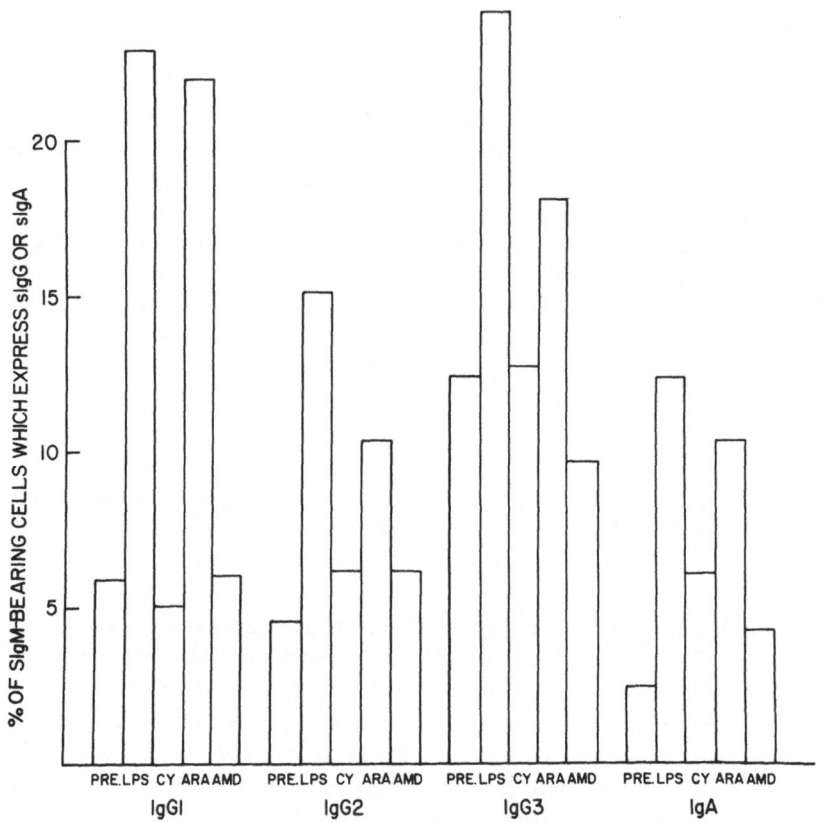

Figure 1. Comparison of the frequences of $sIgG_1$, $sIgG_2$, $sIgG_3$, or sIgA expressed by newborn CBA/J B cells prepared as described in the text and stimulated with LPS in the presence
or absence of metabolic inhibitors. Each experimental culture was divided into aliquots and
then stained with FITC anti-μ and another RITC antiisotype antibody. Each vertical
column represents the percentage of $sIgM^+$ cells which expressed another isotype, before or
after treatment with LPS. PRE represents the percent of $sIgM^+$ cells which expressed a
particular isotype before treatment with LPS; LPS represents the increase in percent of
$sIgM^+$ cells which expressed another isotype after 6 hr of induction with 50 μg/ml of LPS;
CY, cycloheximide (10 μg/ml) completely inhibited the induction of sIgG and sIgA isotypes; ARA, cytosine arabinoside (40 μg/ml) inhibited ^{3}H-thymidine incorporation completely but failed to prevent the increased expression of sIgG- and sIgA-positive cells; AMD,
actinomycin D (0.1 μg/ml) inhibited the induction of increased numbers of sIgG- and sIgA-
positive cells.

However, expression of IgG and IgA on IgM-bearing precursors was prevented by cycloheximide and actinomycin D without affecting the viability or the numbers of sIgM-positive cells.

Other studies in this system showed that cells simultaneously staining with other combinations (e.g., anti-γ1 and anti-γ2) occurred infrequently. Thus (1) during induction, the new expression of usually only one class of Ig occurred, and (2) the increase in frequency of sIgM$^+$ cells staining for sIgG or sIgA was not due to nonspecific uptake of goat antibodies. The results are complementary to the observations made *in vivo*, where only one IgG subclass or IgA appeared on sIgM-bearing cells. Parallel experiments have been performed by exposing the B cells to tritiated thymidine during the induction period. Autoradiographic analysis of these stained cells revealed that sIgM$^+$ cells induced to express a second isotype were rarely labeled, while the occasional single sIgG$^+$ or sIgA$^+$ cells detected were almost always labeled.

When adult nude thoracic duct B lymphocytes (TDL) were treated with LPS for a period of 12 hr, a much smaller increase in the proportion of sIgM$^+$ cells which stained for sIgG or sIgA was seen. However, it has been shown previously that both newborn B lymphocytes and nude TDL will differentiate to give comparable numbers of plasma cells synthesizing all immunoglobulin classes (J. Kearney, unpublished observations). There are several interpretations of these contrasting results, which will be considered below. Fluorescent analysis of nude TDL showed that 95% of these cells were sIgD$^+$, 90% sIgM$^+$, 90% Ia$^+$, 6% IgG$_3$$^+$, 1% sIgG$_1$, 2% sIgG$_2$, and 1% sIgA (Kearney, unpublished). Thus these adult B cells may already express a second isotype at frequencies which preclude detection of a small postinductive increase. Another possible reason for the differences observed between responses of newborn B lymphocytes from these cultures and adult B lymphocytes may be that induction occurs only in a certain phase of the cell cycle. Nude TDL B lymphocytes are resting cells with negligible thymidine incorporation compared to the newborn B-cell preparations, most of them presumably being a Go phase. In other systems (e.g., induction of T1 and Thy-1), the inducible cells reside in large cell fractions (Hammerling *et al.*, 1976). Conceivably, the failure to induce this cell population may be related to the differences between cell cycling properties of the two populations.

An extended kinetic study was then made, using fluorescent antibody techniques, on the isotypes within the cytoplasm and on the membranes of B cells during their progression toward terminally differentiated plasma cells in response to LPS. In newborn LPS-stimulated cultures, as already shown for sIg on freshly isolated newborn B lymphocytes, the cells expressing the first detectable cytoplasmic as well as surface IgG$_1$, IgG$_2$, IgG$_3$, and IgA also expressed sIgM. Subsequent development of immunoglobulin class restriction, characteristic of LPS-stimulated plasma cells, was accompanied by a gradual loss of surface IgM (Kearney *et al.*, 1976*b*, 1977*b*). A detailed kinetic analysis of surface IgM on IgG$_2$ precursors in LPS-stimulated cultures of newborn spleen cells is shown in

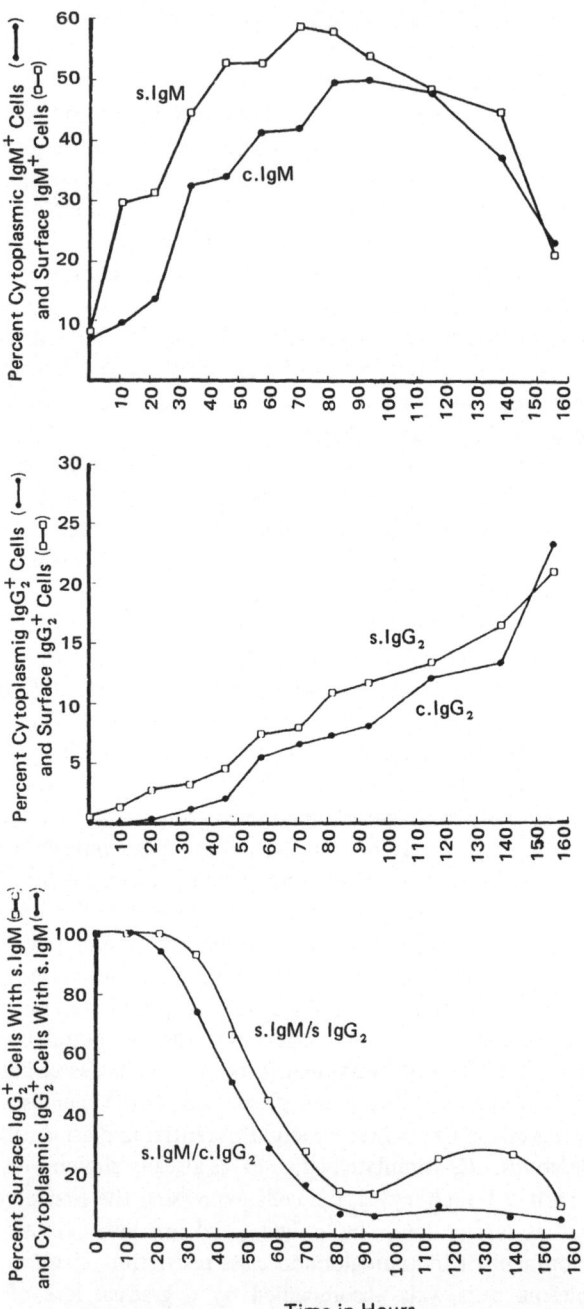

Fig. 2. It can be seen that all surface IgG_2^+ and cytoplasmic IgG_2^+ cells from 0 to 35 hr of culture also expressed sIgM. From 35 to 96 hr, coincident with the period of maximal LPS-stimulated cell proliferation, a population of cells emerged expressing only IgG_2.

A similar response was observed in experiments with adult spleen cells. However, adult spleen cells differed from newborn cells in that of the 4–6% $sIgG_2$-positive cells present in preculture cell suspensions, only 20–30% also stained for sIgM. The proportion of $sIgG_2$ also expressing IgM rose over a 4-day period, which suggested that sIgM-bearing cells were induced to express IgG, although the role of proliferation in this apparent expansion in frequency of IgG-bearing cells was not investigated (Kearney et al., 1976b).

Pernis et al. (1977) obtained similar results to ours with adult cells but also noted that early in LPS-stimulated cultures of adult spleen there were cells which synthesized both cytoplasmic IgG and IgM. These were later replaced by single cytoplasmic IgG-positive cells. We have confirmed their findings and have investigated some of the factors which induce the appearance of these double-isotype producers. We noticed that cultures done with certain batches of fetal calf serum (FCS) contained unusually high frequencies of $cIgG^+$ cells, which were also stained with cIgM at times when normally very few cytoplasmic double cells were observed. These sera also supported low proliferative responses. Adult spleen cells were cultured with LPS in different concentrations of fetal calf serum to alter rates of LPS-stimulated growth. By changing the concentration of FCS from 2.5% to 30%, an approximately twofold increase in cell numbers occurred. The amount of FCS present in the tissue culture medium markedly affected the number of $cIgG_2^+$ or $cIgG_3^+$ cells recovered from the cultures, while the percent of $cIgM^+$ cells was not altered significantly over the same range of FCS concentrations. When cultures were stained with RITC anti-$\gamma2$ or $\gamma3$ and FITC anti-μ and examined for the presence of double-stained cells at 6 days, it was found that at low concentrations of FCS, >40% of $cIgG^+$ cells were also

Figure 2. Kinetics of development of cells expressing IgM and IgG_2 in LPS-stimulated cultures of spleen cells from newborn CBA/J mice. These graphs represent data pooled from five separate experiments. In the top panel the percentages of cytoplasmic and surface IgM-positive cells are plotted against time. In the middle panel the percentages of cytoplasmic or surface IgG_2-positive cells are shown, and in the bottom panel the percentages of surface IgG_2^+ or cytoplasmic IgG_2^+ cells which also express surface IgM are plotted against time. It can be seen that early in culture, all surface or cytoplasmic IgG_2^+ cells also expressed surface IgM. Then the frequency of cells staining for sIgM fell rapidly until at 96 hr only 5–10% of cytoplasmic or surface IgG_2^+ cells stained for surface IgM. At the same time, cells expressing surface or cytoplasmic IgG_2 rose from undetectable levels to ~25% of the total population of cells. Many of the IgG_2^+ cells were blasts, suggesting that they were actively proliferating during this period.

stained for cIgM. As the concentrations of FCS increased, the proportion of cIgG cells which also stained for cIgM decreased. These results indicate that the amount of FCS present in the tissue culture medium had a marked effect on (1) the number of cIgG cells that differentiated in response to LPS and (2) the number of cIgG plasma cells which also stained for cIgM (Kearney et al., 1977b).

Because of the suggestion from these experiments that cell division and proliferation were involved in the loss of IgM-synthesizing potential by IgG and IgA precursors, these studies were then extended to include more specific inhibitors of cell cycling. Thymidine at concentrations greater than 40 μg/ml will markedly affect proliferation of LPS-stimulated B lymphocytes. Another inhibitor of mitogen-induced lymphocyte proliferation is sodium butyrate (Kyner et al., 1976). While greatly reducing cell proliferation, both of these chemicals allowed differentiation of substantial numbers of cells containing cytoplasmic immunoglobulins, even when present for extended periods of time. This is in contrast to an inhibitor of DNA synthesis such as hydroxyurea, which must be used at concentrations of $>10^{-3}$ M to prevent thymidine incorporation but which is also very toxic for LPS-stimulated B cells after ~12 hr of incubation (J. Kearney, unpublished observations). With increased quantities of thymidine, proliferation decreased and the production of IgG-synthesizing plasma cells was markedly inhibited. The great majority of cIgG$^+$ cells which did develop were also cIgM$^+$. In equivalent experiments with newborn liver cultures, almost all cIgG$_1^+$, cIgG$_2^+$, cIgG$_3^+$ and cIgA$^+$ plasma cells were also cIgM$^+$, complementing the early appearance of IgG subclasses and IgA on sIgM-bearing cells. These experiments, and those of Askonas and North (1977), suggested that LPS-induced differentiation of plasma cells restricted to IgG synthesis required LPS-stimulated proliferation of the B-cell precursors.

In a second series of experiments, sodium butyrate was added at 24-hr intervals to LPS-stimulated adult B cells, and at 7 days the blocked cultures were harvested, counted, and the number of cIg$^+$ cells determined. Early addition of sodium butyrate markedly depressed proliferation and production of cIgG cells, while later additions produced a lesser effect on the production not only of single IgG cells but also of double cIgG$^+$.cIgM$^+$ cells (Kearney et al., 1977b). There are two possible interpretations of this experiment: (1) proliferation either results in a recruitment of sIgM$^+$ cells to express cIgG, or (2) the increased incidence of mature double-producing cells results from expansion of the pool of sIgM$^+$.sIgG$^+$ B lymphocytes in the preculture cell population. Addition of sodium butyrate "freezes" the cell in a particular state of differentiation so that even after 7 days, cells expressing cytoplasmic immunoglobulin of both classes can be found.

Removal of 90% of sIgG$_2^+$ cells prior to culture by the use of a fluorescence-activated cell sorter resulted in a failure to deplete LPS-stimulated production of cIgG$_2^+$ plasma cells (M. Loken and J. Kearney, unpublished results). These results suggest that there is recruitment of single sIgM⁺ B lymphocytes as precursors for cIgG₂⁺ cells in this system. Observations from the experiments in which sodium butyrate was used to block proliferation also suggested that there is continued synthesis of cytoplasmic mRNA for cIgM as well as cIgG, or that this message is long-lived. Under normal conditions of proliferation a replicative cycle may be necessary to repress IgM and IgD (see later) synthesis, or a long-lived previously transcribed mRNA for IgM receptor synthesis is diluted into dividing daughter cells. Melchers *et al.* (1974) have provided evidence that continuous DNA-dependent RNA synthesis by small resting B lymphocytes is necessary for maintenance of IgM synthesis, so that the presence of sIgM or sIgD

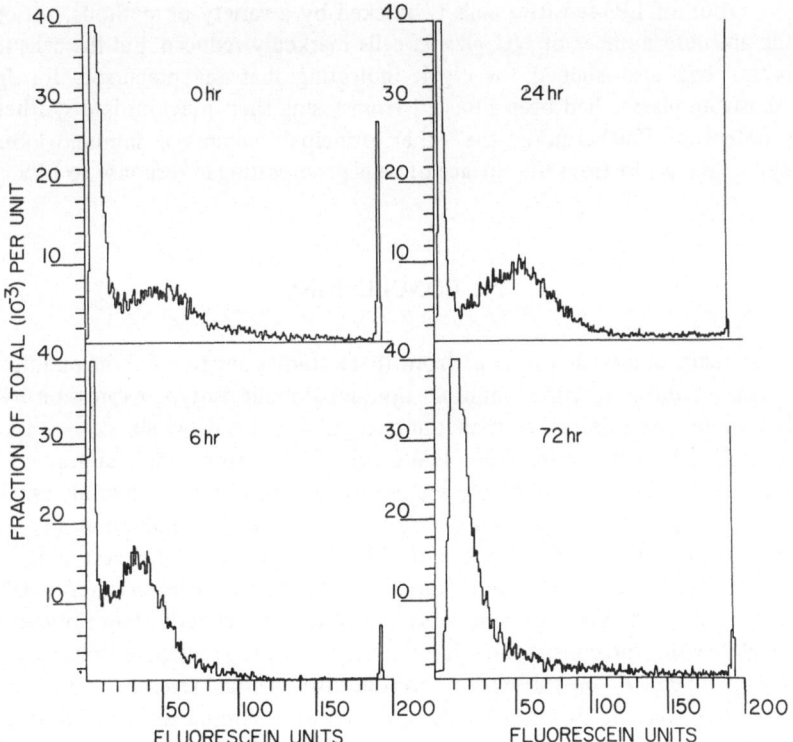

Figure 3. Fluorescence-activated cell-sorter profiles of LPS-stimulated cells taken at intervals after initiation of cultures and stained for surface IgD by incubating with rabbit anti-mouse IgD followed by FITC goat anti-rabbit IgG. It can be seen that with time after stimulation with LPS, the population of cells staining for IgD at 0 hr is replaced by a population which is largely sIgD-negative. At the same time, the mean intensity of staining for sIgM on individual cells increased more than 20-fold (data not shown). These studies were done in collaboration with M. Loken.

on sIgG-positive cells probably means that there must be continuous synthesis of mRNA for all isotypes present on resting B cells.

In collaboration with M. Loken, the fluorescence-activated cell sorter was used to quantitate the relative amounts of sIgD and sIgM on B lymphocytes responding to LPS *in vitro*. In Fig. 3 it can be seen that by 72 hr, virtually all the cells stained for sIgD exhibited only very weak fluorescence. However, a few cells brightly stained for sIgD were still present. At the same time, the mean amount of sIgM on the total population of cells increased by about 20-fold. This increase in the number of surface-located IgM molecules was also observed by Melchers *et al.* (1974) using different methods of detection.

In summary, these results indicate that the LPS-induced development of IgG-synthesizing cells is highly dependent on proliferation and that when the proliferation of LPS-sensitive cells is blocked by a variety of methods, not only is the absolute number of IgG plasma cells markedly reduced, but the cells that express cIgG also stained for cIgM, indicating that the precursors for IgG-synthesizing plasma had been blocked from losing their previous IgM-synthesizing potential. Furthermore, the other principal membrane immunoglobulin isotype, IgD, is lost from the surface of cells proliferating in response to LPS.

IV. CONCLUSIONS

The main points that emerge from these studies are that (1) depending on the stage of differentiation, multiple immunoglobulin isotype expression by B cells may be the rule rather than the exception; (2) cells which express IgG_1, IgG_2, IgG_3, and IgA arise from IgM-bearing precursors which appear to be committed to the synthesis of the second isotype and do not randomly express all other isotypes during normal development or after LPS induction; (3) sIgD expression does not precede, nor is it obligatory for, the expression of IgG or IgA by developing lymphocytes; and (4) while cell division and/or DNA synthesis does not appear to be necessary for the expression of other isotypes by the sIgM-bearing precursors, the development of isotype-restricted plasma cells is highly dependent on subsequent proliferative events. Overall, these results support the concept that most B lymphocytes are committed with respect to the isotype eventually secreted by terminally differentiated plasma cell progeny. This commitment is signaled by the class of membrane immunoglobulin which appears with sIgM and later IgD. These data also support the concept that the development of cells expressing up to three immunoglobulin isotypes is pre-programmed and independent of T cells and antigen. The staining of lympho-cytes from adult, congenitally athymic, antigen-sheltered mice gave basically the same patterns of isotype expression as those observed with conventional mice (Abney *et al.*, 1977). Recently, it has been shown in rats that surface IgE expression by sIgM⁺ B lymphocytes develops normally in T-cell-deficient animals (Urban *et al.*, 1977; Ishizaka *et al.*, 1978) and could also be induced *in vitro* on IgM-bearing cells by extracts of lymphoid tissues from parasite-infested mice (Urban *et al.*, 1977) in a manner very similar to the induction of non-IgM isotypes by LPS on sIgM-bearing cells.

How are these results to be reconciled with the evidence that T lymphocytes may regulate the class of immunoglobulin produced by the daughter antibody-secreting cells of an individual precursor cell (Pierce *et al.*, 1972; Press and Klinman, 1973; Gearhart, 1977)? Using an assay capable of identifying the products of mature progeny of individual clonal precursors, Klinman and associates have shown that one precursor cell may give rise to antibody-forming cells of the same specificity for antigen and idiotype but of different isotypes. They also showed that production of IgG antibodies in this assay was dependent on the presence of carrier primed T cells from syngeneic mice; in the presence of allogeneic T cells, similar numbers of B-cell precursors were detected, but only IgM-producing clones were observed (Pierce and Klinman, 1976). In contrast, B cells from antigen-primed mice appeared to be committed to IgG production and did not require syngeneic T-cell help. This conclusion rests on the observation that clones derived from primed B cells synthesized only one class of antibody (IgG₁) (Pierce and Klinman, 1976). In contrast, unprimed B cells very often gave rise to clones which synthesized several classes of antibody carrying the same idiotypic marker. This implies that many primary B cells may not be irreversibly committed to synthesis of one isotype, and in the presence of appropriate T-cell help may give rise to progeny secreting multiple isotypes, while antigen-experienced secondary B cells are restricted to give rise to progeny secreting only one immunoglobulin class.

The apparent failure of clonal precursors to "switch" to IgG production when allogeneic T cells are used could still be interpreted in the light of the apparent precommitment of B lymphocytes which our results have favored. Because the switch in phenotype as detected in this assay is secretion of antibody by mature plasma cells, the failure of allogeneic cells to provide proliferative signals but still promote some degree of maturation could result in failure of IgG-committed precursors to complete the switch to IgG production but still produce some IgM antibody, in analogy with results of blockage of proliferation in the LPS system. However, the random production of clones of cells from single precursors apparently containing up to four different isotype-secreting cells is obviously incompatible with a precommitment by B lymphocytes to give rise to progeny secreting only one class of immunoglobulin (Gearhart, 1977). Taken together, these results indicate that some B cells are apparently not restricted to isotype expression prior to contact with antigen, while others give rise to progeny secreting only one isotype.

The factors involved in the antigen-induced triggering of B cells are obviously complex; and these, combined with differences in the life history of a particular B cell *in vivo*, e.g., the number of cell cycles through which it has progressed, make a simple explanation for all these observations impossible.

Another caveat in the interpretation of data from LPS-induced differentiation of mouse B lymphocytes *in vitro* concerns the representation of isotypes synthesized by mature plasma cells developing in this system. By far the major isotypes represented are IgM, IgG_2, and IgG_3. In contrast, mature IgG_1 and IgA plasma cells are minor populations, and these have been shown to represent the most thymus-dependent isotypes, as evidenced by their low levels or virtual absence in serum of nude and thymectomized mice (Crewther and Warner, 1972; Luzzatti and Jacobsen, 1972). IgG_1 is represented to the smallest extent on the surface of B cells in normal and athymic mice. On the other hand, substantial numbers of IgG_2 plaque-forming cells can be induced by a thymus-independent antigen (Sharon *et al.*, 1975), and IgG_2 is a relatively prevalent IgG subclass expressed on B cells. IgG_3 is also represented on a large subpopulation of cells, and it is of interest that antibody of this isotype is the most prevalent IgG antibody stimulated in response to polysaccharide antigens, many of which give thymus-independent responses (J. Davie, personal communication).

Therefore it is possible that LPS does not provide maturation signals for the differentiation of $B\gamma1$ and $B\alpha$ precursors to plasma cells secreting these classes. Many attempts to provide nonspecific T-cell help to increase the number of LPS-induced IgG_1- and IgA-synthesizing plasma cells have failed, as have attempts to stimulate their production by prolonged culture times (10–14 days), so it is possible that a similar study with a T-cell-dependent system in which isotype representation by single cells is investigated may give a different picture. LPS will, however, induce comparable numbers of newborn $sIgM^+$ B cells to express surface immunoglobulin of all isotypes, suggesting that the failure of LPS to generate large numbers of plasma cells synthesizing IgG_1 and IgA results from an absence of postinduction maturational signals for their precursors.

There is considerable controversy concerning the question of which isotypes are expressed by IgG-committed memory cells. To date, answers to this question have been: IgM or IgG or IgD (Walters and Wigzell, 1970; Davie and Paul, 1971; Pierce *et al.*, 1972; Abney *et al.*, 1976*b*; Mason, 1976; Okumura *et al.*, 1976; Strober, 1975; Coffman and Cohn, 1977; Jones *et al.*, 1974; Zan Bar *et al.*, 1977). Much of this conflicting data may simply be the result of differences inherent in the model systems used in these studies. For example, although singles, doubles, and trebles can probably all be stimulated by antigen, the relative proportion of these different subsets will vary with the antigenic history of the experimental animal and the immunoglobulin class examined. In general, antigen-driven proliferation will tend to shift lymphocytes from triples to singles, as shown in the LPS model, and this will occur more readily in some cases (e.g.,

IgG$_1$) than in others (e.g., IgG$_3$). In line with this is the reported absence of functional sIgD receptors (Abney *et al.*, 1976*b*) on IgG memory cells taken long after priming.

The fact that there may be single or multiple isotypes on lymphocytes was previously indicated by the experiments of Pierce and his colleagues (Pierce *et al.*, 1972). They found that anti-μ would suppress all classes of Ig (IgM, IgG, IgA) in a primary response *in vitro*, whereas anti-γ and anti-α would only inhibit appearance of the corresponding antibody class. The result is in agreement with our finding of multiple Ig classes on lymphocytes and the consequent suggestion that virgin cells commonly bear two or three isotypes. After priming with antigen, however, Pierce *et al.* (1972) found variable results, depending upon the interval between priming and testing *in vitro*. Thus soon after priming, the IgG response *in vitro* was not inhibited by anti-μ, but when tested after an interval of greater than 1 month, the susceptibility to suppression with anti-μ (of the IgG production) returned. More recently, Strober (1975) has reported experiments which similarly illustrate the heterogeneity of the memory cell pool in rats, and again, serve to show how experimental design may influence the results obtained. In essence he described two general classes of IgG memory cells: one, a small lymphocyte with high density of sIgG and relatively long half-life; the other, a significantly larger lymphocyte with considerably less sIgG and a shorter half-life.

How do these results bear on genetic mechanisms for the regulation of immunoglobulin gene expression? First, the simultaneous synthesis of at least three isotypes by single B lymphocytes makes it unlikely that a simple genetic mechanism for sequentially integrating a selected *V* gene with Cμ, Cγ, and Cα in the progeny of a single stem cell can account for the generation of isotype diversity (Cooper and Lawton, 1974). With this model it was possible to explain the simultaneous presence of sIgM and sIgD or sIgM on IgG-containing plasma cells by invoking persistence of mRNA for μ-chain and continued synthesis of mRNA for the second isotype. However, this possibility is argued against by the long life of sIgM$^+$ .sIgD$^+$ chronic lymphocyte leukemia cells (Pernis *et al.*, 1974; Fu *et al.*, 1975) and made even less likely by our description of triples. The latter requires two *V*-region switches sufficiently close in time to provide the necessary functional pool of heavy-chain mRNAs. If rearrangement of a *V*-region gene so that it becomes contiguous with a constant-region gene is necessary for initiation of transcription of the full *V-C* gene complex (Hozumi and Tonegawa, 1976), then it becomes necessary to invoke simultaneous insertion of multiple copies of *V*-region genes with each *C* gene. Subsequent expression by B cells of one or more immunoglobulins with different constant regions but of the same V region would then result from selective gene activation and repression. The sequence of expression of isotypes we have observed during the development of B lymphocytes probably does not reflect sequential insertion of a *V*-region gene into different *C* genes. However, there is a sequential expression of isotypes on different sublines of B lymphocytes at various times during development which may be linked closely to the number of proliferative cycles that a cell has undergone or the phase of the cell cycle in which a particular B cell appears to be located.

ACKNOWLEDGMENTS

We are grateful to Mrs. Helen Robison, Mrs. Summer King, and Mrs. Diann Gurley for assistance in preparation of this manuscript and to Drs. M. D. Cooper, A. R. Lawton, M. Loken, and R. M. E. Parkhouse for collaborative studies.

Work from our laboratories were supported by grants from the Department of Health, Education and Welfare, National Institutes of Health (AI 11502, CA 16673, and CA 13148).

V. REFERENCES

Abney, E. R., and Parkhouse, R. M. E., 1974, Candidate for immunoglobulin D present on murine B lymphocytes, *Nature* 292:600.

Abney, E. R., Hunter, I. R., and Parkhouse, R. M. E., 1976a, Preparation and characterization of an antiserum to the mouse candidate for immunoglobulin D, *Nature* 259:404.

Abney, E. R., Keeler, K. D., Parkhouse, R. M. E., and Willcox, H. N. A., 1976b, Immunoglobulin M receptors on memory cells of immunoglobulin G antibody-forming cell clones, *Eur. J. Immunol.* 6:443.

Abney, E. R., Cooper, M. D., Kearney, J. F., Lawton, A. R., and Parkhouse, R. M. E., 1978, Sequential expression of immunoglobulins on developing mouse B lymphocytes. A systematic survey which suggests a model for the generation of immunoglobulin isotype diversity, *J. Immunol.* (in press).

Alexander, E. L., and Sanders, S. K., 1977, F(ab')₂ reagents are not required if goat, rather than rabbit antibodies are used to detect human surface immunoglobulin, *J. Immunol.* 119:1084.

Andersson, J., Sjöberg, O., and Möller, G., 1972, Induction of immunoglobulin and antibody synthesis *in vitro* by lipopolysaccharides, *Eur. J. Immunol.* 2:349.

Andersson, J., Coutinho, A., Melchers, F., and Watanabe, T., 1976, Growth and maturation of single clones of normal T and B lymphocytes *in vitro*, in: *Origins of Lymphocyte Diversity*, Cold Spring Harbor Symp. Quant. Biol. 41: 227.

Askonas, B. A., and North, J. R., 1977, The life style of B cells—Cellular proliferation and the invariancy of IgG, *Cold Spring Harbor Symp. Quant. Biol.* 41:749.

Bernier, G. M., and Cebra, J. J., 1964, Polypeptide chains of human gamma globulin: cellular localization by fluorescent antibody, *Science* 114:1590.

Blaese, R. M., and Lawrence, E. C., 1977, Development of macrophage function and the expression of immunocompetence, in: *Development of Host Defences* (M. D. Cooper and D. H. Dayton, eds.), p. 201, Academic Press, New York.

Cebra, J. J., Colberg, J. E., and Dray, S., 1966, Rabbit lymphoid cells differentiated with respect to α, γ, and μ-heavy polypeptide chains and to allotypic markers AA1 and AA2, *J. Exp. Med.* 123:547.

Coffman, R. L., and Cohn, M., 1977, The class of surface immunoglobulin on virgin and memory B-lymphocytes, *J. Immunol.* 118:1806.

Cooper, M. D., and Lawton, A. R., 1974, The development of the immune system, *Sci. Amer.* 231:58.

Cooper, M. D., Lawton, A. R., and Kincade, P. W., 1972, A developmental approach to the biological basis for antibody diversity, in: *Contemporary Topics in Immunobiology*, Vol. 1 (M. G. Hanna, ed.), p. 33, Plenum Press, New York.

Crewther, P., and Warner, N. L., 1972, Serum immunoglobulins and antibodies in congenitally athymic (nude) mice, *Aust. J. Exp. Biol. Med. Sci.* 50:625.

Davie, J. M., and Paul, W. E., 1971, Receptors on immunocompetent cells. II. Specificity and nature of receptors on dinitrophenylated guinea pig albumin-^{125}I-binding lymphocytes of normal guinea pigs, *J. Exp. Med.* 134:495.

Fu, S. M., Winchester, R. J., and Kunkel, H. G., 1975, Similar idiotypic specificity for the membrane IgD and IgM of human B lymphocytes, *J. Immunol.* 114:250.

Gearhart, P. J., 1977, Non-sequential expression of multiple immunoglobulin classes by isolated B cell clones, *Nature* 269:812.

Goding, J. W., and Layton, J. E., 1976, Antigen-induced co-capping of IgM and IgD-like receptors on murine B cells, *J. Exp. Med.* 144:852.

Goding, J. W., Warr, G. W., and Warner, N. L., 1976, A genetic polymorphism of IgD-like cell surface immunoglobulin in the mouse, *Proc. Natl. Acad. Sci. U.S.* 73:1305.

Hammerling, U., Chen, A. F., and Abbott, J., 1976, Ontogeny of murine B lymphocytes: sequence of B-cell differentiation from surface-immunoglobulin-negative precursors to plasma cells, *Proc. Natl. Acad. Sci. U.S.* 73:2008.

Hozumi, N., and Tonegawa, S., 1976, Evidence for somatic rearrangement of immunoglobulin genes coding for variable and constant regions, *Proc. Natl. Acad. Sci U.S.* 73:3628.

Ishizaka, Urban, J. F., Jr., Ishizaka, T., and Ishizaka, K., 1977, IgE formation in the rat following infection with *Nippostrongylus brasiliensis*. III. Soluble factor for the generation of IgE-bearing lymphocytes, *J. Immunol.* 119:583.

Ishizaka, K., Ishizaka, T., Okudaira, H., and Bazin, Hervé, 1978, Ontogeny of IgE bearing lymphocytes in the rat, *J. Immunol.* (in press).

Jones, P. O., Craig, S. W., Cebra, J. J., and Herzenberg, L. A., 1974, Restriction of gene expression in B lymphocytes and their progeny. II. Commitment to immunoglobulin heavy chain isotype, *J. Exp. Med.* 140:452.

Kearney, J. F., and Lawton, A. R., 1975a, B lymphocyte differentiation induced by LPS. I. Generation of cells synthesizing four major immunoglobulin classes, *J. Immunol.* 115:671.

Kearney, J. F., and Lawton, A. R., 1975b, B lymphocyte differentiation induced by LPS. II. Response of fetal lymphocytes, *J. Immunol.* 115:677.

Kearney, J. F., Cooper, M. D., and Lawton, A. R., 1976a, B-lymphocyte differentiation induced by LPS. III. Suppression of B cell maturation by anti-mouse immunoglobulin antibodies, *J. Immunol.* 116:1664.

Kearney, J. F., Cooper, M. D., and Lawton, A. R., 1976b, B cell differentiation induced by lipopolysaccharide. IV. Development of immunoglobulin class restriction in precursors of IgG synthesizing cells, *J. Immunol.* 117:1567.

Kearney, J. F., Cooper, M. D., Klein, J., Abney, E. R., Parkhouse, R. M. E., and Lawton, A. R., 1977a, Ontogeny of *Ia* and IgD on IgM-bearing B lymphocytes in mice, *J. Exp. Med.* 146:297.

Kearney, J. F., Lawton, A. R., and Cooper, M. D., 1977b, Multiple immunoglobulin heavy chain expression by LPS stimulated murine B lymphocytes, in: *ICN-UCLA Symposium*

Proceedings, Immune System II: Regulation and Genetics, Vol. 8 (E. Sercarz, L. A. Herzenberg, and C. F. Fox, eds.), pp. 313–320, Academic Press, New York.

Kincade, P. W., Lawton, A. R., Bockman, D. E., and Cooper, M. D., 1970, Suppression of immunoglobulin G synthesis as a result of antibody mediated suppression of immunoglobulin M synthesis in chickens, *Proc. Natl. Acad. Sci. U.S.* 67:1918.

Knapp, W., Boluis, R. L. H., Radl, J., and Hijmans, W., 1973, Independent movement of IgD and IgM molecules on the surface of individual lymphocytes, *J. Immunol.* 111:1295.

Kubo, R. T., Gray, H. M., and Pirofsky, B., 1974, IgD, a major immunoglobulin on the surface of lymphocytes from patients with CLL, *J. Immunol.* 112:1952.

Kyner, D., Zabos, P., Christman, J., and George, A. C. S., 1976, Effect of sodium butyrate on lymphocyte activation, *J. Exp. Med.* 144:1674.

Lawton, A. R., and Cooper, M. D., 1974, Modification of B lymphocyte differentiation by anti-immunoglobulins, in: *Contemporary Topics in Immunobiology* (M. D. Cooper and N. L. Warner, eds.) p. 193, Plenum Press, New York.

Lobo, P. I., Westervelt, F. B., and Horwitz, D. A., 1975, Identification of two populations of Ig bearing lymphocytes in man, *J. Immunol.* 114:116.

Luzzatti, A. L., and Jacobsen, E. B., 1972, Serum immunoglobulin levels in nude mice, *Eur. J. Immunol.* 2:473.

Manning, D. D., Manning, J. K., and Reed, N. D., 1976, Suppression of reaginic antibody (IgE) formation in mice by treatment with anti-μ antiserum, *J. Exp. Med.* 144:288.

Mason, D. W., 1976, The class of surface Ig on cells carrying IgG memory in rat thoracic duct lymph: The size of the subpopulation mediating IgG memory, *J. Exp. Med.* 143:1122.

Melcher, U., Vitetta, E. S., McWilliams, M., Lamm, M. E., Phillips-Quagliata, J., and Uhr, J. W., 1974, Cell surface immunoglobulin. X. Identification of an IgD like molecule on the surface of murine splenocytes, *J. Exp. Med.* 140:1427.

Melchers, F., Lafeur, L., and Andersson, J., 1974, Immunoglobulin M synthesis in resting (G_0) and in mitogen activated B lymphocytes, in: *Control of Proliferation in Animal Cells (Cold Spring Harbor Conference on Cell Proliferation)*, Vol. 1 (B. D. Clarkson and R. Baserga, eds.), p. 393. Cold Spring Harbor Laboratory, New York.

Melchers, F., von Boehmer, H., and Phillips, R. A., 1975a, B lymphocyte subpopulations in the mouse: Organ distribution and ontogeny of immunoglobulin synthesizing and of mitogen sensitive cells, *Transplant. Rev.* 25:26.

Melchers, F., Coutinho, A., Heinrich, G., and Andersson, J., 1975b, Continuous growth of mitogen reactive B lymphocytes, *Scand. J. Immunol.* 4:853.

Mellors, R. C., and Korngold, L., 1963, The cellular origin of human immunoglobulins gamma 2, gamma 1M and gamma A, *J. Exp. Med.* 118:387.

Mosier, D. E., and Johnson, B. M., 1975, Ontogeny of mouse lymphocyte function. II. Development of the ability to produce antibody is modulated by T lymphocytes, *J. Exp. Med.* 141:216.

Nossal, G. J. V., and Pike, B. L., 1973, Studies on the differentiation of B lymphocytes in the mouse, *Immunology* 25:33.

Nossal, G. J. V., Warner, N. L., and Lewis, H., 1971, Incidence of cells simultaneously secreting IgM and IgG antibody to sheep erythrocytes, *Cell. Immunol.* 2:41.

Okumura, K., Julius, M. H., Herzenberg, L. A., and Herzenberg, L. A., 1976, Demonstration that IgG memory is carried by IgG bearing cells, *Eur. J. Immunol.* 6:467.

Owen, J. J. T., Cooper, M. D., and Raff, M. C., 1974, *In vitro* generation of B lymphocytes in mouse fetal liver—A mammalian "bursa equivalent," *Nature* 249:361.

Pernis, B., Forni, L., and Amante, L., 1971, Immunoglobulins as cell receptors, *Ann. N.Y. Acad. Sci.* 190:420.

Pernis, B., Brouet, J. C., and Seligmann, M., 1974, IgD and IgM on the membrane of lymphoid cells in macroglobulinemia. Evidence for identity of membrane IgD and IgM activity in a case with anti-IgG receptors, *Eur. J. Immunol.* **4**:776.

Pernis, B., Forni, L., and Luzzati, A. L., 1977, Synthesis of multiple immunoglobulin classes by single lymphocytes, *Cold Spring Harbor Symp. Quant. Biol.* **41**:175.

Pierce, C. W., Solliday, S. M., and Asofsky, R., 1972, Immune responses *in vitro*. IV. Suppression of primary γM, γG and γA plaque forming cell responses in mouse spleen cultures by class specific antibody to mouse immunoglobulins, *J. Exp. Med.* **135**:675.

Pierce, S. K., and Klinman, N. R., 1975, The allogeneic bisection of carrier-specific enhancement of monoclonal B-cell responses, *J. Exp. Med.* **142**:1165.

Pierce, S. K., and Klinman, N. R., 1976, Allogeneic carrier specific enhancement of hapten-specific secondary B cell responses, *J. Exp. Med.* **144**:1294.

Press, J. L., and Klinman, N. R., 1973, Monoclonal production of both IgM and IgG_1 anti-hapten antibody, *J. Exp. Med.* **138**:300.

Raff, M. C., Megson, M., Owen, J. J. T., and Cooper, M. D., 1976, Early production of intracellular IgM by B lymphocyte precursors in mouse, *Nature* **259**:224.

Rowe, D. S., Hug, K., Forni, L., and Pernis, B., 1973, Immunoglobulin D as a lymphocyte receptor, *J. Exp. Med.* **138**:965.

Ryser, J. E., and Vassalli, P., 1974, Mouse bone marrow lymphocytes and their differentiation, *J. Immunol.* **113**:719.

Salsano, F., Froland, S., Natvig, J. B., and Michaelsen, T. E., 1974, Same idiotype of B lymphocyte membrane IgD and IgM. Formal evidence for monoclonality of chronic lymphocytic leukemia cells, *Scand. J. Immunol.* **3**:84.

Sharon S., McMaster, P. R. B., Kask, A. M., Owens, J. D., and Paul, W. E., 1975, DNP-Lys-Ficoll: A T-independent antigen which elicits both IgM and IgG anti-DNP antibody secreting cells, *J. Immunol.* **114**:1585.

Strober, S., 1975, Maturation of B lymphocytes in the rat. II. Subpopulations of virgin B lymphocytes in the spleen and thoracic duct, *J. Immunol.* **114**:877.

Urban, J. F., Jr., Ishizaka, T., and Ishizaka, K., 1977, IgE formation in the rat following infection with *Nippostrongylus brasiliensis*. II. Proliferation of IgE-bearing cells in neonatally thymectomized animals, *J. Immunol.* **118**:1982.

van Boxel, J. A., Paul, W. E., Terry, W. D., and Green, I., 1972, IgD bearing human lymphocytes, *J. Immunol.* **109**:648.

Vitetta, E. S., and Uhr, J. W., 1975, Immunoglobulin receptors revisited, *Science* **694**.

Walters, C. S., and Wigzell, H., 1970, Demonstration of heavy and light chains antigenic determinants on the cell bound receptor for antigen, *J. Exp. Med.* **132**:1233.

Wang, A. C., Wang, I. Y. F., McCormick, J. N., and Fudenberg, H. H., 1969, The identity of light chains of monoclonal IgG and monoclonal IgM in one patient, *Immunochemistry* **6**:541.

Wang, A. C., Wilson, S. K., Hopper, J. E., Fudenberg, H. H., and Nisonoff, A., 1970, Evidence for control of synthesis of the variable regions for the heavy chains G and M by the same gene, *Proc. Natl. Acad. Sci. U.S.* **66**:337.

Warner, N. L., 1974, Membrane immunoglobulin and antigen receptors on B and T lymphocytes, *Adv. Immunol.* **19**:67.

Zan Bar, I., Vitetta, E. S., and Strober, S., 1977, The relationship between surface Ig isotype and immune function of murine B lymphocytes II. Surface Ig isotypes on unprimed B cells in the spleen, *J. Exp. Med.* **145**:1206.

Index